Adel Najdowski
775-813-4922

Interventions for Autism Spectrum Disorders

Sam Goldstein • Jack A. Naglieri
Editors

Interventions for Autism Spectrum Disorders

Translating Science into Practice

Springer

Editors
Sam Goldstein
Neurology, Learning and Behavior Center
Salt Lake City, UT
USA

Jack A. Naglieri
University of Virginia
Centreville, VA
USA

ISBN 978-1-4614-5300-0 ISBN 978-1-4614-5301-7 (eBook)
DOI 10.1007/978-1-4614-5301-7
Springer New York Dordrecht Heidelberg London

Library of Congress Control Number: 2012954541

Printed on acid-free paper.

Springer is part of Springer Science+Business Media (www.springer.com)

For all the children with ASD and their families. Thank you for teaching me so much and being so patient as I learned.

Sam Goldstein

For all those who struggle with the behaviors related to ASD and the professionals who work so diligently to ameliorate its impact.

Jack A. Naglieri

This volume is dedicated to the memory of Kenneth W. Merrell who passed away at the age of 53, far too young and too soon. At the time of his passing, Dr. Merrell was in the process of completing a chapter for this volume. The chapter was subsequently completed by his colleagues. Ken's research and scholarly work in social-emotional assessment and interventions has been widely published and has had a significant impact on our understanding of social, emotional learning in children. In 2001, Ken founded the Oregon Resiliency Project. Through this project he developed Strong Start Strong Kids programs, a widely used social-emotional learning curriculum. Ken will be missed. He was a fine scholar, mentor to his students and father to his four children.

Sam Goldstein
Jack A. Naglieri

Preface

Perhaps more so than any other human quality, our drive to connect, socialize, relate, and be with others defines us and provides a solid foundation upon which we build intellectual, emotional, and educational experiences. The capacity to socialize effectively, gain access to peers, and enjoy the company and play of others is a powerful, driving force in human development. Infants deprived of the opportunity to connect to consistent caregivers fail to thrive. Toddlers unable to relate to the social world around them become introverted and disengaged. Preschoolers disinterested or lacking the capacity to develop adequate social skills are quickly ostracized, and they struggle to meet the early challenges of educational and social settings. School-age children who struggle to develop social skills, either because they are withdrawn and neglected or disrupted and rejected, wander the playground at recess. Teenagers and adults unable to relate to the social world struggle to transition successfully to independent living, competitive work, and the normal experiences of adulthood. It is the limited drive to connect, socialize, relate, and be with others that defines Autism Spectrum Disorders (ASD). Helping individuals with ASD overcome these behaviors forms the basis of all intervention programs.

Children with ASD require significantly more assistance, support, and education than other youngsters if they are to transition successfully and happily into adult life. As many of the authors in this volume will attest, the earlier the intervention particularly focused on socialization, the better appears to be the impact and outcome. We have more than adequately demonstrated, however, that symptom relief, while essential, is not the equivalent of changing long-term outcome. Children with ASD require support throughout their childhood into adolescence and adulthood if they are to transition functionally into adult life.

More children are now being diagnosed with ASD than ever before. The Center for Disease Control estimates that of the four million children born in the United States every year, approximately 26,000–27,000 children will eventually be diagnosed with ASD. Assuming a consistent prevalence, about a half a million children under the age of 19 have been diagnosed with ASD. Their outcome, as attested by a number of transitional research studies, speaks of our failure thus far to identify a consistent method/program of socialization and education and to maintain that support into adulthood.

The evolution of the scientific understanding of any clinical diagnosis is often best measured by the number of peer-reviewed scientific articles and text books on the subject. As knowledge about a particular topic such as ASD grows, so do the number of texts, beginning with those that generally cover the topic and eventually evolving to texts that cover specific aspects of the topic. ASD is one such condition on a fast evolutionary track. This is our second scientific volume on autism; the first focused on assessment (Goldstein, Naglieri, and Ozonoff, 2009). It is our belief that this is the first text specifically published focusing on interventions for ASD.

This volume is divided into three parts. In the first part, the chapters cover foundational issues, including an overview of ASD history, assessment, and diagnosis, followed by an important chapter authored by Andrew Livanis focusing on treatment integrity for ASD. Section I concludes with a chapter by co-editor Jack Naglieri providing an examination of issues such as reliability and validity with particular attention to scaling issues related to assessment and intervention.

Section II provides overviews of four widely used comprehensive programs for children with ASD. All focus on young children, a phenomena that very clearly demonstrates the infancy of comprehensive treatment programs for children with ASD.

Section III, the longest in this book, contains nine chapters dealing specifically with strategic interventions. Margaret Semrud-Clikeman and Lori Krasny provide chapters focusing on an overview of strategies for developing social competence. Brooke Ingersoll focuses on adult as well as peer socialization. Chapters additionally cover modifying common symptomatic impairments in autism, including sensory sensitivity, stereotypies, unusual behavior, problems with attention, self-regulation, and pragmatic language. Brenda Smith-Myles provides an overview of classroom strategies for children with ASD. Robert Brooks, along with co-author Sam Goldstein, provides an overview of their resilience model directed at parents raising children with ASD.

Thomas Jefferson wrote, "Nothing can stop the man with the right mental attitude from achieving his goal; nothing on earth can help the man with the wrong mental attitude." We have slowly come to understand the challenges and impairments of children and adolescents with ASD. It is our hope that this volume is to be the first of many to guide this important process.

"On the other hand, I think cats have Asperger's. Like me, they're very smart. And like me, sometimes they simply need to be left alone."

Jodi Picoult, House Rules

"What would happen if the autism gene was eliminated from the gene pool? You would have a bunch of people standing around in a cave, chatting and socializing and not getting anything done."

Temple Grandin, The Way I See It: A Personal Look at Autism and Asperger's

"If they can't learn the way we teach, we teach the way they learn."

O. Ivar Lovaas

Acknowledgments

Our thanks to Kathy Gardner for editorial assistance and our Editor Judy Jones for giving us the opportunity to complete this volume.

Contents

Part III Strategic Interventions

Contributors

Kristie Asaro-Saddler University of Albany, ED 228, Albany, NY 12222, USA
e-mail: ksaddler@albany.edu

Samantha Benvenuto Long Island University, Brooklyn Campus, 1 University Plaza, Brooklyn, NY 11201-5372, USA

Natalie Berger Department of Psychology, Michigan State University, 316 Physics Rd., East Lansing, MI 48824, USA

Mary E. Van Bourgondien Chapel Hill TEACCH Center, The University of North Carolina, Campus Box #6305, Chapel Hill, NC 27599-6305, USA
e-mail: mvan2@email.unc.edu

Brian A. Boyd Division of Occupational Science and Occupational Therapy, University of North Carolina at Chapel Hill, Bondurant Hall, CB#7122, Chapel Hill, NC 27599-7205, USA
e-mail: brian_boyd@med.unc.edu

Robert Brooks Department of Psychiatry, Harvard Medical School, 60 Oak Knoll Terrace, Needham, MA 02492, USA
e-mail: contact@drrobertbrooks.com

Elaine Coonrod Chapel Hill TEACCH Center, The University of North Carolina, Campus Box #6305, Chapel Hill, NC 27599-6305, USA
e-mail: Elaine_Coonrod@med.unc.edu

Melissa DeVries Neurology, Learning and Behavior Center, 230 South 500 East, Suite 100, Salt Lake City, UT 84102, USA
e-mail: Melissa@samgoldstein.com

Sam Goldstein Neurology, Learning and Behavior Center, School of Medicine, University of Utah, 230 South 500 East, Suite 100, Salt Lake City, UT 84102, USA
e-mail: info@samgoldstein.com

Evelyn R. Gould Center for Autism and Related Disorders, 19019 Ventura Blvd Suite 300, Tarzana, CA 91356, USA

Doreen Granpeesheh Center for Autism and Related Disorders, 19019 Ventura Blvd Suite 300, Tarzana, CA 91356, USA
e-mail: doreen@centerforautism.com

Laura Guli University of Texas at Austin, SZB 5800 Austin, TX 78712, USA

Craig A. Hanthorn Long Island University, Brooklyn Campus, 1 University Plaza, Brooklyn, NY 11201-5372, USA

Brooke Ingersoll Department of Psychology, Michigan State University, 316 Physics Rd., East Lansing, MI 48824, USA
e-mail: ingers19@msu.edu

Lori Krasny The Children's Center, 350 South 400 East, Salt Lake City, UT 84111, USA
e-mail: lkrasny@tccslc.org

Amy C. Laurent University of Rhode Island, Kingston, RI, USA

Andrew Livanis Department of Counseling and School Psychology, Long Island University, Brooklyn Campus, 1 University Plaza, Brooklyn, NY 1120-5372, USA
e-mail: andrew.livanis@liu.edu

Linda Mason The Pennsylvania State University, 213 CEDAR, University Park, PA 16802, USA
e-mail: Lhm12@psu.edu

Kenneth W. Merrell University of Massachusetts, Amherst, 360 Hills South, UMASS, 111 Thatcher Rd., Amherst, MA 01003-9361, USA

Ayla Mertturk Long Island University, Brooklyn Campus, 1 University Plaza, Brooklyn, NY 11201-5372, USA

Elizabeth Portman Minne University of Texas at Austin, SZB 5800 Austin, TX 78712, USA

Brenda Smith Myles Ziggurat Group and Ohio Center for Autism and Low Incidence Disabilities, 11400 W. 155th Terrace Overland, Park, KS 66221-2606, USA
e-mail: Brenda_myles@mac.com

Jack A. Naglieri Curry School of Education, Devereux Center for Resilient Children, University of Virginia, Centreville, VA, USA
e-mail: jnaglieri@gmail.com

Adel C. Najdowski Center for Autism and Related Disorders, 19019 Ventura Blvd Suite 300, Tarzana, CA 91356, USA

Dana Princiotta Neurology, Learning and Behavior Center, School of Medicine, University of Utah, 230 South 500 East, Suite 100, Salt Lake City, UT 84102, USA
e-mail: dana@samgoldstein.com

Barry M. Prizant Childhood Communication Services, Center for the Study of Human Development, Brown University, 35 Kent Place, Cranston, RI 02905, USA
e-mail: bprizant@gmail.com

Robert Reid Special Education, University of Nebraska, 202L Barkley, Lincoln, NE 68583-0732, USA
e-mail: Rreid2@unl.edu

Verity L. Rodrigues Division of Developmental and Behavioral Pediatrics, Cincinnati Children's Hospital Medical Center, 3333 Burnet Avenue, Cincinnati, OH 45229, USA
e-mail: verityrodrigues@gmail.com

Emily Rubin Communication Crossroads, 931 Monroe Dr., Suite 102, Box 110, Atlanta, GA 30308, USA
e-mail: Emily@CommXroads.com

Margaret Semrud-Clikeman Division of Pediatric Clinical Neuroscience, University of Minnesota, 420 Delaware Street, Minneapolis, MN 55455, USA
e-mail: semru002@umn.edu

Geralyn R. Timler Speech Pathology and Audiology, Miami University, 2 Bachelor Hall, Oxford, OH 45056, USA
e-mail: timlergr@muohio.edu

Allison Wainer Department of Psychology, Michigan State University, 316 Physics Rd., East Lansing, MI 48824, USA

Linn Wakeford Division of Occupational Science and Occupational Therapy, University of North Carolina at Chapel Hill, Bondurant Hall Suite 2050, CB#7122, Chapel Hill, NC 27599-7122, USA

Katherine Walton Michigan State University, 316 Physics Rd., East Lansing, MI 48824, USA
e-mail: Ktmeyer15@gmail.com

Amy M. Wetherby Department of Clinical Sciences, College of Medicine, Florida State University, Tallahassee, FL, USA

Sara Whitcomb University of Massachusetts, Amherst, 360 Hills South, UMASS, 111 Thatcher Rd., Amherst, MA 01003-9361, USA
e-mail: swhitcomb@educ.umass.edu

About the Editors

Sam Goldstein Ph.D. is a doctoral level psychologist with areas of study in school psychology, child development, and neuropsychology. He is licensed as a psychologist and certified as a developmental disabilities evaluator in the State of Utah. Dr. Goldstein is a Fellow in the National Academy of Neuropsychology and American Academy of Cerebral Palsy and Developmental Medicine. Dr. Goldstein is an Assistant Clinical Instructor in the Department of Psychiatry. Since 1980, Dr. Goldstein has worked in a private practice setting as the Director of a multidisciplinary team, providing evaluation, case management, and treatment services for children and adults with histories of neurological disease and trauma, learning disability, adjustment difficulties, and attention deficit disorder. Dr. Goldstein is on staff at the University Neuropsychiatric Institute. He has served as a member of the Children's Hospital Craniofacial Team. He has also been a member of the Developmental Disabilities Clinic in the Department of Psychiatry at the University of Utah Medical School.

Dr. Goldstein has authored, co-authored, or edited 40 clinical and trade publications, including 21 trade and 19 textbooks dealing with managing children's behavior in the classroom, genetics, attention disorder, and adult learning disabilities. With Barbara Ingersoll, Ph.D., he has co-authored texts dealing with controversial treatments for children's learning and attention problems and childhood depression. With Anne Teeter Ellison, he has authored *Clinician's Guide to Adult ADHD: Assessment and Intervention.* With Nancy Mather, Ph.D., he has completed 3 texts for teachers and parents concerning behavioral and educational issues. With Michael Goldstein, M.D., he has completed two texts on attention deficit hyperactivity disorder. He has edited 3 texts with Cecil Reynolds, Ph.D., on neurodevelopmental and genetic disorders in children. With Robert Brooks, Ph.D., he has authored 11 texts including, *Handbook of Resilience in Children, Understanding and Managing Children's Classroom Behavior – 2nd Edition, Raising Resilient Children, Nurturing Resilience in Our Children, Seven Steps to Help Children Worry Less, Seven Steps to Anger Management, The Power of Resilience, Raising a Self-Disciplined Child and Raising Resilient Children with Autism Spectrum Disorders*. With Jack Naglieri, he has authored a number of texts on autism and assessment of Intelligence and Executive Functioning. He has co-authored a parent training program and is currently completing a number of additional texts on intelligence, executive functioning, and resilience. Dr. Goldstein is the Editor-in-Chief of the *Journal of Attention Disorders* and serves on 7 Editorial Boards. He is also the Co-Editor of the *Encyclopedia of Child Development and Behavior*.

With Jack Naglieri, Ph.D., Dr. Goldstein is the co-author of the *Autism Spectrum Rating Scales, Comprehensive Executive Functioning Inventory, Rating Scales of Impairment and the Cognitive Assessment System – 2nd Edition.*

Dr. Goldstein, a knowledgeable and entertaining speaker and has lectured extensively on a national and international basis to thousands of professionals and parents concerning attention disorders in children, resilience, depression, adjustment and developmental impairments, autism, and assessment of brain dysfunction.

Jack Naglieri Ph.D. is a Research Professor at the University of Virginia, Senior Research Scientist at the Devereux Center for Resilient Children, and Emeritus Professor of Psychology at George Mason University. He is a Fellow of APA Divisions 15 and 16 and recipient of APA Division 16 Senior Scientist Award (2001). He earned degrees in school psychology from St. John's University (1975) and worked as a school psychologist in Bethpage, New York, from 1975 to 1977. He obtained his Ph.D. in Educational Psychology from the University of Georgia in 1979, taught school psychology at Northern Arizona University (1979–1982), The Ohio State University (1982–2000), and George Mason University (2000–2010). Dr. Naglieri's main interest is in the development of psychological and educational tests and the implications these approaches have for diagnosis and academic or emotional interventions.

The author of more than 250 scholarly papers, chapters, books, and tests, he has concentrated his efforts on psychological theory and measurement. His areas of research include fair assessment, cross-cultural issues, cognitive interventions, learning disabilities, ADHD, mental retardation, gifted, and factors related to resilience. He has published several books including *Assessment of Cognitive Processes: The PASS Theory of Intelligence* (1974), *Essentials of CAS Assessment* (1999), *Helping Children Learn: Intervention Handouts for Use in School and at Home* (2003), *Helping Gifted Children Learn* (Naglieri, Brulles, and Lansdowne, 2008), *Assessment of Autism Spectrum Disorders* (Goldstein, Naglieri, and Ozonoff, 2008) and *Essentials of WNV Assessment* (Brunnert, Naglieri, and Hardy-Braz, 2008). He is also the author of *Wechsler Nonverbal Scale of Ability* (2006), *Cognitive Assessment System* (1997, 2013), *CAS Rapid Score* (2002), *General Ability Measure for Adults* (1997), *Naglieri Nonverbal Ability Tests* (1997; 2003; 2008), *Devereux Early Childhood Assessments* (1997; 2003), *Devereux Elementary Student Strength Assessment (DESSA; 2011), DESSA-mini (2011), Devereux Scales of Mental Disorders* (1994), *Devereux Behavior Rating Scales School Form* (1994), *Draw A Person: Screening Procedure for Emotional Disturbance* (1990), *Draw A Person: Quantitative Scoring* System (1988), and *Matrix Analogies Tests* (Naglieri, 1985).

In summary, Dr. Naglieri has an extensive research program that includes scholarly research, books, and psychological tests with an emphasis on uniting sound theory with scientific practice.

Part I
Foundation

Chapter 1
Autism Spectrum Disorder Enters the Age of Multidisciplinary Treatment

Sam Goldstein and Melissa DeVries

The treatments of disorders characterized by patterns of atypical behaviors and development such as those on the autism spectrum are multidimensional, complex, and are often required throughout the life span. Autism spectrum disorder (ASD) contains its share of contradiction, uncertainty, and disagreement. It is still the case that the incidence of "autistic behaviors" in the general population is not fully understood yet continues to rise (Center for Disease Control 2007; Kim et al. 2011). The positive and negative predictive powers of specific behaviors related to autism have not been fully investigated relative to diagnosis and treatment response.

As this book goes to press, the fifth edition of the *Diagnostic and Statistical Manual* of the American Psychiatric Association is about to be published (APA 2013, in press). Major changes have been made in the manner in which autism is viewed, moving from a set of conditions falling under an umbrella referred to as pervasive developmental disorders, to a singular condition referred to as autism spectrum disorder (APA Neurodevelopmental Disorders Work Group 2011). The new diagnosis provides a carefully crafted description of the symptom profile, related criteria, and impairment necessary across diagnostic thresholds. To receive a diagnosis of autism spectrum disorder, individuals will have to demonstrate deficits in four areas; (1) social communication and social interaction patterns including deficits in social-emotional reciprocity; (2) nonverbal communicative behaviors used for social interaction; and (3) in the development and maintenance of developmentally appropriate relationships. A number of example behaviors are provided under each description, but the specific symptom count requirements for those parts of the current DSM-IV-TR criteria have been removed (APA 2000).

S. Goldstein
Neurology, Learning and Behavior Center, School of Medicine, University of Utah,
230 South 500 East, Suite 100, Salt Lake City, UT 84102, USA
e-mail: info@samgoldstein.com

M. DeVries
Neurology, Learning and Behavior Center, 230 South 500 East, Suite 100,
Salt Lake City, UT 84102, USA
e-mail: Melissa@samgoldstein.com

S. Goldstein, J. A. Naglieri (eds.), *Interventions for Autism Spectrum Disorders*,
DOI 10.1007/978-1-4614-5301-7_1, © Springer Science+Business Media New York 2013

The fourth category, restricted, repetitive patterns of behavior, interests, or activities requires that an individual manifests a minimum of two symptoms that may include stereotyped or repetitive speech, motor movements, or use of objects, excessive adherence to routines, ritualized patterns of verbal or nonverbal behavior or excessive resistance to change, highly restricted, fixated interests of abnormal intensity or focus, and hyperreactivity or hyporeactivity to sensory input or unusual interest in sensory aspects of environment. Although the diagnosis will still require that symptoms be present in early childhood, no specific age limit is provided and the proposed criteria acknowledge that for some individuals, full symptom manifestation may not become apparent until the demands of the environment exceed their skills and abilities. Regardless, however, symptoms must impair and limit daily functioning.

It remains to be seen whether the expansion and redefinition of the current diagnostic criteria will lead to more accurate diagnosis; however, as the means of applying these criteria through observation, checklist, and standardized tests present numerous challenges. Further, the means by which treatment effectiveness can be evaluated also remains challenging given the continued heterogeneity of children diagnosed with ASD. As noted, it is still the case that ASD lacks a unifying theory. It is a condition that appears to be composed of social, learning, behavioral, developmental, and cognitive problems. Despite a significant increase in research articles about ASD and the rapid and significant advances, the efficient assessment of the condition and its related problems and, most importantly, effective intervention continues to present challenges. As recognition and prevalence of the condition increases, risks for over and under diagnosis increase in parallel. The need for carefully, crafted guides to inform professionals about research proven treatments is essential. This chapter begins with a brief overview of the history of ASD, discussion of current diagnostic criteria, and a brief overview of a model to comprehensively evaluate and treat youth with ASD first proposed by Odom, Boyd, Hall, and Hume in 2010. The chapter concludes with a brief review of behavioral and medical interventions/treatments and a discussion of a multidisciplinary model.

Historical Overview

Though the famous wild boy of Aveyron was thought to be a feral child living in the woods and purportedly raised by wolves in South Central France at the end of the eighteenth century, it is more likely he suffered from autism. The boy named Victor by the physician Itard reportedly demonstrated classic signs of autism, particularly related to failure to use language or other forms of communication (Lane 1977). In 1867, Henry Maudsley, in a text devoted to the physiology and pathology of the mind, described insanity in children. Some of his descriptions appeared consistent with today's symptoms of autism. Qualities of stubbornness, rigidity, odd and self-centered behavior have also been reported in historical figures throughout time. Interestingly, it was hypothesized by Frith (1989) that a number of fictional historical characters, including Sherlock Holmes, may well have been provided personalities consistent with autism.

The German word *Autismus* was first coined in 1912 by the Swiss psychiatrist, Paul Bleuler. The word is from the Greek *Autos* (self) and *Ismos* a suffix of action or of state. Bleuler, best remembered for his work in schizophrenia, first used this term in 1950 to describe idiosyncratic, self-centered thinking that led to autistic withdrawal into a private fantasy world. In 1943, Leo Kanner, in an article published in the journal *Nervous Child* introduced the modern concept of autism. Kanner borrowed the term autism from the field of schizophrenia as described by Bleuler. Kanner suggested that children with autism also live in their own world cut off from normal social intercourse. Yet he also felt that autism was distinct from schizophrenia, representing a failure of development, not a regression. Kanner also observed in the clinical histories of these children additional features reflecting problems with symbolization, abstraction, and understanding meaning. All had profound disturbances in communication.

In the 1943 article, Kanner described 11 children with "autistic disturbances of affective contact." He suggested that they had been born lacking the usual motivation for social interaction. Kanner described these disturbances as reflecting the absence of the biological preconditions for psychologically metabolizing the social world and making it part of themselves. The condition was noted to lead to severe problems in social interaction and communication as well as a need for sameness. Children with autism were described as rigid, inflexible, and reacting negatively to any change in their environment or routine.

Kanner considered autism as a genetically driven condition. He also observed that parents of some of his patients were successful in academic and vocational realms. Kanner suggested that autism, though a congenital condition, could be influenced by parenting. This led to the characterization at one time that autism was caused by inappropriate parenting. When filtered through psychoanalytic theory of the time it was believed that parents, particularly their child-rearing methods, were the cause of autism. These interactional problem of autism arise from the child, however, not parents has been well demonstrated in the research literature (Mundy et al. 1986). The data today supports the concept that biological and genetic factors convey the vulnerability to autism. Autism is also a condition that is typically observed across many generations and families. In 1956, Kanner and Eisenberg further elaborated on this theory providing case observations collected between 1943 and 1955. During this period it appears Kanner's concept of the condition changed minimally.

Kanner also suggested that many children with autism were not mentally retarded but unmotivated to perform. A body of past research demonstrated that when developmentally appropriate tests are given, intelligence and developmental scores are in the mentally retarded range for the majority of individuals with autism (Rutter et al. 1994). Yet as the concept of autism as reflecting primarily a social learning problem has become more widely accepted, the percentage of individuals on the autism spectrum who have normal intellectual abilities has increased. Though intellectual deficits were traditionally considered a key aspect of autism, the current conceptualization has evolved to appreciate and recognize the differences between general intelligence on the one hand and the social learning problems characteristic of autism on the other.

The year after the publication of Kanner's original paper, Hans Asperger, a physician working in Vienna proposed another autistic condition. Asperger was evidently unaware of Kanner's paper or his use of the word autism. Asperger, however, used a similar term in his description of the social problems these children demonstrated. In 1944, Asperger described a syndrome he referred to as "autistic psychopathy." This condition is now referred to as Asperger's disorder in the DSM-IV-TR. His paper, published in German, was unavailable to English speaking scientists until an account of his work was authored by Wing in 1981 and the paper translated by Frith into English in 1991 (Asperger 1994/1991).

Rutter et al. (1994) reported on Theodore Heller, a special educator in Vienna, who described an unusual condition in which children appeared normal for a number of years and then suffered a profound regression in functioning and development. This condition was originally known as dementia infantalis or disintegrative psychosis. It is currently referred to as childhood disintegrative disorder in the DSM-IV-TR. Further, Rett (1966) first observed females with an unusual developmental disorder characterized by a short period of normal development and a multifaceted form of intellectual and motor deterioration with many symptoms similar to autism. In the DSM-IV-TR this is now referred to as Rett's disorder. Autism is also associated with many other genetic and medical conditions occurring at a higher than expected rate in conditions such as fragile X, tuberous sclerosis, Williams syndrome, and neurofibromatosis (Gillberg 1990).

Until the 1970's, autism was considered a form of schizophrenia. In the first and second editions of the *Diagnostic and Statistical Manual* (APA 1968, 1968) only the term childhood schizophrenia was available to describe children with autism. It has become abundantly clear with further research that although young children with autism suffer in many other areas of their development, their behavior is very different from the psychotic problems of later childhood or teenage years (Kolvin 1971; for review see Cohen and Volkmar 1997). The work of Cantwell et al. (1980) and DeMyer et al. (1981) was influential in differentiating the field such that autism was identified as a condition separate and apart from schizophrenia. There is now a general consensus on the validity of autism as a diagnostic category and on the majority of features central to the definition. This consensus has been contributed to by the convergence of the two major diagnostic systems that include psychiatric and developmental disorders, the DSM and the World Health Organization International Classification of Diseases (ICD). Although there continue to be some differences between these two sets of diagnostic criteria, they have become more alike than different with each text revision (Volkmar 1998). In fact, autism probably offers the best empirical basis for cross cultural, diagnostic criteria.

Autism was first included in the DSM in its third edition (APA 1980), then called infantile autism. The criteria were limited in their descriptions, specific symptoms were not outlined, and the criteria needed to be met for the diagnosis to be made (Volkmar 1998). Major changes occurred in the text revision of DSM-III (Factor et al. 1989), known as DSM-III-R, included detailed and concrete descriptions of specific behaviors and guidelines for number and patterns of symptoms that needed to be present, increasing the reliability of diagnosis. The lifelong nature of the disorder was acknowledged in the change in name from infantile autism to autistic disorder. Deficits were defined relative to the child's mental age and subjective words and phrases ("bizarre," "gross deficits") that may have limited applicability to older or higher functioning individuals were removed. Both verbal and nonverbal communication difficulties, including social use of language, were highlighted, rather than simply structural language deficits. Changes were much smaller from the DSM-III-R to the DSM-IV but a major one was the inclusion for the first time of Asperger's disorder. The current diagnostic protocol for autism as it appears in the DSM-IV-TR (APA 2000) has been recognized and slightly modified as previously reviewed for DSM-V set to be published sometime in 2013 will remain active for at least the next 5 years.

Current Conceptualization of ASD

Because of the unusual combination of behavioral weaknesses and the lack of biological models to understand this disorder, autism is a most perplexing condition (Schopler and Mesibov 1987). It is best conceptualized as a biologically determined set of behaviors that occurs with varying presentation and severity, likely as the result of varying cause. Autism occurs significantly more often in boys (Smalley et al. 1988) and presents across all social classes (Gillberg and Schaumann 1982). It is estimated that one out of four children with autism experiences physical problems, including epilepsy (Rutter 1970). Up to 75 % are generally found to experience intellectual deficiencies, although this proportion appears to be dropping in recent years. Lotter (1974) first suggested that level of intellectual functioning and amount of useful language by 5 years of age were the best predictors of outcome and these findings have been consistently supported by later research (Gillberg and Steffenburg 1987; Howlin et al. 2004; Venter et al. 1992).

Autism is a spectrum disorder in which individuals can present problems ranging from those that cause almost total impairment to others that allow the individual to function but not optimally. Children on the autism spectrum experience a wide variety of developmental difficulties involving communication, socialization, thinking, cognitive skills, interests, activities, and motor skills. Although critics suggest that the diagnosis of pervasive developmental disorder is poorly defined and inconsistent because it does not refer to all pervasive developmental disorders (e.g., mental retardation) and because some children experience only specific or partial impairments (Gillberg 1990), the term seems to well define the breadth of difficulties experienced by most of these children.

Rutter (1983) found that the pattern of cognitive disabilities in autistic children is distinctive and different from that found in children with general intellectual handicaps. Language and language-related skills involving problems with semantics and pragmatics are present (Rutter 1983). Other difficulties frequently include perceptual disorders (Ornitz and Ritvo 1968), cognitive problems (Rutter 1983), specific types of memory weaknesses (Boucher 1981), and impairment in social relations (Fein et al. 1986). Consistent with Kanner's description of autism, social impairments have been found to be the strongest predictors of receiving a diagnosis (Siegel et al. 1989). Dimensionally measured variables such as those related to interpersonal relationships, play skills, coping, and communication are consistently impaired areas for youth with a pervasive developmental disorder. Hobson (1989) found that higher functioning autistic children are unable to make social or emotional discriminations or read social or emotional cues well. These deficits appear to impact social relations and likely stem from cognitive weaknesses. The inability to read social and emotional cues and understand others' points of view leads to marked interpersonal difficulties (Baron-Cohen 1989; MacDonald et al. 1989). Since Rutter's (1978) first description of social impairments, absent cognitive deficits, in some higher functioning youth with autism, diagnostic criteria for these conditions have expanded to include deficits in nonverbal behavior, peer relations, lack of shared enjoyment and pleasure, and problems with social and emotional reciprocity (APA 1994; World Health Organization 1993). Relative to their cognitive abilities, children with autism exhibit much lower than expected social skills, even compared to a mentally handicapped group (Volkmar et al. 1987). Delays in social skills are strong predictors of receiving a diagnosis of autism, even when compared to delays in communication (Volkmar et al. 1993). Clearly, impairments in social skills among those receiving diagnoses of any PDD are greater than expected relative to overall development (Loveland and Kelley 1991).

Current Diagnostic Criteria

The DSM-IV-TR (APA 2000) criteria include a group of pervasive developmental disorders. The three criteria for autistic disorder include three sets of behavioral descriptions. To qualify for the diagnosis, the child must present at least two from the first set of criteria and one from each of the second and third sets of criteria. The first set of criteria features qualitative impairment in social interaction as manifested by impairment of nonverbal behaviors, including eye contact, facial expression, body postures, and gestures of social interaction; failure to develop peer relationships appropriate to developmental level; markedly impaired sharing of emotional states or interests with others, expression of pleasure in other people's happiness, and lack of social or emotional reciprocity. The second set of criteria refers to qualitative impairment in communication as manifested by a delay or total lack of the development of spoken language without efforts to compensate through gestures; marked impairment in the ability to initiate or sustain conversation despite adequate speech; repetitive or stereotyped use of language or idiosyncratic language; and lack of varied, spontaneous make-believe play or social imitative play appropriate for the child's developmental level. The third set of criteria involves repetitive and stereotypic patterns of behavior; restricted interest or activities, including preoccupation in a certain pattern of behavior that is abnormal in intensity or focus; compulsive adherence to specific nonfunctional routines or rituals; repetitive motor mannerisms (self-stimulatory behavior), or persistent preoccupation with parts of objects. The second two sets of criteria include delay prior to the age of 3 years in social interaction, language as used in social communication, or symbolic or imaginative play. Finally, the child's clinical description should not be better accounted for by Rett's disorder or childhood disintegrative disorder.

DSM-IV-TR criteria describe Rett's disorder as being manifested by normal development for at least the first 5 months of life, including normal prenatal and perinatal development, apparently normal psychomotor development through the first 5 months, and normal head circumference at birth. Between 5 and 48 months there is deceleration of head growth, loss of previously acquired purposeful hand movements with the development of stereotypic hand movements (e.g., hand-wringing), loss of social engagement, appearance of poorly coordinated gait or trunk movements, and marked delay as well as impairment of expressive and receptive language with severe psychomotor retardation.

Childhood disintegrative disorder in the DSM-IV-TR is defined as normal development for at least the first 2 years and then loss of skills in at least two areas including expressive or receptive language, social skills or adaptive behavior, bowel or bladder control, play or motor skills. In addition, the child begins to manifest qualitative impairments in social interaction, including at least two of the following: impaired use of nonverbal behaviors, failure to develop peer relationships, markedly impaired expression of pleasure in other people's happiness, and a lack of social or emotional reciprocity. There are also qualitative impairments in communication as manifested by at least one symptom involving delay or total lack of spoken language, an inability to sustain and initiate conversation despite adequate speech, stereotyped or repetitive use of language or idiosyncratic language and a lack of varied, spontaneous make-believe play or social, imitative play. The child with childhood disintegrative disorder also demonstrates restrictive, repetitive, and stereotypic patterns of behavior, interests, and activities. The child's behavior should not be accounted for by another specific developmental disorder or by schizophrenia. Thus, childhood disintegrative disorder reflects an autistic diagnosis that occurs after a longer and clearer period of normal development. Autism can also involve a regression in behavior but it usually occurs before the child's second birthday (Kurita et al. 2004).

DSM-IV defined the criteria for a new diagnosis, Asperger's disorder, which remained unchanged in DSM-IV-TR. Included in the diagnostic criteria are deficits in the qualitative impairment in social interaction, including at least two criteria involving: (1) marked impairment in the use of nonverbal behaviors such as body posture; failure to develop appropriate peer relations; (2) a lack of spontaneous seeking to share enjoyment, interests, or achievements and lack of social or emotional reciprocity. A second set of criteria involves restricted repetitive and stereotyped behaviors, interests or activities, including at least one symptom of the following: Restricted or stereotyped pattern of interest that is abnormal in intensity or focus; inflexible adherence to specific rituals or routines; repetitive motor mannerisms; or persistent preoccupation with parts of objects. This disturbance must cause clinically significant impairment in social, academic, and other areas of functioning. Further, for this diagnosis to be made, the child should not exhibit a delay in early language development or a significant delay in language or cognitive development or in the development of age appropriate self-help skills and adaptive behavior. Most critically, children diagnosed with Asperger's disorder cannot also meet criteria for autism. This exclusion was added to make the diagnoses mutually exclusive and thus more reliable but has been controversial (Frith 2004; Mayes et al. 2001; Miller and Ozonoff 1997) and other systems may be entertained for future DSM editions (Klin et al. 2005).

Assessment

As Cohen noted in 1976, the clinical provision of a diagnosis is only part of a diagnostic process. Assessment is more than the simple application of a set of criteria to a particular individual. Assessment must provide an overview of the individual's history, change over time, as well as relevant information about development, life course, socialization and, equally important, the environment in which the individual lives and functions. The diagnostic process, as Cohen noted, should provide a thorough overview of the individual person, their assets, liabilities, and needs. History is likely the best assessment tool. In most clinical assessments, history is often supported by specialized checklists and standardized instruments (Goldstein and Naglieri 2009b). It is the rule rather than the exception that most autism evaluations screen broadly for comorbid developmental, emotional, and behavioral problems (Odom et al. 2010). A comprehensive assessment for autism thus typically evaluates a child's intellectual, neuropsychological, language, behavioral, and emotional functioning in addition to the administration of observational questionnaires to parents and teachers specific for ASD (Goldstein and Naglieri 2009a). Readers interested in a review of comprehensive assessment for ASD are directed to Goldstein et al. (2008).

Overview of Current Treatment

This volume contains both comprehensive and symptom focused treatment interventions. Those treatments with demonstrated effectiveness as well as those that hold promise based on initial report and case studies are given equal space. In 2010, Odom, Boyd, Hall, and Hume identified 30 comprehensive treatment models, the majority based on an applied behavior analysis (ABA) framework with others following a developmental or relationship-based model for the treatment of ASD. The authors reported that these 30 were strong in the operationalization of their models although weaker in the measurement of implementation and weak in evidence of efficacy.

This book is organized in a manner similar to the professional literature in which there are two classifications of intervention. One set of interventions focus on specific interventions designed to produce certain behavioral or developmental outcomes for children with ASD. Such examples would include reinforcement, discrete trial teaching, peer mediated interventions, prompting, and strategies such as social stories. These types of interventions are used with children with ASD for a limited time period with the intent of demonstrating a specific change in targeted behavior. Many focused intervention practices have evidence of efficacy for ASD (Hall 2009; Odom et al. 2003). Comprehensive treatment models form the second classification of intervention approaches for ASD. These models are designed to achieve a broader learning or developmental impact on the core deficits of ASD typically administered over a longer period of time and focus upon a broader range of target behaviors (National Research Council 2001). Many of these interventions have been referred to as branded (Rogers and Vismara 2008) and are often identified, as in this text, by a consistently used name (e.g., TEACCH, etc.). Some models have been disseminated widely, others are less well known. In 2001, a committee convened by the National Academy of Sciences to review the research on effective practices for children with ASD identified a set of proven interventions. Their review primarily described the modular approach focused almost exclusively on young children, finding limited evidence of efficacy for all but the Lovaas model used with very severely impaired children and some limited support for a program referred to as pivotal response treatment (Koegel et al. 1999). The authors concluded that their analysis of comprehensive treatment models for autism noted some with well-established evidence for the model, others with mixed evidence while still others with very weak evidence.

ASD is associated with a wide range of internalizing and externalizing behavioral problems as well. Young children with ASD typically exhibit patterns of hyperactivity, noncompliance, and frequent aggression. Latency age and teenagers with ASD often manifest internalizing symptoms related to anxiety and depression as the stresses of everyday life combined with an inability to understand, appreciate and function well within a social environment takes its toll on their psychological well being. Typically the more disruptive a particular behavior may be the more likely it is to become a target for intervention and modification. Thus, more severe patterns of tantrums, stereotypies, noncompliance, self-injury, and aggression, often observed at young ages and initially targeted for modification.

These patterns of internalizing and externalizing problem behaviors are part of the clinical presentation of ASD. Some are very consistent with the symptom profile. Others appear to be a consequence of associated but not diagnostic symptoms involving language, communication, emotional dysregulation, and sensory sensitivities (Gadow et al. 2004; Lecavalier 2006). Serious behavioral problems, including those related to violent aggression or self-injury not only pose immediate safety risks for the individual child and care givers but have been associated with broader functional impairments (RUPP Autism Network 2007). They typically interfere with opportunities to gain emotional and academic knowledge as well as increase independence and maturity (Horner et al. 2002). Absent direct intervention, these behavioral difficulties frequently shift and modify but nearly always lead to greater impairment as these children mature (Horner et al. 2002; Tonge and Einfeld 2003). Disruptive behaviors, particularly in ASD, have been associated with higher levels of parental stress, perception of parents' isolation and unsupport, and decreased family cohesion (Lecavalier et al. 2006; Schieve et al. 2007).

Table 1.1 Evidence-based practice briefs for children and youth with ASD

Antecedent-based interventions (ABI)
Computer-aided instruction
Differential reinforcement
Discrete trial training
Extinction
Functional behavior assessment
Functional communication training
Naturalistic intervention
Parent-implemented intervention
Peer-mediated instruction and intervention
Picture exchange communication system (PECS)
Pivotal response training
Prompting
Reinforcement
Response interruption/redirection
Self-management
Social narratives
Social skills groups
Speech generating devices/VOCA
Structured work systems
Task analysis
Time delay
Video modeling
Visual supports

Given this pattern of prevalence, chronicity, and adverse impact on the child and environment, these problems have been the impetus driving the development of effective and feasible interventions as part of an overall treatment plan for autism. As such they have become an increasing focus of research and applied practice. There is an increasing body of research (for review see Livanis et al. 2012) demonstrating the effectiveness of behavioral interventions in assessing and treating disruptive behavior in ASD as well as targeting core social and communication deficits. The Center for Autism Research recently published a table and accompanying analysis of effective treatments (The National Professional Development Center on Autism Spectrum Disorders n.d.). Thus, behavioral and social interventions have become a predominant treatment approach for the related symptoms and impairments associated with autism (Bregman et al. 2005) (Table 1.1).

The majority of empirically based behavioral interventions are rooted in the principles of applied behavioral analysis (ABA) (Johnson et al. 2007). There is a wide range of research supporting the use of focused ABA strategies for enhancing social and functional communication skills and treating behavior problems in children with ASD (National Research Council 2001; Schreibman and Ingersoll 2005). Although much of this research is based on single subject design (Johnson et al. 2007), there are at least some randomized controlled studies completed to date (for review see Tonge et al. 2006). These interventions have reflected a shift from consequence driven approaches to more preventive antecedent approaches (Horner et al. 2002). Positive behavior support (PBS) underlies the most current treatment approach and has been supported by extensive research (e.g., Dunlap et al. 1999, 2008; Fox et al. 2002; Koegel and Keogel 2006). PBS focuses on modifying situations and environmental context that precipitate problem behavior, thus creating a prosthetic environment in which the child with ASD is more likely to function well and benefit from experience. Concomitantly, there is also a focus on teaching adaptive and appropriate behaviors with the goal of reducing impairment and helping children experience greater success. PBS has been shown to be effective in reducing a range of negative behaviors in children and adults with autism (Koegel et al. 1996, Van Bourgondien et al. 2003).

These behavioral approaches have also evolved in that rather than focusing on reductions in very specific targeted behavior change they take a more global view attempting to impact motivation and communication providing the child with a greater chance of generalizing learned skills. This pattern of pivotal response training (Koegel et al. 1996) attempts to use intrinsic motivation within the child to teach functional social skills and communication. This pattern of child initiated learning in children with ASD has demonstrated positive outcomes that may be more generalizable across settings (Koegel et al. 1996).

There has also been an equal shift away from treatment within highly controlled clinical settings to more natural contexts with caregivers and teachers acting as agents of change. This has allowed for collaborative treatment and opportunities to teach skills within the context of children's daily routines (Smith et al. 2010). This approach, known as family centered intervention, has also been demonstrated to lead to positive outcomes for ASD (Smith et al. 2010). Intensive community based interventions based on PBS and positive support strategies have yielded positive outcomes with respect to enhanced language and communication as well as reductions in problem behavior (Perry et al. 2008; Smith et al. 2010).

Concomitantly, there is an increased interest in functional behavioral analysis (Gresham et al. 2001), for example, this model has become the central part of assessment within the schools for all children with developmental challenges. Problem behaviors associated with ASD are often complex, difficult to operationalize, and guided by multiple variables. Functional behavioral analysis involves direct and indirect clinical observation and data collection to determine the function, purpose, or outcome of such behaviors. This information is then utilized to develop efficient and effective treatment plans. There has been an increased focus on attempting to collect specific, quantified data concerning symptoms and impairments as part of the assessment process to guide treatment planning (Goldstein and Naglieri 2009b).

Numerous single case studies have demonstrated the positive effects of parent training and parent directed interventions for reducing problem behaviors in children with ASD's (Aman et al. 2009). Parents are taught behavioral principles and strategies for defining and shaping positive behaviors. Many of the current comprehensive training programs for children with ASD include parent components, including TEACCH (Mesibov et al. 2005), SCERTS (Prizant et al. 2003), and Star Denver (Arick et al. 2005). In 2007, the RUPP Autism Network developed a manualized training program for parents of children 4–16 years of age with ASD and severe behavior problems. A multisite, randomized controlled treatment study was developed as an adjunct to medication treatment. Primary treatment goals included improving child compliance and adaptive functioning and decreasing disruptive behaviors. Sessions included empirically based behavioral techniques such as direct instruction, modeling, role play, homework, and activity sheets for behavior tracking as well as a review of video vignettes. Autism specific strategies were employed. The feasibility of this parent training program was carefully evaluated. Rates of parental attendance and adherence as well as satisfaction with the program were high as was treatment integrity. Parents reported reduced rates of child noncompliance and irritability as well as enhanced child daily living skills and reductions in parenting stress (RUPP Autism Network 2007). In 2009, Aman et al. completed a randomized controlled trial examining the effects of this program combined with medication in children with ASD and serious behavioral problems. They demonstrated significant improvements in hyperactivity/noncompliance, stereotypic behavior, and irritability symptoms beyond the medication only effect.

The effectiveness of medications particularly focused on hyperactivity and impulsivity being well demonstrated (Aman et al. 2009). Although medications have been demonstrated to be helpful in managing severe disruptive behaviors in ASD, these medicines offer symptom relief but do not target core symptoms of the disorder. Typically challenging behaviors associated with ASD reemerge when medications are missed or discontinued (Aman et al. 2009). The pharmacotherapy of particularly disruptive and to some extent nondisruptive behavioral problems associated with ASD has primarily focused on associated impairments and not necessarily attempted to directly treat autistic symptoms. Particularly, physical aggression and self-injurious behaviors have been of greatest concern to treating physicians. As such, targeted behaviors involving irritability, aggression, and self-injurious behavior that are thought to be beyond capacity for efficient behavioral management and shaping are often treated with a variety of atypical antipsychotic agents. Further, problems of hyperactivity, impulsiveness, and inattention are found to be highly associated with ASD if not a part of the diagnostic condition (Goldstein and Naglieri 2009b). Pharmacotherapy has become increasingly a part of the treatment regime for children with autism spectrum disorders. Some community surveys have suggested a prevalence of medication use in this population of at least 40–80 % (Aman et al. 2005; Oswald and Sonenkler 2007; Witwer and Lacavalier 2005). Most common medications include the selective serotonin reuptake inhibitors, antipsychotics Alpha 2 adronergic agonists, psychostimulants, and anticonvulsants. Empirical support for the use of medications in children with ASD varies widely. Multiple researchers have demonstrated that the antipsychotic Risperidone can reduce serious behavioral problems in children with ASD including tantrums, aggression, and self-injury. The Food and Drug Administration has approved Risperidone as a treatment for children with autism accompanied by irritability such as tantrums, aggression, and self-injury. However, this medication clearly does not improve the core symptoms of the condition. Stimulants have also been widely used in children with ASD, particularly in light of their common attention, impulse, and hyperactive behaviors (Research Units on Pediatric Psychopharmacology Autism Network 2002; Shay et al. 2004).

References

Aman, M. G., Lamb, K. L., & Van Bourgondien, M. E. (2005). Medication patterns in patients with Autism: Temporal, regional and demographic influences. *Journal of Adolescent Psychopharmacology, 15,* 116–126.

Aman, M. G., McDougle, C. J., Scahill, L., Handen, B., Arnold, L. E., Johnson, C., Stigler, K. A., Bearss, K., Butter, E., et al. (2009). Medication and parent training in children with pervasive developmental disorders and serious behavior problems: Results from a randomized clinical trial. *Journal of the American Academy of Child and Adolescent Psychiatry, 48*(12), 1143–1154.

American Psychiatric Association. (1952). *Diagnostic and statistical manual of mental disorders.* Washington, DC: Author.

American Psychiatric Association. (1968). *Diagnostic and statistical manual of mental disorders* (2nd ed.). Washington, DC: Author.

American Psychiatric Association. (1980). *Diagnostic and statistical manual of mental disorders* (3rd ed.). Washington, DC: Author.

American Psychiatric Association. (1994). *Diagnostic and statistical manual of mental disorders* (4th ed.). Washington, DC: Author.

American Psychiatric Association. (2000). *Diagnostic and statistical manual of mental disorders* (4th ed., text rev.). Washington, DC: Author.

American Psychiatric Association. (2013). *Diagnostic and statistical manual of mental disorders* (5th ed.). Washington, DC: Author (in press).

American Psychiatric Association Neurodevelopmental Disorders Work Group. (2011). Autism Spectrum Disorder. Retrieved from http://www.dsm5.org/ProposedRevisions/Pages/proposedrevision.aspx?rid=94#. 26 Jan 2011.

Arick, J., Loos, L., Falco, R., & Krug, D. (2005). *The STAR program: Strategies for teaching based on autism research.* Austin: Pro-Ed.

Asperger, H. (1991). 'Autistic psychopathy' in childhood (U. Frith, Trans). In U. Frith (Ed.), *Autism and asperger syndrome* (pp. 37–92). Cambridge, UK: Cambridge University Press. (Original work published 1944).

Baron-Cohen, S. (1989). Do autistic children have obsessions and compulsions? *British Journal of Clinical Psychology, 28*(3), 193–200.

Bregman, J. D., Zager, D., & Gerdtz, J. (2005). Behavioral interventions. In F. Volkmar, R. Paul, A. Klin, & D. Cohen (Eds.), *Handbook of autism and pervasive developmental disorders* (3rd ed., pp. 897–924). Hobokin: Wiley.

Boucher, J. (1981). Memory for recent events in autistic children. *Journal of Autism and Developmental Disorders, 11,* 293–302.

Cantwell, D. P., Baker, L., & Rutter, M. (1980). Families of autistic children and dysphasic children: Family life and direction patterns. *Advances in Family Psychiatry, 2,* 295–312.

Center for Disease Control and Prevention. (2007). *Prevalence of the autism spectrum disorders in multiple areas of the United States, surveillance years 2000 and 2002: A report from the autism and developmental disabilities monitoring network* (February 8, 2007). Atlanta: Author.

Cohen, D. J., & Volkmar, F. R. (1997). *Handbook of autism and pervasive developmental disorders.* New York: Wiley.

DeMyer, M. K., Hingtgen, J. N., & Jackson, R. K. (1981). Infantile autism reviewed: A decade of research. *Schizophrenia Bulletin, 7,* 388–451.

Dunlap, G., Clarke, S., & Steiner, M. (1999). Intervention research in behavioral and developmental disabilities: 1980–1997. *Journal of Positive Behavior Interventions, 1*(3), 170–180 (1999). doi:10.1177/109830079900100305.

Dunlap, G., Iovannone, R., & Kincaid, D. (2008). Essential components for effective educational programs. In J. Luiselli, D. C. Russo, W. P. Christian, & S. M. Wilczynski (Eds.), *Effective practices for children with Autism: Educational and behavior support interventions that work* (pp. 111–136). New York: Oxford University Press.

Factor, D. C., Freeman, N. L., & Kardash, A. (1989). A comparison of DSM-III and DSM-III-R criteria for autism. *Journal of Autism and Developmental Disorders, 19,* 637–640.

Fein, D., Pennington, B., Markowitz, P., Braverman, M., & Waterhouse, L. (1986). Towards a neuropsychological model of infantile autism: Are the social deficits primary? *Journal of the American Academy of Child Psychiatry, 25,* 198–212.

Fox, L., Benito, N., & Dunlap, G. (2002). Early intervention with families of young children with Autism and behavior problems. In J. M. Lucyshyn, G. Dunlap, & R. W. Albin (Eds.), *Families, family life, and positive behavior support: Addressing the challenge of problem behavior in family contexts* (pp. 251–269). Baltimore: Brookes.

Frith, U. (1989). *Autism: Explaining the enigma.* Oxford: Blackwell.

Frith, U. (2004). Confusions and controversies about Asperger syndrome. *Journal of Child Psychology and Psychiatry, 45,* 672–686.

Gadow, K. D., DeVincent, C. J., Pomeroy, J., & Azizian, A. (2004). Psychiatric symptoms in preschool children with PDD and clinic and comparison samples. *Journal of Autism and Developmental Disorders, 34,* 379–393.

Gillberg, C. (1990). Autism and pervasive developmental disorders. *Journal of Child Psychology and Psychiatry, 31,* 99–119.

Gillberg, C., & Schaumann, H. (1982). Social class and autism: Total population aspects. *Journal of Autism and Developmental Disorders, 12,* 223–228.

Gillberg, C., & Steffenburg, S. (1987). Outcome and prognostic factors in infantile autism and similar conditions: A population-based study of 46 cases followed through puberty. *Journal of Autism and Developmental Disorders, 17,* 273–287.

Goldstein, S., Naglieri, J., & Ozonoff, S. (Eds.) (2008). *Assessment of Autism.* New York: Guilford.

Goldstein, S., & Naglieri J. (2009a). *Autism Spectrum Rating Scales.* Toronto: MHS Publishers.

Goldstein, S. & Naglieri, J. (Eds.) (2009b). *Practitioner's Guide to Assessing Intelligence and Achievement.* New York: Wiley.

Gresham, F. M., Watson, T. S., & Skinner, C. H. (2001). Functional behavioral assessment: Principles, procedures, and future directions. *School Psychology Review, 30,* 156–172.

Hall, L. (2009). Autism spectrum disorders: *From theory to practice.* Upper Saddle River, NJ: Pearson Merrill Prentice Hall.

Hobson, R. P. (1989). Beyond cognition: A theory of autism. In G. Dawson (Ed.), *Autism: Nature, diagnosis, and treatment* (pp. 22–48). New York: Guilford Press.

Horner, R. H., Carr, E. G., Strain, P. S., Todd, A. W., & Reed, H. K. (2002). Problem behavior interventions for young children with autism: A research synthesis. *Journal of Autism and Developmental Disorders, 32*(5), 423–446.

Howlin, P., Goode, S., Hutton, J., & Rutter, M. (2004). Adult outcome for children with autism. *Journal of Child Psychology and Psychiatry, 45,* 212–229.

Johnson, C. R., Handen, B. L., Butter, E., Wagner, A., Mulick, J., Sukhodolsky, D. G., et al. (2007). Development of a parent training program for children with pervasive developmental disorders. *Behavioral Interventions, 22,* 201–221.

Kim, Y. S., Leventhal, B. L., Koh, Y. J., Fombonne, E., Laska, E., Lim, E. C., Cheon, K. A., Kim, S. J., Kim, Y. K., Lee, H., Song, D. H., & Grinker, R. R. (2011). Prevalence of autism spectrum disorders in a total population sample. *American Journal of Psychiatry, 168,* 904–912.

Klin, A., Pauls, D., Schultz, R., Volkmar, F. (2005). Three diagnostic approaches to Asperger syndrome: Implications for research. *Journal of Autism and Developmental Disorders,* 35, 221–234.

Koegel, R. L., & Koegel, L. K. (2006). *Pivotal response treatments for Autism.* Baltimore: Brookes.

Koegel, L. K., Koegel, R. L., & Dunlap, G. (1996). *Positive behavioral Support: Including people with difficult behavior in the community.* Baltimore: Paul H. Brookes.

Koegel, L. K., Koegel, R. L., Shoshan, Y., & McNerney, E. (1999). Pivotal response intervention II: Preliminary long-term outcome data. *Journal of the Association for Persons with Severe Handicaps, 24,* 186–198.

Kolvin, I. (1971). Studies in the childhood psychoses: I. Diagnostic criteria and classification. *British Journal of Psychiatry, 118,* 381–384.

Kurita, H., Osada, H., & Miyake, Y. (2004). External validity of childhood disintegrative disorder in comparison with autistic disorder. *Journal of Autism and Developmental Disorders, 34,* 355–362.

Lane, H. (1977). *The wild boy of Aveyron*. London: Allen & Unwin.

Lecavalier, L. (2006). Behavioral and emotional problems in young people with pervasive developmental disorders: Relative prevalence, effects of subject characteristics, and empirical classification. *Journal of Autism and Developmental Disorders, 36,* 1101–1114.

Lecavalier, L. (2006). Behavioral and emotional problems in young people with pervasive developmental disorders: Relative prevalence, effects of subject characteristics, and empirical classification. *Journal of Autism and Developmental Disorders, 36,* 1101–1114.

Lecavalier, L., Leone, S., Wiltz, J., (2006). The Impact of behaviour problems on caregiver stress in young people with autism spectrum disorders. *Journal of Intellectual Disability Research, 50,* 172–183.

Livanis, A., Benvenuto, S., Mertturk, A., & Hanthorn, C. (2012). Treatment integrity in autism spectrum disorders. In S. Goldstein & J. A. Naglieri (Eds.), *Interventions for autism spectrum disorders: Translating science into practice*. New York: Springer.

Lotter, V. (1974). Factors related to outcome in autistic children. *Journal of Autism and Child Schizophrenia, 4,* 263–277.

Loveland, K. A., & Kelley, M. L. (1991). Development of adaptive behavior in preschoolers with autism and Down syndrome. *American Journal on Mental Retardation, 96*(11), 13–20.

MacDonald, H., Rutter, M., Howlin, P., Rios, P., LeConeur, A., Evered, C., & Folstein, S. (1989). Recognition and expression of emotional cues by autistic and normal adults. *Journal of Child Psychology and Psychiatry, 30*(6), 865–877.

Mayes, S. D., Calhoun, S. L., & Crites, D. L. (2001). Does DSM-IV Asperger's disorder exist? *Journal of Abnormal Child Psychology, 29,* 263–271.

Mesibov, G. B., Shea, V., & Schopler, E. (2005). *The TEACCH approach to autism spectrum disorders*. New York: Springer.

Miller, J., & Ozonoff, S. (1997). Did Asperger's cases have Asperger disorder? *Journal of Child Psychology and Psychiatry, 38,* 247–251.

Mundy, P., Sigman, M. D., Ungerer, J., & Sherman, T. (1986). Defining the social deficits of autism: The contribution of non-verbal communication measures. *Journal of Child Psychology and Psychiatry, 27,* 657–669.

National Research Council. (2001). C. Lord & J. McGee (Eds.), *Educating children with autism*. Washington, DC: National Academy.

Odom, S. L., Brown, W. H., Frey, T., Karasu, N., Smith-Carter, L., & Strain, P. (2003). Evidence-based practices for young children with autism: Evidence from single-subject research design. *Focus on Autism and Other Developmental Disabilities, 18,* 176–181.

Odom, S. L., Boyd, B. A., Hall, L. J., & Hume, K. (2010). Evaluation of comprehensive treatment models for individuals with Autism Spectrum Disorders. *Journal of Autism and Developmental Disorders, 40,* 425–436.

Ornitz, E. M., & Ritvo, E. R. (1968). Neurophysiological mechanisms underlying perceptual inconstancy in autistic and schizophrenic children. *Archives of General Psychiatry, 19,* 22–27.

Oswald, D. P., Sonenkler, N. A. (2007). Medication use among children with Autism Spectrum Disorders. *Journal of Adolescent Psychopharmacology, 17,* 348–355.

Perry, A., Cummings, A., Dunn Geier, J., Freeman, N. L., Hughes, S., LaRose, L., et al. (2008). Effectiveness of intense behavior intervention in a large, community-based program. *Research in Autism Spectrum Disorders, 2,* 621–642.

Prizant, B. M., Wetherby, A. M., Rubin, E., & Laurent, A. C. (2003). The SCERTS model: A transactional, family-centered approach to enhancing communication and socioemotional abilities of children with Autism Spectrum Disorder. *Infants and Young Children, 16,* 296–316.

Research Units on Pediatric Psychopharmacology Autism Network. (2002). Risperidone in children with autism and serious behavior problems. *New England Journal of Medicine, 347,* 314–321.

Rett, A. (1966). Uber ein eigenartiges hirnatrophisces Syndrome bei Hyperammonie im Kindersalter. *Wein Medizinische Wochenschrift, 118,* 723–738.

Rogers, S., & Vismara, L. (2008). Evidence-based comprehensive treatments for early autism. *Journal of Clinical Child and Adolescent Psychology, 37,* 8–38.

Rutter, M. (1970). Autistic children. *Seminars in Psychiatry, 2,* 435–450.
Rutter, M. (1978). Diagnostic validity in child psychiatry. *Advances in Biological Psychiatry, 2,* 2–22.
Rutter, R. (1983). Cognitive deficits in the pathogensis of autism. *Journal of Child Psychology and Psychiatry, 24*(4), 513–531.
Rutter, M., Bailey, A., Bolton, P., & Le Conteur, A. (1994). Autism in known medical conditions: Myth and substance. *Journal of Child Psychology and Psychiatry, 35,* 311–322.
RUPP Autism Network. (2007). Parent training for children with pervasive developmental disorders: A multi-site feasibility trial. *Behavioral Interventions, 22,* 179–199.
Schieve, L. A., Blumberg, S. J., Rice, C., Viser, S. N., & Boyle, C. (2007). The relationship between autism and parenting stress. *Pediatrics, 119,* s114–s121.
Schreibman, L., & Ingersoll, B. (2005). Behavioral interventions to promote learning in individuals with autism. In F. Volkmar, R. Paul, A., Klin, & D. Cohen (Eds.), *Handbook of autism and pervasive developmental disorders* (3rd ed., pp. 882–896). Hoboken: Wiley.
Schoper, E., & Mesibov, G. B. (Eds.). (1987). *Neurobiological issues in autism.* New York: Plenum Press.
Seigel, B., Vukicevic, J., Elliot, G. R., & Kraemer, H. C. (1989). The use of signal detection theory to assess DSM-III-R criteria for autistic disorder. *Journal of the American Academy of Child and Adolescent Psychiatry, 28*(4), 542–548.
Shay, S., Turgay, A., Carroll, A., et al. (2004). Risperidone in the treatment of disruptive behavioral symptoms in children with autistic and other pervasive developmental disorders. *Pediatrics, 115,* 634–641.
Smalley, S., Asarnow, R., & Spence, M. (1988). Autism and genetics: A decade of research. *Archives of General Psychiatry, 45,* 953–961.
Smith, I. M., Koegel, R. L., Koegel, L. K., Openden, D. A., Fossum, K. L., & Bryson, S. E. (2010). Effectiveness of a novel community based early intervention model for children with autistic spectrum disorder. *American Association on Intellectual and Developmental Disabilities, 115*(6), 504–523.
The National Professional Development Center on Autism Spectrum Disorders (n.d.). *Evidence-based practices for children and youth with ASD.* Retrieved from http://autismpdc.fpg.unc.edu/content/briefs.
Tonge, B. J., & Einfeld, S. L. (2003). Psychopathology and intellectual disability: The Australian child to adult longitudinal study. In L. M. Glidden (Ed.), *International review of research in mental retardation.* San Diego: Academic.
Tonge, B., Brereton, A., Kiomall, M., MacKinnon, A., King, N., & Rinehart, N. (2006). Effects on parental mental health of an education and skills training program for parents of young children with autism: A randomized controlled trial. *Journal of the American Academy of Child and Adolescent Psychiatry, 45,* 561–569.
Van Bourgondien, M. E., Reichle, N. C., & Schopler, E. (2003). Effects of a model treatment approach on adults with autism. *Journal of Autism and Developmental Disorders, 33*(2), 131–140.
Venter, A., Lord, C., & Schopler, E. (1992). A follow-up study of high-functioning autistic children. *Journal of Child Psychology and Psychiatry, 33,* 489–507.
Volkmar, F. (1998). Categorical approaches to the diagnosis of autism: An overview of DSM-IV and ICD-10. *Autism, 2,* 45–59.
Volkmar, F., Carter, A., Sparrow, S. S., & Cicchetti, D. V. (1993). Quantifying social development in autism. *Journal of the American Academy of Child and Adolescent Psychiatry, 32*(3), 627–632.
Volkmar, F. R., Sparrow, S. S., Goudreau, D., Cicchetti, D. V., Paul, R., Cohen, D. J. (1987). Social deficits in autism: An operational approach using the Vineland Adaptive Behavior Scales. *Journal of the American Academy of Child and Adolescent Psychiatry, 26*(2), 156–161.
Witwer, A., & Lacavalier, L. (2005). Treatment incidence in patterns in children and adolescents with Autism Spectrum Disorders. *Journal of Adolescent Psychopharmacology, 15,* 671–681.
World Health Organization. (1993). *The ICD-10 classification of mental and behavioural disorders: Diagnostic criteria for research.* Geneva: Author.

Chapter 2
Treatment Integrity in Autism Spectrum Disorder Interventions

Andrew Livanis, Samantha Benvenuto, Ayla Mertturk and Craig A. Hanthorn

The last few years have seen a remarkable proliferation of treatment programs to ameliorate the symptoms of autism spectrum disorders (ASD; National Autism Center 2009). In addition, there is an increasing legal and ethical burden placed on the practitioner working with an ASD population to use evidence based interventions (EBI) that have been evaluated in the scientific literature (Detrich 2008). The vast database of interventions and added pressures make the job of the clinician quite difficult—they must sift through competing evidence bases, spectacular statistical claims, and treatments that "wrap themselves in the cloak of science" (Wilczynski et al. 2008, p. 37) in order to find treatment programs that will be effective. Fortunately, there exist a variety of resources to help the practitioner identify an EBI. In fact, this book will serve as a very useful guide to help parents and professionals select potentially effective interventions for children with ASD.

The selection and implementation of EBIs require that professionals consider the construct of *treatment integrity*, both during the research development and dissemination stages. During the selection process, the practitioner will obviously review a good deal of research documenting a variety of experimental research where the EBI is investigated. These studies follow a very typical format: a treatment is outlined a priori, implemented with one or several children, and the effects of the EBI on various symptoms or quality of life indicators is then discussed. However, most research studies do not provide the assurance that the study was carried out in a controlled and prespecified manner, without deviations to the a priori treatment descriptions (i.e., the protocol). Deviations from this protocol cast doubt on the relationship between the treatment and the outcomes, and as such, would decrease the confidence that the reader would have in the strength of that treatment.

After a treatment program has been selected, the practitioner must implement the package as written or as close to its original design as possible. An EBI that is

A. Livanis (✉)
Department of Counseling and School Psychology, Long Island University,
Brooklyn Campus, 1 University Plaza, 11201–5372 Brooklyn, NY USA
e-mail: andrew.livanis@liu.edu

S. Benvenuto · A. Mertturk · C. A. Hanthorn
Long Island University, Brooklyn Campus, 1 University Plaza, Brooklyn,
NY 11201–5372, USA

S. Goldstein, J. A. Naglieri (eds.), *Interventions for Autism Spectrum Disorders*,
DOI 10.1007/978-1-4614-5301-7_2, © Springer Science+Business Media New York 2013

applied in a radically different way than how it was described in the literature ceases to be based in evidence and is no better than a haphazard combination of treatments. Treatment integrity, as a construct, factors considerably in the implementation of an intervention.

Treatment Integrity

A critical issue which needs to be demonstrated by researchers and practitioners is the reliable and accurate implementation of an intervention and how true the treatment is to the theoretical and procedural components of the overall treatment model or as intended by the developers of the treatment package (Reed and Codding 2011; Nezu and Nezu 2008; Dusenbury et al. 2003). This phenomenon is what is typically referred to as *treatment integrity* (also known as *treatment fidelity, procedural fidelity, or intervention integrity*). The failure to control for treatment integrity can lead to one of three major problems: an inability to evaluate the effects of a program or intervention; the potential lack of improvement among clients and/or consumers; and a host of related ethical and potential legal problems.

First, and most importantly, if the treatment is not implemented with integrity, practitioners and researchers cannot realistically evaluate the effects of the independent variable upon the dependent variable (Kazdin 2011; Cooper et al. 2007). In other words, a lack of treatment integrity decreases confidence in the ability of the treatment to effect changes in the symptomology and quality of life of children with ASD. An unsystematic or careless manipulation of the independent variable can lead to errors in inferential reasoning due to the fact that a distorted or diluted version of the treatment may have been applied (Nezu and Nezu 2008). In these instances, the intervention takes on multiple "lives"—one which exists on paper and one which is actually implemented—both of which may be similar to one another but not exactly the same (Livanis and Mercer 2011).

Second, the implementation of interventions with high rates of treatment integrity is associated with positive treatment outcomes (Hogue et al. 2008; DiGennaro et al. 2005, 2007; Erhardt et al. 1996). Treatment integrity appears to serve to mediate on the effect that the intervention plans had on student outcomes (Cook et al. 2010). In other words, good treatments, when implemented correctly, tend to have positive effects on clients and consumers.

Lastly, within certain systems, the failure to follow a treatment protocol in written form can potentially constitute a denial of certain state and/or federal rights. For instance, under IDEA (2004) it is federally mandated that administrators, teachers, service personnel, and other school staff are trained in the implementation of evidence-based curriculum, practices, and interventions. Within the field of psychology, the push for EBIs has increased tremendously over the past decade and a wide variety of governmental agencies and professional organizations have sought to define EBIs for children with ASD (Reichow and Volkmar 2011). However, an EBI, when not implemented as intended, ceases to be an EBI. Therefore, when considering intervention plans within school systems for children with ASD, a lack of treatment integrity can potentially be considered to be a deprivation of constitutionally protected due process rights (Cook et al. 2010; Etschdeit 2006), due to the fact that an EBI was technically not provided to the child.

Various professional organizations address treatment integrity within their ethical codes or in collections of best practices for treatment implementation. The American Psychological Association's (APA) policy statement on evidence-based practice in psychology (APA 2005) states that in order to ensure the effectiveness and validity of intervention strategies, systematic review and assessment is necessary; a lack of such evaluation would otherwise be viewed as unethical. The code of ethics mandated by the American Speech-Language-Hearing Association (ASHA 2010) finds that it is ethically necessary for consistent evaluation of services and products to ensure effectiveness and to sufficiently maintain research records of professional services performed. The National Association of School Psychologists (NASP) principles for professional ethics (NASP 2010a) states that, "school psychologists use assessment techniques and practices that the profession considers to be responsible, research-based practice" (p. 7). The NASP model for comprehensive and integrated school psychological services (NASP 2010b) urges school psychologists to use multisource data collection and assessment procedures to ensure effective implementation of EBIs.

Despite the problems that can result from a lack of treatment integrity, the construct is often not measured effectively in studies that evaluate psychological and educational interventions (McLeod et al. 2009; Dusenbury et al. 2003), and in too many instances, not at all. In fact, the measurement and demonstration of treatment integrity often serves as a much more challenging process than the development of effective treatment programs (Foxx 1996). Wheeler et al. (2006) found that only 18 % of the studies of interventions for children actually assessed and reported treatment integrity data. This is a problem for clinicians because the literature that they are reading fails to demonstrate that the protocol was followed reliably and can translate to a lack of adherence by clients, staff, and consumers (Allen and Warzak 2000). In fact, only 1–2 % of practicing school psychologists regularly measured rates of treatment integrity (Cochrane and Laux 2008).

Dimensions of Treatment Integrity

Treatment integrity is described as a multidimensional construct (McLeod et al. 2009), typically consisting of three components (Perepletchikova and Kazdin 2005): treatment adherence, agent competence, and treatment differentiation.

Treatment Adherence

Adherence refers to the reliable use of the procedures as specified a priori by the clinician or researcher. Adherence has been demonstrated to improve dramatically when those who are implementing the treatment are exposed to some form of consistent and ongoing training or supervision. For example, Hogue et al. (2008) found that the provision of weekly supervision to therapists increased fidelity to the manualized treatment protocols, which in turn led to significant decreases in problem behaviors in an outpatient setting. Codding et al. (2005) implemented biweekly direct observations and immediate feedback to increase the level of integrity to the treatment plan in a school setting.

Adherence to the treatment protocol is a complex issue, and may be dependent upon the setting that the treatment will be administered as well as the functional levels of the client. The adoption of programs in real-world settings such as clinics, hospitals, and schools often requires some form of protocol flexibility to meet the individual needs of children with ASD or the systemic constraints of the agency that serves children with ASD (Schulte et al. 2009; Dusenbury et al. 2003). As such, treatment protocols (or follow-up research studies) should strive to identify the amount that each component can vary, as well as the relative contribution of each component to the overall outcome. For example, Taylor and Miller (1997) identified which components could be modified in their application of a functional analysis protocol (designed for use in a university clinic setting) for use in a residential hospital setting for the treatment of children with ASD. While the original protocol called for initial assessment to be conducted in a room with which the child was unfamiliar with novel materials, Taylor and Miller conducted the assessment in the classroom with familiar materials, with commensurate results. The researchers still maintained the same conditions that the original protocol highlighted (i.e., the provision of alternating assessment conditions).

Even in situations where some level of individualization was called for, the absolute lack of treatment integrity still poses a problem. Barber et al. (2006) in their evaluation of the treatment integrity of drug treatment found that very high levels, as well as very low levels, of adherence were associated with negative client outcomes, and some level of protocol adaptation was necessary depending on the client's unique situation, as well as the amount and intensity of their symptomologies (Perepletchikova and Kazdin (2005). However, too much deviation may lead to a situation in which the EBI loses its essential core components. On the basis of this line of reasoning, adherence to ASD interventions may be dependent on the severity of client functioning; perhaps the same interventions need to be applied to children with high and low levels of functioning with different levels of integrity. For example, the use of a token economy to increase desired routines in the home and in the school might need stricter adherence for children with lower levels of functioning (e.g., children with lesser cognitive and language abilities) than when used for children with high levels of functioning. Aspects of the intervention, such as the immediacy of reinforcement, can be allowed to deviate from the protocol, which is useful when the treatment is applied to multiple children simultaneously.

Agent Competence

Agent competence refers to the knowledge base and skill that the individual who is implementing an intervention exhibits (Perepletchikova and Kazdin 2005). Competence may be a dimension whose importance is dependent on the complexity of the intervention—if the intervention procedures are simple, competence may become less of an issue (Schulte et al. 2009; Gresham 2005). For example, competence may not be as important when evaluating an intervention where notes are exchanged between the home and in school but may be important when implementing a school-based behavior plan in nontraditional settings such as a school trip. Since treatment programs designed for children with ASD tend to be more complex and labor-intensive (Livanis and Mercer 2011; Yeaton and Sechrest 1981), the consideration of agent competence should be routine. Researchers must constantly demonstrate that agents have been trained effectively to implement the treatment program at hand. In the field, client and consumer comprehension of the intervention can be conceptualized as a function of agents' access to preservice and continuous inservice training opportunities and the agent's establishment of solid communication patterns with the client or consumer.

The issue of continuous inservice training for agents is a pressing matter. In many situations, the treatment agent may not have had access to preservice opportunities that would have prepared them for program implementation. For instance, parents, teachers, paraprofessionals, as well as hospital and group home workers, might all be asked to implement the same program although each individual may have different educational backgrounds. Therefore, time-efficient methods must be implemented to rapidly develop and maintain competence. Especially in situations where multiple agents are used, the intervention is only as strong as the most limited treatment agent, so it is important that all agents are trained to deliver the intervention.

Sterling-Turner et al. (2001) compared a variety of methods to train undergraduate volunteers in a protocol for issues related to tics: didactic methods, modeling, and a combination of staff rehearsal and feedback were compared and contrasted. The investigating team found that modeling, rehearsal, and feedback worked best to train undergraduates with no particular psychological training to use particular protocols in their interventions. Leblanc et al. (2005) looked at techniques to teach classroom paraprofessionals to implement a behavioral protocol for children with ASD and found that the use of corrective feedback increased competence rapidly. In fact, corrective feedback, or the process of observing agents' in vivo implementation and delivering feedback as to correctly and incorrectly applied components, has been demonstrated to be quite an effective and time-efficient manner to deliver inservice training opportunities to a wide variety of agents (Codding et al. 2005, 2008; DiGennaro et al. 2005, 2007; DiGennaro-Reed et al. 2010; Mortensen and Witt 1998; Mouzakitis 2010; Noell et al. 1997).

The client's comprehension of the intervention has been shown to increase as a function of the treatment agent's communication strategies (Barber et al. 2006; Cowan and Sheridan 2003; DiGennaro et al. 2005; Gresham 1996). Cowan and Sheridan (2003) found that the highest levels of integrity resulted when all parties engaged in clear communication patterns, which led to an understanding that the treatment program was under joint ownership. The agent's communication patterns can serve to make the components of the intervention meaningful to the client, thus establishing a better rapport. An agent's knowledge and experience in working with children with ASD may help to modify *how* the intervention is described when the client is the child himself or herself. For example, a competent treatment agent might use some of the child's idiosyncratic language patterns to explain the goals and the processes of the treatment, which may lead to increased comprehension. Teachers and parents appear to prefer interventions to be described to them in practical, common sense terms as opposed to psychological jargon (Elliot 1988; Witt et al. 1984). Overall, while time is a factor that can potentially impact treatment implementation and integrity (Elliot 1988; DiGennaro et al. 2005), there must also be time set aside for communication among all stakeholders.

Treatment Differentiation

Treatment differentiation refers to the extent that the treatment, intervention, or program that is implemented is "pure" and other treatments are not implemented in addition to or instead of the intervention (Perepletchikova and Kazdin 2005). Treatment differentiation is particularly important when two or more treatment programs are compared to one another in the research literature. Specifically, treatment protocols must be reliably distinguished from one another in order to ensure that potential differences in the dependent variable can be attributed to differences in the independent variable (Kazdin 1986).

An issue that can potentially affect differentiation in both the field and in research studies is *therapist drift* (Gresham 2005), where agents may modify the treatment in minor ways over a continuous period of time, thus producing a gradual shift in the independent variable over time. Such drift is often not purposeful but may result due to decreasing levels of diligence, supervision, or boredom. Therapist drift can serve to artificially overestimate or underestimate treatment effects.

Associated Variables

Treatment Complexity

The complexity of a treatment—which is operationally defined as the number of components of a treatment program—can be a very consistent predictor of treatment integrity (Perepletchikova and Kazdin 2005; Allen and Warzak 2000; Gresham 1996; Meichenbaum and Turk 1987; Yeaton and Sechrest 1981). Treatment complexity has the potential to impact programs for children with ASD since these interventions typically include more components and may require more preservice and ongoing inservice training. At one extreme, complex programs may be applied without integrity but in other situations, treatment programs may not be implemented at all due to their complexity (Yeaton and Sechrest 1981). The second extreme is quite troubling since a good deal of EBIs may not be implemented due to their complexity (or perceived complexity).

Livanis and Mercer (2011) described a procedure in which they taught school staff, with minimal preservice training, to implement a set of complex treatment programs to three children with ASD. Treatment integrity was achieved rapidly when a complex program was divided into smaller sections and the staff was presented with these smaller sections in a gradual manner, only when they demonstrated 100 % treatment adherence in previous sections. In essence, the study suggests that a graduated method of program presentation to staff can be useful to guard against the threats of complexity on treatment integrity.

Time Required to Deliver Intervention

Interventions for children with ASD tend to be more complex and as a result, require significantly more time to implement than interventions with children diagnosed with other conditions. The more time needed to learn the procedures in a program and implement them, the greater the threat to treatment integrity (Gresham 1996). Some procedures may not require an inordinate amount of time to implement but may require intensive levels of ongoing supervision and inservice training to maintain at effective levels (Happe 1982). Other treatments require extended periods of administration (typically referred to as *dosage*) due to the severity of the targeted social, communication, or stereotypical behaviors, or due to the comorbid psychiatric issues that also need to be addressed (Perepletchikova and Kazdin 2005). Time is an important variable because it introduces more opportunities for the treatment agent to implement aspects of a program without integrity.

Materials

The materials that are used in various treatment programs can potentially impact treatment integrity. In essence, the more materials needed, the greater the potential threat to treatment integrity (Gresham 1996). However, even a modest amount of expensive or highly technical materials can compromise treatment integrity (Perepletchikova and Kazdin 2005). Limited access to materials that are not commonly found in the school, home, or community can lower treatment integrity. In practical settings, such as hospitals, schools, and other therapeutic facilities, the budget cuts and ongoing financial constraints could potentially impact agents' abilities to access materials. For example, after an agency cuts their budget, the burden for purchasing and maintaining treatment materials will unfortunately fall on the treatment agents, such as teachers, therapists, hospital workers (Mouzakitis 2010), and without systemic support, there is no guarantee that supplies will be replenished in appropriate quality and quantity. Such issues are important to consider as most programs for children with ASD require a fair amount of materials (e.g., rewards, program sheets, special furniture, therapeutic aides, etc.).

Rate of Change

Treatments that result in rapid changes may be implemented with greater integrity than those that take longer to achieve an effect. Typically, treatments for ASD that demonstrate a broad evidence base will have documented rates of change. It may be helpful to maintain intervention persistence if the treatment agents have a realistic understanding of how long it might take to see any socially significant changes. Fortunately, there are public documents that are available to help program developers identify interventions for autism that have a substantial evidence base. One such document—the National Autism Center's (2009) National Standards Report (NSR)—is designed to help parents and professionals identify the research base for interventions, and make more informed decisions as to treatments to be used. The NSR categorizes interventions into three broad categories—*established, emerging,* and *unestablished.* Interventions in the established category refer to those studies that have a solid research base to demonstrate effectiveness across various age ranges, target difficulties, and diagnostic categories. Emerging interventions are those that show some limited but promising evidence of effectiveness and unestablished interventions show no evidence of effectiveness—in fact, in some instances the interventions are harmful. Established interventions may show improvements in overall functioning much more rapidly than those treatments in the emerging and unestablished categories, and may lead to fewer problems with treatment integrity.

Number of Agents

Most interventions with children with ASD often require that multiple agents implement the same treatment program. In general, the more agents that a treatment requires, the greater the risks to treatment integrity (Perepletchikova and Kazdin 2005; Gresham 1989). This threat can be reliably dealt with if all the agents are in one setting. For example, Koegel et al. (1977) highlighted a procedure to rapidly assess and train 11 teachers of children with ASD by providing in vivo individualized instruction, modeling, and feedback. Later in the study, the authors worked to help the staff members generalize these skills to other situations and groups of children.

However, if the agents are situated in different settings, such threats are difficult to manage. Gresham (1996) indicates that the lack of communication between agents among settings can potentially compromise program integrity—parents, teachers, and individual therapists might not understand which aspects of the program have been or need to be implemented. Additional problems arise when parents are asked (with little supervision) to implement aspects of a program. In these instances, parents may experience certain procedures as difficult to manage over a continuous period of time, which may cause them to drift from the originally stated procedure (Allen and Warzak 2000). This may be especially true in case of interventions that target more challenging difficulties, such as self-injurious behaviors. Inservice training that places an inordinate focus on the use of verbalizations for training may contribute to this drift. Such a focus on didactic training assumes that parents will develop adequate rules for program implementation based solely on instruction and follow them perfectly, which is an unrealistic assumption (Hayes and Wilson 1993). It is for this reason that a fair amount of training programs for parents (and all treatment agents) should include modeling, role-play, and rehearsal—ultimately, these training techniques need to be implemented on an ongoing basis, in situ.

Treatment Acceptability

Acceptability refers to the degree that a particular treatment program is evaluated as fair and reasonable to the referral question (Sterling-Turner et al. 2001), and has been typically implicated as a factor that can potentially impact treatment integrity (Perepletchikova and Kazdin 2005; Lentz et al. 1996; Gresham 1989; Elliot 1988). A number of variables can affect treatment acceptability. For example, acceptability appears to increase for interventions that are suggested for severe problems (Frentz and Kelley 1986; Elliot 1988), even when the interventions are complex and contain a large number of components. It may be the case, that desperation moves clients and consumers to be willing to attempt extreme interventions. In addition, when information is presented regarding the effectiveness of an intervention, acceptability tends to increase (Tingstrom et al. 1989). In fact, simply informing clients and consumers of the nature of the treatment, goals, and potential side effects in simple, everyday language can serve to increase acceptability significantly (Elliot 1988; Singh and Katz 1985; Witt et al. 1984).

However, a study conducted by Sterling-Turner et al. (2001) calls into question the relationship between treatment acceptability and treatment integrity. A central problem of most studies that examined this relationship is that they tended to correlate self-report measures of treatment acceptability and treatment outcome data. In order to correct this deficit in the literature, they collected data on treatment acceptability pretreatment and posttreatment implementation but conducted direct observations of student functioning. They found that clients' treatment acceptability before the intervention and after the intervention was not correlated with treatment integrity.

The relationship between acceptability and integrity appears logical: If an individual does not find a treatment acceptable, they will not implement it faithfully. However, there is a line of research that highlights the incongruence between what people say they will do and what they actually do. From a research perspective, it would not be unexpected to have a low correlation between self-report data of what people say they will do and actual observations of actions in an environment or what people actually do. In one instance, we are tapping into individuals' verbal reports of one (of many) potential future sequences of behaviors while in the other we measure an actual sequence of behaviors (Lloyd 1994), and such multiple assessment methods rarely result in high correlations (Gresham 1996).

However, the treatment acceptance may still affect integrity in other ways. Acceptance may play a role in the process of treatment selection. Agents that are allowed to select their own treatment, or feel as if they are valued during the treatment development stage, may be more motivated to implement an EBI with higher rates of integrity. Acceptance may serve as a mediator or moderator of treatment integrity in these instances. These agents may feel more committed to the treatment plan and seek out training opportunities or supervision on their own, thus working independently to increase treatment integrity. However, in some instances, the treatment agent may not necessarily agree with the treatment, and may be forced to implement the intervention against their will, based on their employment in a setting that has adopted a particular theoretical orientation (and the interventions that result from it conceptually) in a wholesale fashion. For example, paraprofessionals in school systems and group home workers often have little to no input during the treatment development process.

Measuring Treatment Integrity

Operational Definition of the Treatment and its Components

The treatment and its components should have clear, concise, and specific operational definitions that identify or describe which specific actions that the treatment agent and the client should perform (Cooper et al. 2007). A good operational definition of an independent variable (e.g., the treatment and/or its components) should include four dimensions: verbal (descriptions of scripts to be presented at various times), physical (descriptions of what actions should be performed), spatial (the positioning of materials such as furniture, papers, etc.), and temporal (which actions should follow which environmental events in the program sequence). Such descriptions allow for an easy replication of the intervention, both as a research study as well as in applied settings. However, it is possible that by overspecifying treatments and its individual components, a treatment can be made to appear overly complex, thus potentially affecting treatment integrity (Gresham 1996). One way to minimize this threat is to create two separate operational definitions that target varying levels of specification. The first operational definition would be presented to treatment agents and clients and include a description of each component of the intervention in everyday practical language; the second would include a series of behaviors identified from a task analysis of each component within the larger treatment. In this way, we can maintain the integrity of the intervention without introducing too much complexity.

Direct Assessment of Treatment Integrity

The direct assessment of treatment integrity is conducted similarly to traditional behavioral assessment (Cooper et al. 2007). The components of the treatment plan should be operationally defined and a system should be developed to monitor the presence or absence of the component. This direct assessment can take place at the point of treatment delivery or at a later time using video technology (Perepletchikova and Kazdin 2005).

As with all direct observations, it is important that the data are valid and representative of the component and treatment as a whole. The literature generally agrees that there should be multiple observations periods of sufficient length, but there are some differences among researchers as to how many times and how long treatment agents should be observed. Gresham (1996) offers a rough practical guideline of 3–5 observational sessions of 20–30 min duration each. During the nonexperimental conditions of their studies (i.e., baseline), Leblanc et al. (2005) and DiGennaro-Reed et al. (2010) observed treatment agents for 10–15 min, while Codding et al. (2005) observed treatment agents for 55–60 min. There is also variability in the amount of distinct observations that are conducted as well, ranging from 3 sessions (Leblanc et al. 2005) to 12 sessions (Codding et al. 2008). Reviews of these studies suggest that the number of observations may be the result of significant issues with establishing a baseline that was level. In order to establish an adequate control for the experimental condition of the study, the experimenters waited until they observed a sequence of data points that evidenced minimal variability. In studies that were conducted in controlled settings (i.e., special schools) such as in DiGennaro-Reed et al. (2010) and LeBlanc et al. (2005), the investigators obtained a baseline that had little to no variability rather quickly; in Codding et al. (2008), which was conducted in a public school setting, a level number of data points took much longer to obtain. Indeed, Codding et al. (2008) suggested that factors such as less training and more variability may necessitate more observational periods in order to better establish treatment integrity rates.

Treatment agents may change their behavior if they are aware that they are the subjects of observation—this is referred to as *reactivity* (Cooper et al. 2007). Reactivity has the potential to change a good deal of up to one-third of all behaviors for the duration of time that they are observed (Foster and Cone 1986). In certain settings, such as schools, hospitals, or group homes, staff may evidence concerns that a lack of treatment integrity may lead to a demotion or, in some instances, loss of a job. They may work harder when they know that they are being observed but may not necessarily implement the plan with much integrity at other times.

However, Codding et al. (2008) investigated observer reactivity in a particularly novel manner. The investigators observed classroom staff's implementation of a treatment program in two conditions: first, with an observer in the classroom and second, through a one-way mirror. The data during the experimental and nonexperimental conditions suggest that there were no differences between the two sets of observation. In this study, however, one of the researchers had worked closely with the staff in their classroom for several years prior to the start of the study, which implies that one key way to minimize reactivity is to spend a considerable amount of time in the environment prior to beginning observation. In addition, the research team took many of the precautions noted in Gresham (1996), such as observing staff on a randomized schedule, positioning themselves as unobtrusively as possible in the classroom (e.g., in corners of the room), and not indicating which staff member was going to be observed.

Although the majority of studies that examine treatment integrity focus on the assessment of treatment adherence, Perepletchikova and Kazdin (2005) stress that the other two dimensions of treatment integrity need to be assessed as well: agent competence and treatment differentiation. Measures of competence should assess the quality of the delivery. Factors that should be examined should include the level of concordance between training and agent activities, and client or consumer comprehension of the purposes, goals, and procedures of the treatment. Measures of treatment differentiation should focus on an assessment of procedures that are not prescribed, that are delivered in addition to or instead of the prescribed intervention (Perepletchikova and Kazdin 2005).

Indirect Assessment of Treatment Integrity

Treatment integrity can also be monitored via the use of indirect assessment methods, such as therapist self-reports, an evaluation of permanent products (e.g., completed worksheets or data collection sheets), rating scales, and self-monitoring (Perepletchikova and Kazdin 2005). Self-monitoring has received a good deal of attention, both as an assessment tool as well as a method to help increase and improve treatment integrity (Petscher and Bailey 2006; Coyle and Cole 2004; Richman et al. 1988; Burgio et al. 1990). Self-monitoring is difficult to implement—in essence, the process creates a concurrent choice situation where the rater must stop the activity that they are engaged in, rate the behavior, and then continue with their activity. Gresham (1996) suggests that complex environments, such as classrooms, may not be amenable to the collection of extended self-monitoring data. Following this line of reasoning, it might be difficult for agents to collect accurate self-monitoring data for interventions for ASD that are quite complex.

It is possible that the self-monitoring method is simply not an effective method to collect data on adherence (McLeod et al. 2009; Coyle and Cole 2004; Richman et al. 1988). Self-monitoring data may still be a useful ancillary data collection technique when combined with prompts to collect data (Petscher and Bailey 2006) or visual representations of data (Burgio et al. 1990). However, ultimately, self-monitoring data should be treated cautiously as the assessment may be due to a subtle demand characteristic that pulls for social approval and may cause treatment agents to overreport treatment integrity (Perepletchikova and Kazdin 2005).

Interpretation of Treatment Integrity Data

In essence, measurements of treatment integrity are quantitative methods used to identify therapist drift (Gresham 1996), as well as their effects on the dependent

Table 2.1 Interpretative issues that can arise from effects of varying levels of treatment integrity on the dependent variable

Dependent variable change	Levels of integrity	
	High	Low or none
Desired direction	Confidence that the treatment package has an effect	No confidence that the treatment package has any effect Increased risk of making a type I error (*false positive*) if treatment integrity data are not collected
No change	Confidence that the treatment package has no effect	No confidence that the treatment package has any effect Increased risk of making a type II error (*false negative*) if treatment integrity data are not collected
Undesired direction	Confidence that the treatment package has no effect and may even be potentially harmful	No confidence that the treatment package has any effect Increased risk of making a type II error (*false negative*) if treatment integrity data are not collected

variable or the treatment outcome (which should be operationalized similarly to the independent variable). Therapist drift or low levels of treatment integrity often cause a variety of difficulties that call into question the functional relationship of the independent and dependent variables.

Table 2.1 highlights some of the interpretative issues that can arise from differing levels of treatment integrity. In conditions where there are high levels of treatment integrity, decisions can be made with a fair amount of confidence relating to the potential effects of the independent variable on the dependent measures. However, in conditions where there are low levels of treatment integrity (or none), the drift may actually serve to artificially improve outcomes, thus creating a situation where the treatment procedure is inappropriately deemed to be effective (type I error). In this instance, one could hypothetically argue that a change was effected on the child with ASD in the desired direction (e.g., an increase in social skills or a decrease in stereotypy). From a research perspective, however, nothing has been added to the scientific literature in this condition. In fact, Gresham (1996) suggests that the majority of published research might simply be cases of false positives, which is a sobering thought, given that very few studies offer evidence of treatment integrity. From a practitioner perspective, a false positive would unfortunately not add to the body of knowledge that is collected about a particular child. For example, agents implementing a treatment at home which demonstrates good effects but low levels of treatment integrity would not be able to realistically inform school staff as to what can be done to deal with the same symptoms.

In other conditions, the lack of treatment integrity coupled with no changes (e.g., a lack of an increase in social skills) or undesired changes in the dependent variables (e.g., an increase in stereotypical behaviors) may lead practitioners or researchers to conclude that the procedures were not effective. Procedures that are not effective should clearly be discontinued; however, it is possible that the treatment, had it been applied with integrity, might have been effective in that instance (in the field) or for all children evidencing a particular profile (in the research literature). Rejecting an intervention when it may actually be effective is considered to be a type II error. A lack of treatment integrity in these conditions would hinder the identification of potentially effective treatments.

Methods to Increase Treatment Integrity

The most commonly reported method to increase treatment integrity is performance feedback (PFB; Codding et al. 2005, 2008; DiGennaro et al. 2005, 2007; DiGennaro-Reed et al. 2010; Mortensen and Witt 1998; Mouzakitis 2010; Noell et al. 1997). Performance feedback typically consists of a meeting between a treatment agent and a supervisor, evaluator, or consultant. During this meeting, a variety of information can be shared. Feedback and praise can be delivered on the amount of correctly implemented components. The treatment agent and the observer can also discuss aspects of a plan that were not followed. Finally, some training method can be employed to ensure correct component implementation in the future. The failure to implement a plan with integrity may be due to potential skill deficits or a lack of fluency or automaticity. At times, the treatment agent may simply forget to implement all the steps of the intervention or they may have begun the process of drift. PFB is a method that can allow these issues to be addressed via the use of review, modeling, rehearsal, and role-play, if needed. A typical PFB session can last anywhere between 5 and 20 min (Reed and Codding 2011), with initial PFB sessions lasting much longer than later sessions.

Various components of PFB have been manipulated to examine how to make the process more efficient and effective. For example, Guercio et al. (2005) varied PFB private meetings with public postings of treatment integrity to train 30 staff members at a residential facility. Although the results of the study showed dramatic increases of integrity among all staff, it is unclear which PFB condition was superior. The amount of time between the observation period and the delivery of PFB has also been investigated. Noell et al. (1997) delivered PFB immediately after observation, while Codding et al. (2005) delivered PFB every other week—others have examined varying lengths of time in between. PFB is an effective way to increase treatment integrity, despite its distance from the initial observation; however, stronger, faster increases of treatment integrity were associated with shorter time lapses (Mortenson and Witt 1998).

While PFB has been demonstrated to be effective, investigations into the removal of this intervention evidence decreases in levels of treatment integrity (Noell et al. 1997; Witt et al. 1997). In order to deal with this issue, the process of fading (also referred to as systematic fading or dynamic fading) is recommended (Reed and Codding 2011; DiGennaro et al. 2005; Noell et al. 2000). Fading refers to the gradual decrease of PFB (i.e., *thinning*) over time that is contingent upon the demonstration of treatment integrity at specified criterion levels. For example, if a treatment agent is receiving a daily schedule of PFB and demonstrates integrity rates of 90 % or better for three consecutive observation sessions, then the schedule is *thinned* to once every other day.

Some investigation has been conducted into the essential components of PFB. While PFB is a procedure employed to ensure treatment integrity, PFB itself must be scrutinized for treatment integrity. Some have indicated that the essential components of PFB are praise and corrective feedback (Mouzakitis 2010). Corrective feedback refers to the process of delivering feedback on components that were incorrectly applied (or not applied at all) and the provision of training procedures to help correct skill deficits or improve automaticity. However, DiGennaro et al. (2005) conceptualized the PFB process as one that was aversive. In this conceptualization, treatment agents worked to obtain high rates of integrity in return for the removal of PFB. This is in contrast to Codding et al. (2008), in which the treatment agents rated the PFB process as rewarding and beneficial. However, these discrepant results can be due to the setting (e.g., an inner city private school vs. a suburban public school), the person delivering PFB (e.g., a university faculty member vs. agency supervisor), how PFB is used by the setting (e.g., as a teaching tool or as a way to evaluate staff dismissal), and perhaps even the personality characteristics of the individual delivering PFB himself or herself.

Self-monitoring as an intervention has also been investigated as a procedure to improve treatment integrity. Self-monitoring as a procedure would be attractive because it would decrease the reliance on other individuals observing and intervening with treatment agents, thus saving time for staff and resources for the agency as a whole. Self-monitoring as an intervention to improve treatment integrity shows some good results (Richman et al. 1988; Coyle and Cole 2004) and more rapid increases when paired with environmental prompts (Petscher and Bailey 2006; Burgio et al. 1990); however, overall, these results do not approach the speed and total amount of improvement that the PFB procedure offers.

Conclusions

Issues related to treatment integrity are of critical importance to treatment programs designed for children with ASD. Given the course and symptomology of the disorder, treatments targeting ASD tend to be intricate, and often have deep roots in theory that may not necessarily be apparent to many treatment agents. Given these issues, there needs to be considerable work to ensure treatment adherence, improve competence, and establish differentiation. Unfortunately, treatment integrity is an important construct that is not measured as often as it should be in both research and practice.

The recent interest in the application of EBI's to treat ASD has the potential to increase awareness and interest in treatment integrity. Detrich (2008) suggests that environmental factors (such as the agency or stress levels of the family in the home) may play a considerable role in the selection and implementation of EBIs, to the point where various pieces of interventions might be combined to form unique treatment plans. While this may appear to be intuitively attractive to the clinician, the process does not necessarily equal a "mix-and-match" strategy—on the contrary, practitioners will need to work much harder in defining the treatment (i.e., independent variable), as well as the treatment outcomes (i.e., dependent variable) and a measurement strategy. This newly developed treatment protocol will need to be assessed for treatment integrity, so that agents can make an informed decision as to the effectiveness of the treatment.

Over the last 30 years, there has been an ever-increasing focus on the measurement of and interventions to improve treatment integrity. Direct observation and PFB appear to be the most commonly used (and most successful) measurement and assessment strategy. Attempts have been made to examine components of PFB to see how the process can be improved; however, it would be helpful to investigate what types of situations hinder PFB. For example, it is within the authors' clinical experience that observations conducted by external individuals tend to be better received than those conducted by administrators or supervisors. This may partially explain some of the discrepancies in the field, but as of yet, there have been no investigations of the status of the observer upon the effectiveness of PFB.

In conclusion, the demonstration of treatment integrity within the context of the evidence-based movement in identifying interventions for ASD will serve to be a challenge that needs to be dealt with both in scientific literature as well as in practice. The level of treatment integrity adds another interpretative layer that deepens inferences made from outcome data. Ultimately, efforts to improve treatment integrity serve to develop better researchers and professionals that can make a difference in the lives of children diagnosed with ASD.

References

Allen, K. D., & Warzak, W. J. (2000). The problem of parental non-adherence in clinical behavior analysis: Effective treatment is not enough. *Journal of Applied Behavior Analysis, 33*(3), 373–391. doi:10.1901/jaba.2000.33-373.

American Psychological Association. (2005). *Policy statement on evidence-based practice in psychology.* http://www.apapracticecentral.org/ce/courses/ebpstatement.pdf. Accessed 15 Oct. 2012.

American Speech-Language-Hearing Association. (2010). *Code of ethics* [Ethics]. doi:10.1044/policy.ET2010-00309.

Barber, J. P., Gallop, R., Crits-Chirstoph, P., Frank, A., Thase, M. E., Weiss, R. D., et al. (2006). The role of therapist adherence, therapist competence, and alliance in predicting outcome of individual drug counseling: Results from the National Institute Drug Abuse Collaborative Cocaine Treatment Study. *Psychotherapy Research, 16,* 229–240. doi:10.1080/10503300500288951.

Burgio, L. D., Engel, B. T., Hawkins, A. M., McCormick, K., Schieve, A, & Jones, L. T. (1990). A staff management system for maintaining improvements in continence with elderly nursing home residents. *Journal of Applied Behavior Analysis, 23,* 111–118. doi:10.1901/jaba.1990.23-111.

Cochrane, W. S., & Laux, J. M. (2008). A survey investigating school psychologists' measurement of treatment integrity in school-based interventions and their beliefs in their importance. *Psychology in the Schools, 45,* 499–507. doi:10.1002/pits.20319.

Codding, R. S., Feinberg, A. B., Dunn, E. K., & Pace, G. M. (2005). Effects of immediate performance feedback on implementation of behavior support plans. *Journal of Applied Behavior Analysis, 38,* 205–219. doi:10.1901/jaba.2005.98-04.

Codding, R. S., Livanis, A., Pace, G., & Vaca, L. (2008). Using performance feedback to improve treatment integrity of classwide behavior plans: An investigation of observer reactivity. *Journal of Applied Behavior Analysis, 41,* 417–422. doi:10.1901/jaba.2008.41-417.

Cook, C. R., Mayer, G. M., Wright, D. B., Kraemer, B., Wallace, M. D., Dart, E., Collins, T., & Restori, A. (2010). Exploring the link among behavior intervention plans, treatment integrity, and student outcomes under natural educational outcomes. *Journal of Special Education, 20,* 1–14. doi:10.1177/0022466910369941.

Cooper, J. O., Heron, T. E., & Heward W. L. (2007). *Applied behavior analysis* (2nd ed.). New Jersey: Merrill Prentice Hall.

Cowan, R. J., & Sheridan, S. M. (2003). Investigating the acceptability of behavioral interventions in applied conjoint behavioral consultation: Moving from analog conditions to naturalistic settings. *School Psychology Quarterly, 18*(1), 1–21.

Coyle, C., & Cole, P. (2004). A video-taped self-modeling and self-monitoring treatment program to decrease off-task behaviour in children with autism. *Journal of Intellectual and Developmental Disability, 29,* 3–15. doi:10.1080/08927020410001662642.

Detrich, R. (2008). Evidence-based, empirically supported, or best practice? A guide for the scientist-practitioner. In J. K. Luiselli, D. C. Russo, W. P. Christian, & S. M. Wilczynski (Eds.), *Effective practices for children with autism* (pp. 3–25). New York: Oxford University Press.

DiGennaro, F. D., Martens, B. K., & McIntyre, L. L. (2005). Increasing treatment integrity through negative reinforcement: Effects on teacher and student behavior. *School Psychology Review, 34*(2), 220–231.

DiGennaro, F. D., Martens, B. K., & Kleinman, A. E. (2007). A comparison of performance feedback procedures on teachers' treatment implementation integrity and students' inappropriate behavior in special education classrooms. *Journal of Applied Behavior Analysis, 40,* 447–461. doi:10.1901/jaba.2007.40-447.

DiGennaro-Reed, F. D., Codding, R., Catania, C. N., & MaGuire, H. (2010). Effects of video modeling on treatment integrity of behavioral interventions. *Journal of Applied Behavior Analysis, 43,* 291–295. doi:10.1901/jaba.2010.43-291.

Dusenbury, L., Brannigan, R., Falco, M., & Hansen, W. B. (2003). A review of research on fidelity of implementation: implications for drug abuse prevention in school settings. *Health Education Research: Theory and Practice, 18*(2), 237–256. doi:10.1093/her/18.2.237.

Elliot, S. N. (1988). Acceptability of behavioral treatments in educational settings. In J. C. Witt, S. N. Elliott, & F. M. Gresham (Eds.), *Handbook of Behavior Therapy* (pp. 121–150). New York: Plenum.

Erhardt, K. E., Barnett, D. W., Lentz, F. E., Stollar, S. A., & Raifin, L. H. (1996). Innovative methodology in ecological consultation: Use of scripts to promote treatment acceptability and integrity. *School Psychology Quarterly, 11,* 149–168. doi:10.1037/h0088926.

Etchdeit, S. K. (2006). Behavioral intervention plans: Pedagogical and legal analysis of themes. *Behavior Disorders, 31*(2), 223–243.

Foster, S., & Cone, J. (1986). Design and use of direct observation. In A. Ciminero, K. Calhoun, & H. Adams (Eds.), *Handbook of behavioral assessment* (2nd ed., pp. 253–324). New York: Wiley Interscience.

Foxx, R. M. (1996). Twenty years of applied behavior analysis in treating the most severe problem behavior: Lessons learned. *The Behavior Analyst, 19*(2), 225–235.

Frentz, C., & Kelley, M. L. (1986). Parents' acceptance of reductive treatment methods: The influence of problem severity and perception of child behavior. *Behavior Therapy, 17*(1), 75–81. doi:10.1016/S0005-7894(86)80116-2.

Gresham, F. M. (1989). Assessment of treatment integrity in school consultation and prereferral intervention. *School Psychology Review, 18,* 37–50.

Gresham, F.M. (1996). Treatment integrity in single-subject research. In R. D. Franklin, D. B. Allison, B. S. Gorman (Eds.), *Design and analysis of single-case research* (pp. 93–117). Mahwah: Lawrence Erlbaum Associates.

Gresham, F. M. (2005). Treatment integrity and therapeutic change: Commentary on Perepletchikova and Kazdin. *Clinical Psychology: Science and Practice, 12*(4), 391–394. doi:10.1093/clipsy/bpi048.

Guercio, J. M., Dixon, M. R., Soldner, J., Shoemaker, Z., Zlomke, K., Root, S., & Small, S. (2005). Enhancing staff performance measures in an acquired brain injury setting: Combating the habituation to organizational behavioral interventions. *Behavioral Interventions, 20,* 91–99. doi:10.1002/bin.174.

Happe, D. (1982). Behavior intervention: It doesn't do any good in your briefcase. In J. Grimes (Ed.), *Psychological approaches to problems of children and adolescents* (pp. 15–41). Des Moines: Iowa Department of Public Instruction.

Hayes, S. C., & Wilson, K. G. (1993). Some applied implications of a contemporary behavior-analytic account of verbal events. *The Behavior Analyst, 16*(2), 283–301.

Hogue, A., Henderson, C. E., Dauber, S., Barajas, P. C., Fried, A., & Liddle, H. A. (2008). Treatment adherence, competence, and outcome in individual and family therapy for adolescent behavior problems. *Journal of Consulting and Clinical Psychology, 76*(4), 544–555. doi:10.1037/0022-006X.76.4.544.

IDEA. (2004). P.L. 108–446, § 665 [b][1][B], 118 Stat. 2787 [2005].

Kazdin, A. E. (1986). Comparative outcome studies of psychotherapy: Methodological issues and strategies. *Journal of Consulting and Clinical Psychology, 54,* 95–105. doi:10.1037/0022-006X.54.1.95.

Kazdin, A. E. (2011). *Single-case research designs*. New York: Oxford University Press.

Koegel, R. L., Russo, D. C., & Rincover, A. (1977). Assessing and training teachers in the generalized use of behavior modification with autistic children. *Journal of Applied Behavior Analysis, 10*(2), 197–205. doi: 10.1901/jaba.1977.10-197.

LeBlanc, M., Ricciardi, J. N., & Luiselli, J. K. (2005). Improving discrete trial instruction by paraprofessional staff through an abbreviated performance feedback intervention. *Education and Treatment of Children, 28*(1), 76–82.

Lentz, F. E., Allen, S. J., & Erhardt, K. E. (1996). The conceptual elements of strong Interventions in school settings. *School Psychology Quarterly, 11,* 118–136. doi:10.1037/h0088924.

Livanis, A., & Mercer, S. H. (2011). The effects of graduated treatment introduction and performance feedback on treatment integrity for complex behavior intervention plans. *School Psychology Review*. (Manuscript submitted for publication)

Lloyd, K. E. (1994). Do as I say, not as I do. *The Behavior Analyst, 17*(1), 131–139.

McLeod, B. D., Southam-Gerow, M. A., & Weisz, J. R. (2009). Conceptual and methodological issues in treatment integrity measurement. *School Psychology Review, 38*(4), 541–546.

Meichenbaum, D., & Turk, D. C. (1987). *Facilitating treatment adherence: A practitioner's guidebook*. New York: Plenum.

Mortensen, B. P., & Witt, J. C. (1998). The use of weekly performance feedback to increase teacher implementation of a prereferral intervention. *School Psychology Review, 27,* 613–627.

Mouzakitis, A. (2010). *The effects of self-monitoring training and performance feedback on the treatment integrity of behavior support plans for children with autism*. Unpublished doctoral dissertation, The Graduate Center of the City University of New York, New York.

National Association of School Psychologists. (2010a). *Principles for professional ethics*. http://www.nasponline.org/standards/2010standards/1_%20Ethical%20Principles.pdf. Accessed 15 Oct. 2012.

National Association of School Psychologists. (2010b). *Model for comprehensive and integrated school psychological services*. http://www.nasponline.org/standards/2010standards/2_PracticeModel.pdf. Accessed 15 Oct. 2012.

National Autism Center. (2009). *The National Autism Center's National Standards Report*. Massachusetts: Author.

Nezu, A. M., & Nezu, C. M. (2008). Treatment integrity. In D. McKay (Ed.), *Handbook of research methods in abnormal and clinical psychology* (pp. 351–363). New York: Sage.

Noell, G. H., Witt, J. C., Gilbertson, D. N., Ranier, D. D., & Freeland, J. T. (1997). Increasing teacher interventions implementation in general education settings through consultation and performance feedback. *School Psychology Quarterly, 12,* 77–88. doi:10.1037/h0088949.

Noell, G. H., Witt, J. C., LaFleur, L. H., Mortenson, B. P., Ranier, D. D., & LeVelle, J. (2000). Increasing intervention implementation in general education following consultation: A comparison of two follow-up strategies. *Journal of Applied Behavior Analysis, 33,* 271–284.

Perepletchikova, F., & Kazdin, A. E. (2005). Treatment integrity and therapeutic change: Issues and research recommendations. *Clinical Psychology: Science and Practice, 12*(4), 365–383. doi:10.1093/clipsy/bpi045

Petscher, E. S., & Bailey, J. S. (2006). Effects of training, prompting and self-monitoring on staff behavior in a classroom for students with disabilities. *Journal of Applied Behavior Analysis, 39,* 215–226. doi:10.1901/jaba.2006.02-05.

Reed, F. D., & Codding, R. S. (2011). Intervention integrity assessment. In J. K. Luiselli (Ed.), *Teaching and behavior support for children and adults with autism spectrum disorder* (pp. 38–47). New York: Oxford University Press.

Reichow, B., & Volkmar, F. R. (2011). Evidence-based practices in autism: Where we started. In B. Reichow, P. Doehring, D. V. Cicchetti, & F. R. Volkmar (Eds.), *Evidence-based practices and treatments for children with autism* (pp. 3–24). New York: Springer. doi:10.1007/978-1-4419-6975-0_1.

Richman, G. S., Riordan, M. R., Reiss, M. L., Piles, D. A. M., & Bailey, J. S. (1988). The effects of self-monitoring and supervisor feedback on staff performance in a residential setting. *Journal of Applied Behavior Analysis, 21,* 401–409. doi:10.1901/jaba.1988.21-401.

Schulte, A. C., Easton, J. E., & Parker, J. (2009). Advances in treatment integrity research: Multidisciplinary perspectives on the conceptualization, measurement, and enhancement of treatment integrity. *School Psychology Review, 38*(4), 460–475.

Singh, N. N., & Katz, R. C. (1985). On the modification of acceptability ratings for alternative child treatments. *Behavior Modification, 9*(3), 375–386. doi:10.1177/01454455850093006.

Sterling-Turner, H. E., Watson, T. S., Widmon, M., Watkins, C., & Little, E. (2001). Investigating the relationship between training type and treatment integrity. *School Psychology Quarterly, 16*(1), 56–67. doi:10.1521/scpq.16.1.56.19157.

Taylor, J., & Miller, M. (1997). When timeout works some of the time: The importance of treatment integrity and functional assessment. *School Psychology Quarterly, 12*(1), 4–22. doi:10.1037/h0088943.

Tingstrom, D. H., McPhail, R. L., & Bolton, A. B. (1989). Acceptability of alternative school-based interventions: The influence of reported effectiveness and age of target child. *The Journal of Psychology, 123,* 133–140.

Wheeler, J. J., Baggett, B. A., Fox, J., Blevins, L. (2006). Treatment integrity: A review of intervention studies conducted with children with autism. *Focus on Autism and Other Developmental Disabilities, 21*(1), 45–54. doi:10.1177/10883576060210010601.

Wilczynski, S. M., Christin, L., & National Autism Center. The National Standards Project: Promoting evidence-based practice in autism spectrum disorders. In J. K. Luiselli, D. C. Russo, W. P. Christian, & S. M. Wilczynski (Eds.), *Effective practices for children with autism* (pp. 37–60). New York: Oxford University Press.

Witt, J. C., Elliott, S. N., & Martens, B. K. (1984). Acceptability of behavior interventions used in classrooms: The influence of teacher time, severity of behavior program, and type of intervention. *Behavioral Disorders, 10,* 204–209.

Witt, J. C., Moe, G., Gutkin, T. B., & Andrews, L. (1984). The effect of saying the same thing in different ways: The problem of language and jargon in school-based consultation. *Journal of School Psychology, 22,* 361–367. doi:10.1016/0022-4405(84)90023-2.

Witt, J. C., Noell, G. H., LaFleur, L. H., & Mortenson, B. P. (1997). Teacher use of interventions in general education: Measurement and analysis of the independent variable. *Journal of Applied Behavior Analysis, 30,* 693–696. doi:10.1901/jaba.1997.30-693.

Yeaton, W. H., & Sechrest, L. (1981). Critical dimensions in the choice and maintenance of successful treatments: Strength, integrity, and effectiveness. *Journal of Consulting and Clinical Psychology, 49*(2), 156–167. doi:10.1037/0022-006X.49.2.156.

Chapter 3
Evaluation of Treatment Effectiveness in the Field of Autism

Psychometric Considerations and an Illustration

Jack A. Naglieri and Sam Goldstein

Introduction

Evidence-based treatment and the assessment of treatment effectiveness are dependent upon the collection of data during the evaluation process providing information about symptoms, impairment, and abilities. Such an assessment allows for a seamless transition from assessment and diagnosis to effective treatment. Evaluating the effectiveness of a treatment strategy or program is important for interventions designed to address symptoms related to any psychological or developmental disorder. The validity of this entire process is closely related to the tools used during the diagnostic and treatment process. More specifically, the reliability and validity of the tools used will be directly related to the psychometric attributes of the instruments. As in all areas of science, what is learned depends upon the quality of the data generated and the manner in which the findings are interpreted. Scientifically developed diagnostic and assessment instruments yield accurate and informative data. Tests and rating scales developed to provide valid and reliable information about the examinee better informs researchers and clinicians. Tools chosen for diagnostic decision-making and treatment planning have a profound impact on the information obtained and the conclusions reached. The better the tools, the more valid and reliable the decisions and most importantly, the more helpful the gathered information will be in developing a treatment plan, monitoring progress, and documenting treatment effectiveness.

Determining the effectiveness of any treatment program for individuals with Autism Spectrum Disorders (ASDs) should be accomplished using methods that

J. A. Naglieri (✉)
Curry School of Education, Devereux Center for Resilient Children,
University of Virginia, Centerville, Virginia, USA
e-mail: jnaglieri@gmail.com

S. Goldstein
Neurology, Learning and Behavior Center, School of Medicine, University of Utah, 230 South 500 East, Suite 100, Salt Lake City, UT 84102, USA
e-mail: info@samgoldstein.com

S. Goldstein, J. A. Naglieri (eds.), *Interventions for Autism Spectrum Disorders*,
DOI 10.1007/978-1-4614-5301-7_3, © Springer Science+Business Media New York 2013

reflect specific behaviors as well as larger conceptualizations of the disorder (e.g., social, communication, and atypical behavior problems). Four key questions in this process are:

1. how are these behaviors identified?
2. how are these behaviors measured?
3. how does the behavior change with intervention? and
4. to what reference point or points will behavior change be calibrated?

Clarification of the last point is particularly important—is behavior change determined in relation to the individual's baseline, or in reference to a control group, or in contrast to a national norm? In this chapter, we will examine all these questions taking into consideration psychometric as well as practical issues. We will begin with a discussion of the impact that psychometric characteristics of the tools, used for assessment and treatment evaluation, have on the information obtained. Next, we provide a practical illustration of how to assess behaviors related to autism, how those results can be used to identify the focus of an intervention plan, how data obtained during treatment can be examined, and how pre- and posttreatment results can be evaluated.

Psychometric Characteristics and Treatment Outcomes

Calibration of Scores

Naglieri and Chambers (2009) provided summaries of the characteristics of rating scales, used to assess behaviors associated with autism, and the psychometric qualities that such measures possess. They concluded that the methods used to calibrate rating scale scores differed considerably. For example, some rating scales provide only raw scores whereas others yield derived scores, based upon the particular group the scale is intended to identify i.e., some authors provide T-scores based on a comparison to individuals with an ASD. Naglieri and Chambers questioned the utility of a comparison group comprised of children referred for or having the disorder of interest, and Naglieri (2012) explored this issue further using data from the Autism Spectrum Rating Scale (ASRS; Goldstein and Naglieri 2009).

Naglieri (2012) examined the differences in T-scores that would be obtained when using a nationally representative sample versus a sample of children identified as having autism as a reference group. He constructed a raw score to T-score conversion table based on a sample of children with ASD ($N = 243$) and compared those results to T-scores obtained from the ASRS standardization sample. This group ($N = 1,828$) was representative of the US population, included males and females from each of the four geographic regions of the US and four racial-ethnic groups (Asian, Black, White-Not Hispanic, and Hispanic Origin) aged 6–18 years. [See Naglieri (2012) for more details about the procedures that were used.] The results are summarized in Table 3.1.

Table 3.1 Comparison of *T*-scores based on a national normative group and a sample of individuals with ASD

Total scale raw score	*T*-scores based on comparison to others with ASD	*T*-scores based on comparison to national normative group
150	54	77
140	52	74
130	50	71
120	48	69
110	46	66
100	44	63
90	42	60
80	40	57
70	37	55
60	35	52
50	33	49
40	31	46
Mn	117.8	53.1
SD	50.3	36.1

Table 3.1 provides a raw score to *T*-score conversion table based on the means and standard deviations (*SD*) for the national and ASD reference groups. What is most remarkable about the results is that a raw score of 80 on the ASRS would yield a *T*-score of 40 if the reference groups were individuals who had previously been identified as having ASD. This would suggest that a child who earned this score would be one *SD* below the mean for the reference group of individuals with ASD. It would be reasonable to conclude that an individual who obtained such a score was not like those with ASD. The raw score of 80, however, is equal to a *T*-score of 57 in relation to the national norm, nearly one *SD above* the national mean. These results illustrate how different conclusions may be reached when the same rating scale is calibrated against two different samples. We suggest that the comparison with the national norm is more informative and the score that should be used to understand the extent to which an individual evidences behaviors associated with ASD. The use of a national norm also has considerable impact on evaluation of behavior change as a function of intervention.

Calibration of Change

In recent years, practitioners and researchers in educational and psychological settings have compared raw scores from a test to evaluate the effectiveness of some academic instruction or other treatment. Naglieri (2012) illustrated how the comparison of raw scores over time can be misleading when students' progress over time was monitored using words read per minute as a measure of reading skill. The issue is that some tests of skills, like reading or vocabulary, show a very strong age-to-age progression of raw scores. This progression reflects the typical changes in skills

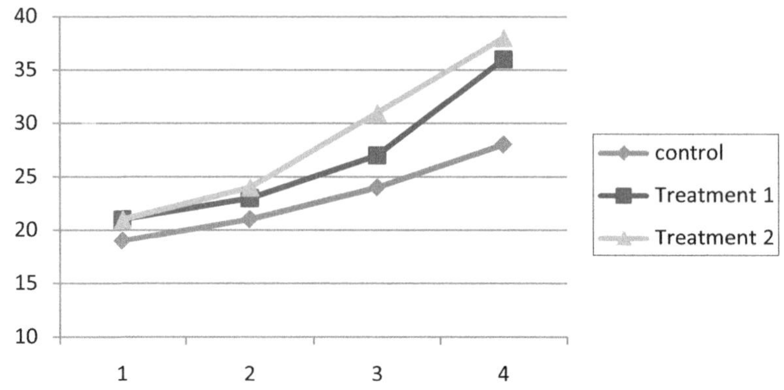

Fig. 3.1 Performance from time 1 through time 4

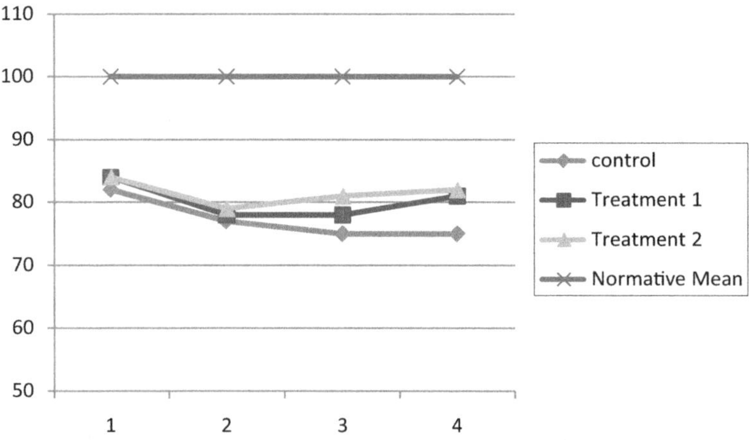

Fig. 3.2 Conclusion on the basis of examination of standard scores associated with the raw scores

that occur as a child grows older as a combination of factors including maturation, learning from the environment as well as school. In order to calibrate change as a function of some specific instruction or intervention, the amount of change should be calibrated to the normal growth curve, not only the pretreatment level. This is a particularly important issue in treatment programs for individuals with ASD.

Expressive vocabulary is one variable that is often studied as a way to demonstrate improvement over time (e.g., Kasari et al. 2008). The choice of which expressive vocabulary test and score to use, has a profound impact on the result. Using the Kasari et al. study results as a guide, we obtained the standard scores using the normative tables from the Expressive Vocabulary Test (Williams 1997). The results shown in Fig. 3.1 suggest that there were changes in performance from Time 1 through Time 4 (12 month interval). Both treatment groups appear to have higher scores at Time 4. The interpretation of these data could lead to the conclusion that the treatments were effective but examination of the standard scores associated with these raw scores suggests a different conclusion as shown in Fig. 3.2.

When the raw scores are converted to standard scores (mean of 100 and *SD* of 15) shown in Fig. 3.2, the results suggest that although the raw scores increased over the 12-month interval the standard scores associated with these raw scores actually showed *no* improvement. That is, even though the two treatment (as well as the control) groups' raw scores increased, the difference between those scores and the mean for the standardization group remained large. In fact, the average raw scores for the four age groups are 41, 48, 52, and 56. Therefore, we suggest that raw score improvement alone is insufficient to show treatment effectiveness. Standard score improvement provides an additional reference point that *must* be taken into consideration in order to determine if a treatment is sufficiently effective.

Reliability of Measurement

Consideration of the role reliability plays in evaluation of treatment change is essential because all measurements have some degree of error. In classical test theory, an obtained score is comprised of the true score plus error (Crocker and Algina 1986). For this reason, we should always report an obtained score with a range of values within which the person's true score likely falls with a particular level of confidence. The size of the range is determined by the level of confidence and the reliability of the measurement; the higher the reliability the smaller the range. When reporting a T-score, for example, we state that a child earned a score of 50 ($\pm$ 7); meaning that there is a 95 % likelihood that the child's true IQ score falls within the range of 43–50. The range of scores (called the confidence interval) is computed by first obtaining the standard error of measurement (SEM) from the reliability coefficient and the *SD* of the score in the following formula (Crocker and Algina 1986):

$$SEM = SD \times \sqrt{1 - reliability}$$

The SEM is considered the average *SD* (68 % of the normal curve is in this range) of the theoretical distribution of a person's scores around the true score. If one *SEM* is added to and subtracted from an obtained score, there is a 68 % chance (the percentage of scores contained within $\pm$ 1 *SD*) that the person's true score is contained within that range. The SEM is multiplied by a z value of, for example 1.64 or 1.96, to obtain a confidence interval at the 90 or 95 % levels, respectively. The resulting value is added to and subtracted from the obtained score to yield the confidence interval. For example, the 95 % confidence range for a test score with a reliability of .95 and an obtained T-score of 60 (recall that a T-score is set to have a mean of 50 and *SD* of 10) is 57 ($60 - 3$) to 63 ($60 + 3$). It is important to note that the higher the reliability the smaller the interval of scores that can be expected to include the child's true score. The smaller the range, the more precise the practitioners can be in their interpretation of the results, resulting in more accurate decisions regarding the child. The relationships between reliability and size of the confidence interval is provided in Fig. 3.3 for T-scores ($M = 50$; $SD = 10$). Confidence intervals should

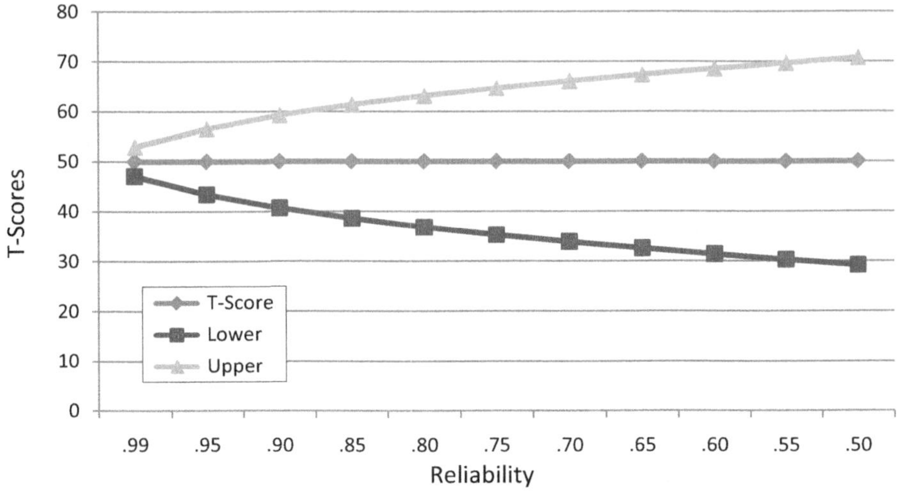

Fig. 3.3 Relationship between reliability and confidence intervals for *T*-scores

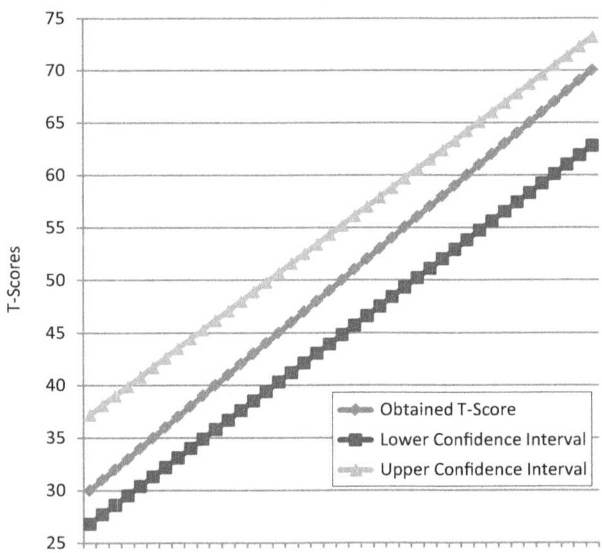

Fig. 3.4 Upper and lower values of estimated true score-based confidence intervals for *T*-scores

always be used for interpretation of *all* scores because they take measurement error into account at a specific level of probability.

The method of computing confidence intervals described above has been modified in recent years by some test authors (e.g., Wechsler and Naglieri 2006) to be theoretically more accurate than the approach of basing confidence intervals around obtained scores (Nunnally 1978). The modification involves centering the confidence interval on the estimated true score. This approach accounts for measurement error associated with the scores to provide a band of error that is centered on the estimated true score and thereby takes into account regression to the mean (Salvia and Ysseldyke 1981).

Figure 3.4 shows the relationships between obtained scores from 30 to 70 and the confidence intervals associated with those scores using estimated true score-based method. This is the method used in most ability tests and some rating scales.

Reliability and Comparison of Scores

The SEM is also particularly important when scores from different raters are compared. When comparing scores earned on the same scale, it is critical to recognize that the lower the reliability the larger the SEM, and the more likely scores will differ as a function of measurement error i.e., the lower the reliability, the more likely there will be differences among scores. Inconsistent results that reflect measurement error can complicate the interpretation of pre- and postfindings, and make a clear understanding of an individual's treatment progress more difficult to interpret. For example, when a researcher or practitioner is attempting to determine whether the several scores an individual has received are similar or significantly different, the answer to that question is directly related to each score's reliability because the calculation of the SEM is based on reliability. In fact, the formula for the difference between two scores earned by an individual is calculated using the SEM of each score.

$$Difference = Z \times \sqrt{SEM\,1^2 + SEM\,2^2}$$

Applying this formula to T-scores, as shown in Fig. 3.5, we see that as the reliability goes down, the differences needed when comparing two scores increases dramatically. This means that scores from measures with reliability of .70 from two different teachers would have to differ by 15 T-score points to be significant at the 95 % level. This means that test scores with higher reliability reduce the influence of *measurement error* on the different scores. Clearly, in both research and clinical settings, variables with high reliability are needed for precision of measurement, but how are these coefficients evaluated?

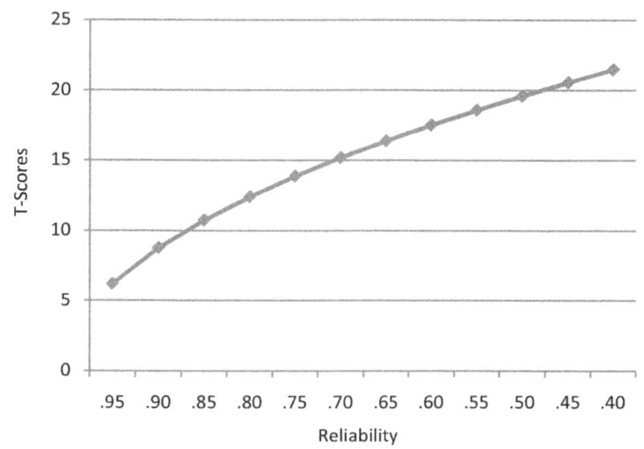

Fig. 3.5 Relationship between reliability and the difference required for significance when comparing two T-scores

Evaluation of Reliability Coefficients

Bracken (1987) provided suggested levels for acceptable for test reliability. He stated that scales that comprise a complete instrument should have at least an internal reliability estimate of .80 or greater and total test scales should have an internal consistency of .90 or greater. These guidelines should be further considered in light of the decisions being made. For example, if a score is used for screening purposes where over identification is preferred to under identification, a .80 reliability standard for a Total Score may be acceptable. If, however, scores from a scale contribute to important decisions then a higher (e.g., .95) standard should be deemed more appropriate (Nunnally and Bernstein 1994). We suggest that professionals evaluating the treatment of symptoms related to ASD use scores that have internal reliability estimates of .80 or higher. For scores comprised of several variables that have been combined, an internal reliability estimates of .90 or greater. Clinicians are advised not to use measures that do not meet these standards because there will be too much error in the measurement to allow for confidence in the result. This is especially important because the decisions clinicians make can have significant impact on the life of a child. Therefore, we urge the reader to carefully examine the reliability findings of any measure they choose to use.

Implications

We have stressed the need for norm-referenced measurement of symptoms related to ASD as well as the advantages of using measures that have high reliability so that greater accuracy can be achieved. The overarching goal is to use well-developed psychological tools when assessing individuals with ASD and particularly when evaluating the effects of any treatment. We will now illustrate how these measurement issues can be operationalized with a rating scale. Although all the issues related to reliability are well established, the issues surrounding psychometrics of treatment effectiveness are much more complex. There are many questions and an evolving set of possible solutions. Typically, researchers have studied both global changes in symptoms associated with a particular condition as well as specific behaviors, some of which may or may not be associated with a particular condition. In clinical practice, treatment goals are rarely set at the disorder level, instead, the focus is typically on general symptoms (e.g., improve peer socialization) and specific behaviors associated with a general symptom (e.g., increase ability to initiate conversation with peers).

Treatment Evaluation Illustration

In this section, we present a way to evaluate symptoms related to ASD on both global and specific levels, identify areas for treatment, and evaluate the effects of treatment. To do so, we will illustrate using information from the ASRS (Goldstein and Naglieri 2009). We choose to illustrate using this tool because it is nationally normed and provides several different types of global scores as well as measures of specific behaviors. In addition, the reliability of the scales is well documented and guidelines for assessing treatment change are also provided. We will begin with a brief explanation of the ASRS and then describe the steps needed to determine the current status of the individual who was rated, which scales and individual behaviors warrant attention, and how to assess treatment effectiveness.

Autism Spectrum Rating Scale

The ASRS (Goldstein and Naglieri 2009) is a rating scale for assessing behaviors associated with ASD. Children aged 2–5 years (N of items = 70) and youth aged 6–18 years (N of items = 71) can be rated by parents and teachers. Each of the items is scaled using a 5-point Likert scale (0 = Never, 1 = Rarely, 2 = Occasionally, 3 = Frequently, 4 = Very Frequently) and scored so that higher scores are indicative of behaviors associated with ASD. Initial item generation was based on a comprehensive review of both current theory and literature on the assessment of ASDs (autistic disorder, Asperger's disorder, and Pervasive Developmental Disorder, Not Otherwise Specified), the DSM-IV-TR (APA 1994), and ICD-10 (World Health Organization 2007) diagnostic criteria, as well as the authors' clinical and research experiences. The ASRS scale structure includes three factorially defined scales (Social/Communication, Unusual Behaviors, Self-Regulation), eight content-derived Treatment Scales (Peer Socialization, Adult Socialization, Social/Emotional Reciprocity, Atypical Language, Stereotypy, Behavioral Rigidity, Sensory Sensitivity, Attention), a DSM-IV-TR Scale based on the DSM-IV-TR symptomatic criteria for autistic disorder and Asperger's disorder, and a Total Score. The structure of the ASRS scales is shown in Fig. 3.6.

The ASRS was normed using samples obtained from parents (N = 1,280) and teachers (N = 1,280). The normative samples closely match the US population according to age, sex, race/ethnicity, parental educational level (for parent raters), and geographic region. The ASRS internal reliability coefficients are summarized in Table 3.2. The median reliabilities for the Total Scale (.97) and the empirical scales (range from .92 to .94) are all high. The median reliabilities for the Treatment Scales range from .69 to .91, suggesting that some of these scale which were built according to the content of the items have higher reliability than others. This is important to recognize when comparing scores across raters or over time. There is considerable evidence about validity of the ASRS which can be found in the test manual (Goldstein and Naglieri 2009). The goal of this section was to provide a brief overview of the ASRS so that the sections which follow will be more easily understood.

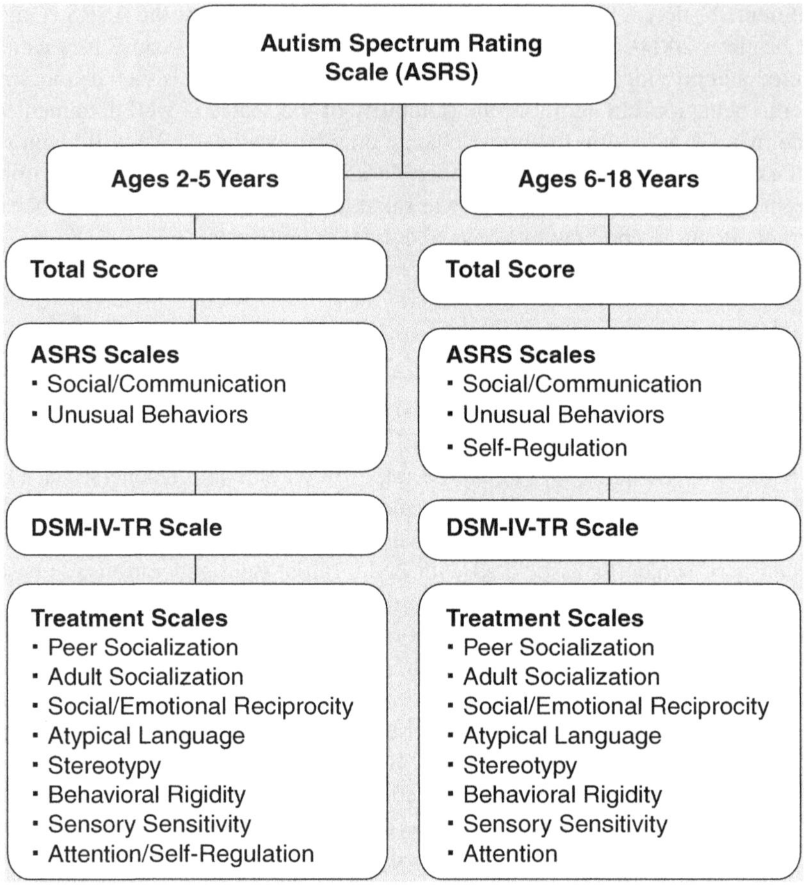

Fig. 3.6 Structure of the autism spectrum rating scale

Identify Areas of Concern

The first step in determining treatment for behaviors related to ASD is to clarify the specific area or areas of need. We suggest that any nationally normed standard score from a scale like the ASRS that is above one *SD* (e.g., a *T*-score of 60 or more) indicates that the individual rated has many behavioral characteristics similar to individuals diagnosed with an ASD. Users should begin with an examination of the Total Score and the ASRS Scales. The illustration in Table 3.3 pertains to a 6-year-old boy, fictitiously given the name Donny, who has an overall Total Score of 73 which is consistent with the finding for individuals with ASD reported by Goldstein and Naglieri (2009). The Total Score is, however, insufficient for treatment planning because it is too general. Analyzing the separate Social Communication, Unusual Behavior, and Self-Regulation scales provides more information about symptomology. Ratings provided by his mother indicate that Donny has considerable problems

Table 3.2 Reliability Coefficients for the Autism Spectrum Rating Scales (ASRS) by Age in Years and Rater

	Parent raters				Teacher raters			
	2–5	6–11	12–18	Median	2–5	6–11	12–18	Median
Total Scale	.95	.97	.97	.97	.94	.97	.97	.97
Social/Communication	.94	.91	.92	.92	.95	.93	.92	.93
Unusual Behaviors	.91	.94	.93	.93	.85	.93	.94	.93
Self-Regulation	–	.92	.93	.93	–	.94	.93	.94
Treatment Scales								
Peer Socialization	.77	.84	.84	.84	.85	.84	.83	.84
Adult Socialization	.67	.77	.79	.77	.78	.80	.77	.78
Social/Emotional Reciprocity	.83	.85	.88	.85	.88	.89	.89	.89
Atypical Language	.71	.81	.82	.81	.59	.75	.80	.75
Stereotypy	.75	.79	.77	.77	.67	.69	.72	.69
Behavioral Rigidity	.85	.89	.86	.86	.82	.90	.90	.90
Sensory Sensitivity	.71	.79	.77	.77	.59	.77	.84	.77
Attention/Self-Regulation (2–5) or Attention (6–18)	.83	.90	.89	.89	.83	.92	.91	.91

Note The ASRS form for ages 2–5 years has two empirically derived scales (Social/Communication and Unusual Behaviors)

Table 3.3 Case of Donny: Parent and Teacher ASRS *T*-Scores, Differences Between Raters, and Values Needed for Significance

	Parent	Teacher	Difference	Difference needed[a]	Significance
Total Score	*73*	*73*	0	5	NS
Social Communication	*77*	*78*	1	6	NS
Unusual Behavior	*60*	53	−7	6	Sig
Self-Regulation	*70*	*74*	4	7	NS
DSM-IV Scale	*69*	*68*	−1	6	NS
Treatment Scales					
Peer Socialization	*70*	*73*	3	9	NS
Adult Socialization	58	*63*	5	12	NS
Social/Emotional Reciprocity	*77*	*76*	−1	8	NS
Atypical Language	52	44	−8	11	NS
Stereotypy	49	54	5	13	NS
Behavioral Rigidity	*72*	48	−24	8	Sig
Sensory Sensitivity	*44*	48	4	12	NS
Attention	*71*	*73*	2	7	NS

T-scores greater than 59 appear in italic text
[a]*Note* Differences needed for significance when comparing Parent and Teacher ratings are found in Table 4.5 of the ASRS Manual

with appropriate use of verbal and nonverbal communication requiring him to initiate, engage in, and maintain social contact (Social Communication *T*-score of 77) and he struggles with maintaining control over his behavior (i.e., he is very argumentative) and attending in complex settings (Self-Regulation score of 70). Donny has trouble tolerating changes in routine. He also engages in apparently purposeless odd and atypical behaviors (Unusual Behavior score of 60).

Differences Between Raters

Donny's Total ASRS T-score as rated by his Teacher was the same as his mother's and ratings on all the scales except two did not differ significantly. The difference between Donny's Unusual Behavior scores as rated by his mother (60) and teacher (51) is significant ($p = .10$) as determined by the method described earlier in this chapter and using the values provided in the ASRS manual (Table 4.5, p. 34). This suggests that Donny's behaviors in the home and the classroom are different; which implies that the exploration of the environmental impact on his odd behaviors could lead to good intervention options. There was also a significant difference between Donny's Behavioral Rigidity scores as rated by his mother (72) and teacher (48), which also warrants further exploration. Despite these few inconsistencies Donny's score clearly show that he has many behaviors associated with ASD and these behavioral manifestations of the disorder are pervasive. The two raters consistently rated him as having considerable problems with Peer Socialization, Social/Emotional Reciprocity, and Attention. His mother's ratings also yielded a high score on Behavioral Rigidity (72) and his teacher reported problems with Adult Socialization (63). These results also indicate that Donny's ratings were typical to the normative sample (T-scores ranging from 44 to 54) on the ASRS scales Atypical Language, Stereotypy, and Sensory Sensitivity.

Intervention Planning

Considering all the ratings by parents and teachers as a whole, the next step is to identify an intervention plan based on the profile of T-scores on the ASRS Treatment Scales. To illustrate using the case of Donny, we would begin by prioritizing the areas of need based on the magnitude of the T-scores. Donny's highest T-scores were on the Social/Emotional Reciprocity scale rated by both parents and teachers. This scale involves specific behaviors such as looking at others appropriately while talking with them, understanding the feelings of others, recognizing social cues, responding appropriately to other people's statements, interests, or feelings, and enjoying interacting with others. In order to have a more precise understanding of the exact behaviors that contributed to this high score, or a high score on any of the Treatment Scales, practitioners can use an item level analysis to identify the greatest need for improvement. This can be accomplished by determining when an item rating is substantially higher than the item mean from the normative group. This approach is similar to the technique used by Naglieri et al. (1991) and LeBuffe and Naglieri (2003). They suggested that when an individual item score falls at, or above, the 85th percentile rank the item can be considered to be substantially elevated. The values needed to meet this rule for the ASRS are provided in Appendix B of the test Manual and are automatically provided in the computerized ASRS interpretive report (see Fig. 3.7). Analysis of the Treatment Scales and the items included on those scales can be used to identify which specific behaviors warrant intervention. A Quick Solution

Fig. 3.7 Item level analysis from ASRS interpretive report (shaded items indicate scores that are more than 1 *SD* from the normative mean)

Peer Socialization	
Item	**Score**
3. seek the company of other children? (R)	1
14. have trouble talking with other children?	3
19. have social problems with children of the same age?	2
31. play with others? (R)	1
45. understand age-appropriate humor or jokes? (R)	0
50. talk too much about things that other children don't care about?	4
64. choose to play alone?	3
69. show good peer interactions? (R)	2
70. respond when spoken to by other children? (R)	1
Peer Socialization Raw Score =	**17**

Guide (see Appendix) is also provided to select interventions associated with each behavioral need.

The Quick Solution Guide provides the correspondence of behaviors associated with ASD and specific interventions provided by authors in the chapters that appear in this book. For example, Donny had a high ASRS *T*-score on the Social/Emotional Reciprocity scale and one of the items that addressed "looking at others when spoken to" was very high. According to the Quick Solution Guide Interventions that address this behavior are provided on pages 54 and 55 of this book. The next scale that warrants intervention is Peer Socialization which Donny's parent and teacher rated 70 and 73, respectively. The behaviors in this ASRS scale involve seeking the company of other children, talking with other children, choosing to play with peers, and responding when spoken to all of which were very highly scored by both raters. Interventions for these behaviors are also included in the Quick Solution Guide. For example, the guide indicates that interventions for "encouraging a child to play with peers" is addressed on pages 50 and 51. Next, the items that contributed to Donny's high scores on Adult Socialization (at school) and Behavioral Rigidity (at home) would be examined and specific intervention identified.

Progress Monitoring and Treatment Effectiveness

Once treatment has begun, it is important to monitor the effect of the interventions over time. We assume that treatment of a youngster such as Donny would take some time and, therefore, progress toward the goals should be evaluated as frequently as possible during treatment. This may include traditional methods of specific behavior change (e.g., Applied Behavior Analysis) but should also include normative data from a rating scale to calibrate change from the pretreatment period. When using a rating scale the minimum time interval will be based on the time period indicated in the administration instructions. For example, raters who complete the ASRS are informed to evaluate the individual based upon the behaviors observed during the

Table 3.4 Parent T-Scores for ASRS Scales Obtained Over Three Time Periods

	Time 1	Time 2	Time 3	Progress monitoring (Time 2 – 1)	Significance	Progress monitoring (Time 3 – 1)	Significance
Total Score	*73*	*70*	*63*	−3	NS	10	Sig
Social Communication	*77*	*77*	*66*	0	NS	11	Sig
Unusual Behavior	*60*	58	58	−2	NS	2	NS
Self-Regulation	*70*	*67*	*62*	−3	NS	8	NS
DSM-IV Scale	*69*	*68*	*63*	−1	NS	6	NS
Treatment Scales					Sig	0	Sig
Peer Socialization	*70*	*69*	*68*	−1	NS	2	NS
Adult Socialization	58	58	58	0	NS	0	NS
Social/Emotional Reciprocity	*77*	*77*	*63*	0	NS	14	Sig
Atypical Language	52	52	52	0	NS	0	NS
Stereotypy	49	49	49	0	NS	0	NS
Behavioral Rigidity	*72*	*67*	*67*	−5	NS	5	NS
Sensory Sensitivity	44	44	44	0	NS	0	NS
Attention	*71*	*68*	58	−3	NS	13	Sig

T-scores greater than 59 appear in italic text

Note Differences needed for significance when comparing scores over time for Parent and Teacher ratings are found in Table 4.11 of the ASRS Manual ($p = .10$ with Bonferroni correction)

previous 4 weeks. The combination of specific behavior change and standard scores from a norm referenced measure will provide a well balanced view of progress.

We suggest that evidence of effective treatments is strongest when the pre- and postintervention behaviors related to ASD are evaluated using nationally calibrated T-scores for the reasons as discussed earlier in this chapter. Just how to assess these changes, however, has been an area of controversy (see Jensen 2001; Tingey et al. 1996). The approach we recommend here is based on the dual criteria of statistically reliable differences and clinically meaningful change (see Jacobsen and Truax 1991). In order to determine if the differences are related to measurement error or actual change brought about by treatment, the statistical difference between the two scores should be determined using the methods described earlier in this chapter. The values needed for significance when comparing pretest with posttest scores are obtained from Goldstein and Naglieri (2009, Tables 4.10–4.13). The values provided there are used to determine the significance when two ratings by the same rater are compared at various levels of significance.

In the illustration involving Donny, for example, Table 3.4 provides ratings obtained over time. The differences between ratings suggest that Donny's overall level of behaviors associated with ASD has declined significantly (Time 3 T-score of 63 is significantly lower than the score of 73 for Time 1). Closer examination of the Time 3 score shows that the change in the Total Score was related to the significant decrease in the Social/Emotional Reciprocity and Attention Treatment Scale changes. The Attention scale showed the most substantial change because the final T-score was significantly lower than the initial score *and* the final score was below 60. The

Social/Emotional Reciprocity score posttreatment was also significantly lower than the first evaluation but the posttreatment score of 63 suggests that additional treatment is needed. The small differences in pre- and postratings on the Behavioral Rigidity and Peer Socialization scales indicate that the strategies chosen to address these behaviors were ineffective to this point and should be reconsidered. Special attention should be paid to the item level scores for fine tuning the treatment targets and alternate treatments should be considered.

Conclusions

The process of assessment of ASD requires more than just a diagnostic pronouncement. It requires the collection of well-defined behavioral data facilitating a smooth transition between assessment, treatment planning, and ultimately the evaluation of treatment effectiveness. In this chapter, we addressed a number of important issues regarding the quality and effectiveness of the tools used to evaluate the symptoms and impairments related to ASD. We reviewed important psychometric issues related to the diagnostic process, treatment design and evaluation of treatment effectiveness. Finally, we offered a case example to illustrate these important ideas.

References

American Psychiatric Association. (1994). *Diagnostic and statistical manual of mental disorders* (4th ed.). Washington, DC: Author.

Arick, J., Young, H., Falco, R., Loos, L., Krug, D., Gense, M., & Johnson, S. (2003). Designing an outcome study to monitor the progress of students with autism spectrum disorders. *Focus on Autism and Other Developmental Disabilities, 18*(2), 75–87.

Bracken, B. A. (1987). Limitations of preschool instruments and standards for minimal levels of technical adequacy. *Journal of Psychoeducational Assessment, 5*(4), 313–326.

Crocker, L., & Algina, J. (1986). *Introduction to classical and modern test theory*. New York: Harcourt.

Goldstein, S., & Naglieri, J. A. (2009). *Autism spectrum rating scale*. Toronto: Multi Health Systems.

Jacobson, N. S., & Truax, P. (1991). Clinical significance: A statistical approach to defining meaningful change in psychotherapy research. *Journal of Consulting and Clinical Psychology, 59*(1), 12–19.

Jensen, P. S. (2001). Clinical equivalence: A step, a misstep, or just a misnomer? *Clinical Psychology: Science and Practice, 8*(4), 436–440.

Kasari, C., Paparella, T., Freeman, S., & Jahromi, L. (2008). Language outcome in autism: Randomized comparison of joint attention and play interventions. *Journal of Consulting and Clinical Psychology, 76*(1), 125–137.

LeBuffe, P. A., & Naglieri, J. A. (2003). *Devereux early childhood assessment clinical form (DECA-C)*. Lewisville: Kaplan Press.

Naglieri, J. A. (2012). Psychological assessment by school psychologists: Opportunities and challenges of a changing landscape. In K. Geisinger & B. A. Bracken (Eds.), *APA handbook of testing and assessment in psychology*. Washington, DC: APA.

Naglieri, J. A., & Chambers, K. (2009). Psychometric issues and current scales for assessing autism spectrum disorders. In S. Goldstein, J. A. Naglieri, & S. Ozonoff (Eds.), *Assessment of autism spectrum disorders* (pp. 55–90). New York: Springer.
Naglieri, J. A., McNeish, T. J., & Bardos, A. N. (1991). *Draw a person: Screening procedure for emotional disturbance*. Austin: Pro-Ed.
Nunnally, J. C. (1978). *Psychometric theory* (2nd ed.). New York: McGraw-Hill.
Nunnally, J. C., & Bernstein, I. H. (1994). *Psychometric theory* (3rd ed.). New York: McGraw-Hill.
Salvia, J., & Ysseldyke, J. E. (1981). *Assessment in special and remedial education* (2nd ed.). Boston: Houghton Mifflin.
Tingey, R. C., Lambert, M. J., Burlingame, G. M., & Hansen, N. B. (1996). Clinically significant change: Practical indicators for evaluating psychotherapy outcome. *Psychotherapy Research, 6*(2), 144–153.
Wechsler, D., & Naglieri, J. A. (2006). *Wechsler nonverbal scale of ability*. San Antonio: Pearson.
Williams, K. T. (1997). *Expressive vocabulary test* (2nd ed.). Minneapolis: Pearson Assessments.
World Health Organization. (2007). *International statistical classification of diseases and related health problems—10th Revision*. Geneva: Author.

Appendix

Quick Solution Guide

Peer Socialization

Adult Socialization

Social/Emotional Reciprocity

Atypical Language

Use language appropriate for age 81
Speak with normal, pitch, tone and rhythm 284
Avoid echolalia 111
Maintain a topic when speaking 297
Use appropriate pronouns 297

Stereotypy

Reduce repetitive behavior such as hand flapping 234
Shift focus of discussion easily 346
Avoid fascination with parts of objects 234
Avoid repetitive activities with objects such as twirling, spinning or banging 113

Behavioral Rigidity

Increase ability to handle change in routine 241
Avoid obsession with details 240
Avoid insistence on doing things the same way each time 241

Sensory Sensitivity

Desensitize to fabrics and tags in clothing 341
Desensitize to touch 247
Avoid smelling, tasting or eating inedible objects 234
Become comfortable with touch 247
React normally to sound in the environment 234

Attention/Self-Regulation

Stick with boring tasks 284
Continue working with surrounding noise 246
Sustain effort during work 265
Stay focused when reading 90
Maintain an on task conversation 269
Sustain attention and concentrate for long periods of time 111
Listen to instructions 112

Part II
Comprehensive and Related Programs

Chapter 4
Early Start Denver Model

An Intervention for Young Children with Autism Spectrum Disorders

Dana Princiotta and Sam Goldstein

Introduction and Overview of Chapter

While an increasing number of children with Autism Spectrum Disorder (ASD) are being identified at younger ages, most early interventions are targeted at older preschoolers. The necessity for early interventions for toddlers has increased as the gap widens between age of identification and age of available intervention. Further, few studies or sources have compared the effectiveness of present interventions. Interventions including Applied Behavioral Analysis (ABA); the Lovaas Model; the Treatment and Education of Autistic and Related Communication-Handicapped Children (TEACCH); and Social Communication, Emotional Regulation, and Transactional Support (SCERTS®) have received support in the treatment of ASD. A promising intervention developed by Sally Rogers and Geraldine Dawson comprises elements of ABA and relationship-based approaches to target the younger children now being identified as having ASD as infants and toddlers (Rogers and Dawson 2010). With origins from the Denver Model of 1981, the Early Start Denver Model (ESDM) is the only early intervention model validated in a randomized clinical trial for children as young as 18 months (Dawson et al. 2010). A manualized treatment, ESDM has gained acceptance as an efficacious program (Rogers and Dawson 2010). Published in 2010, the ESDM will require further longer term follow-up studies and replications to demonstrate consistency of results over time.

D. Princiotta (✉) · S. Goldstein
Neurology, Learning and Behavior Center, School of Medicine, University of Utah, 230 South 500 East, Suite 100, Salt Lake City, UT 84102, USA
e-mail: dana@samgoldstein.com

S. Goldstein
e-mail: info@samgoldstein.com

S. Goldstein, J. A. Naglieri (eds.), *Interventions for Autism Spectrum Disorders*,
DOI 10.1007/978-1-4614-5301-7_4, © Springer Science+Business Media New York 2013

Early Markers of ASDs

The emergence of early symptomology of an ASD plays an integral role in the early identification and treatment of children with developmental delays. Displayed in the early stages of life, social communication deficits can be observed between the ages of 12 and 24 months (Baranek 1999; Warren et al. 2011). More specifically, children may demonstrate lack or loss of skills, including, but not limited to, vocalization, pointing, playing with a variety of toys, and responses to contextual cues (CDC 2009; Ghaziuddin 2005). While symptomology in the domain of atypical behaviors may surface, including repetitive movements with objects or body parts, these behaviors typically emerge later than those within social and communicative functioning (Ghuman et al. 1998). Early indicators of an ASD may include: lack of pointing, sharing interest, response to name, coordinating gestures, vocalizations, or eye contact. These indicators may suggest the presence of an emerging pervasive developmental disorder (Ghuman et al. 1998).

The majority of children with ASD do not receive a formal diagnosis until 4–5 years of age (Stone et al. 2000). In alliance with this figure, most interventions are designed for these older preschoolers. This trend does not reflect current research studies suggesting an ASD diagnosis can be made prior to 2 years of age, possibly as early as 12–18 months of age (CDC 2009; Ghaziuddin 2005). Identifying deficits in social interaction has been validated in identifying young children with autism (Ghuman et al. 1998). Many parents of children with ASD detect signs of ASD within the first 12 months of age (Baranek 1999). Children identified at earlier stages have demonstrated deviance in social or language development when compared to typically developing peers (Baranek 1999). With recent trends suggesting earlier identification, the need for interventions for children recently diagnosed as infants or toddlers has increased.

Why Earlier Intervention?

The discord between age of identification and age of treatment creates an urgent search for efficacious treatments for these youngsters. If able to diagnose ASD earlier and earlier, it is imperative that efficacious treatment programs are available to utilize with children of all ages. Few published studies have discussed the efficacy of intervention models for children less than 2 years (Warren et al. 2011). Can interventions utilized with older preschoolers be modified for use with toddlers? Recent trends have provided some promising results, including psychosocial, pharmacological, and behavioral interventions. Interventions may take many forms and be directed to treat comorbid conditions as well. Few existing sources compare the effectiveness of behavioral treatment interventions. The consequences include clinicians and families choosing among interventions based on availability, insurance coverage, or affordability (Warren et al. 2011). Thus, fragmented interventions are being provided to young children with ASD (Warren et al. 2011).

Multiple intervention approaches exist within various areas of child development. Children with ASD require intervention in the realms of communication and behavior, minimally (Warren et al. 2011). Communication interventions may include the assistance of speech/language pathologists in the form of enhancing social communication and interactions. Positive behavior support systems aim to identify environmental contingencies to focus on positive aspects of the environment and the child's behavior. This approach is particularly helpful in the development of adaptive skills (Warren et al. 2011). While pharmacological and medical interventions exist for ASD, the focus will be placed upon behavioral interventions for purposes of this review.

In recent years, ABA, TEACCH, and SCERTS® demonstrated efficacy in the treatment of ASD. While these models and others have gained acceptance in the field of autism, challenges remain in the early intervention of ASD. One of the greatest difficulties in the field of autism involves the varying range of possible outcomes for diverse children receiving "identical" interventions (Howlin et al. 2009). Reviews of early interventions for autism highlight concerns of limitations. Howlin et al. (2009) conducted a systematic review of controlled studies of early intensive behavioral interventions (EIBIs) for young children with ASD. Through inclusion criteria, 11 studies were included. When examining group changes, EIBI yielded improvements in IQ scores when compared to comparison groups; yet at the individual level, a high level of variability was present (Howlin et al. 2009).

Current Intervention Programs

Methods in ABA have been utilized with children with ASD since the early 1960s. In 1987, Ivar Lovaas published findings for a group of children demonstrating improvements in both cognitive abilities and educational placement in response to intensive interventions (Warren et al. 2011). ABA is widely recognized as a helpful treatment for autism. Interventionists teach children with ASD by breaking a target skill into smaller components, performing each part in isolation. Once criterion is reached for components, teachers gradually add the components together to build a complex behavior (Warren et al. 2011).

Other supported interventions include the TEACCH program and the SCERTS® Model. Through Structured Teaching, the TEACCH model emphasizes building new skills as well as creating strategies to compensate for difficulties (Van Bourgondien and Coonrod 2012). TEACCH is based on the following general components: physical organization/structure, daily schedules, work systems, and task structure (Van Bourgondien and Coonrod 2012). Research studies utilizing the TEACCH program suggest children in the TEACCH program demonstrated greater improvements in development of cognitive, motor, and imitation skills (Van Bourgondien and Coonrod 2012).

The SCERTS® Model incorporates a focus upon SCERTS® (Rubin et al. 2012). The SCERTS® Model states it is implemented across a wider breadth of settings and "teachers" than other programs (e.g., family members, peers, teachers). The highlighted goal of the SCERTS® Model is in shifting the focal point to improving the quality of life for individuals with ASD over time that are predictable of long-term positive outcomes (Rubin et al. 2012). The SCERTS® Model supports child-initiated communication in "everyday" activities, differentiating it from a model of ABA (Rubin et al. 2012).

Trends in Interventions

While medical interventions of risperidone and aripiprazole have demonstrated decrease in problematic behaviors for some children, side effects are often considerable (Warren et al. 2011). Behavioral interventions attempt to elicit positive responses from children as they develop skill sets. Warren et al. (2011) identified 78 early behavioral interventions for ASD in a systematic review. The systematic review uncovered few studies of "adequate" quality. Most studies utilize small sample sizes and varying duration/frequencies of administration (Warren et al. 2011). At the present time, a dearth of studies exists directly comparing different treatment modality outcomes (Warren et al. 2011).

Currently, ABA coupled with TEACCH approaches is recommended as a service delivery model in which significant results can be gained (Van Bourgondien and Coonrod 2012). According to Warren's 2011 review, Lovaas-based interventions reported improvements in language, adaptive behavior, and cognitive skills in comparison to "eclectic" treatments found in the community (Warren et al. 2011). While some evidence exists that suggests change in IQ in Lovaas-based interventions, it is not clear whether these changes predict long-term consequences. Currently, the literature does not provide a wealth of information regarding baseline information of children to predict long-term outcomes (Warren et al. 2011).

A promising intervention developed by Sally Rogers and Geraldine Dawson joins elements of ABA and "relationship-based approaches" to target children identified with ASD as infants and toddlers (Dawson et al. 2010). With origins from the Denver Model, the ESDM was created to be implemented with children as young as 18 months (Dawson et al. 2010). With similarities and differences between ESDM and other models, the model possesses characteristics akin to SCERTS® (Rubin et al. 2012), Relationship Development Intervention (Gutstein 2005), Pivotal Response Training (PRT), and Developmental Individual-difference Relationship (DIR)/Floortime (Rogers and Dawson 2010; Greenspan and Wieder 2005). The authors claim that the model is differentiated from aforementioned models due to explicit behavioral lessons, the incorporation of data, and the incorporation of "all developmental domains" (Rogers and Dawson 2010, p. 33). This promising new model may respond to the need for earlier interventions reflecting age of identification in the field of ASD.

Introduction to the ESDM

Can researchers determine if intervention earlier than 24 months is effective for children in reducing or eradicating language impairments and social deficits associated with ASD? A promising intervention program developed by principal investigators,

Sally Rogers and Geraldine Dawson, targets infants, toddlers, and preschoolers with ASD. Developed through collaborators at the University of Washington, the M.I.N.D. Institute, and University of Colorado Health Sciences Center, the ESDM is based on ABA techniques coupled with a more naturalistic, relationship-based approach that highlights decades of research on typical child development. ESDM integrates social-communicative development, imitation skills, social motivation, and naturalistic behavioral intervention approach (Rogers and Dawson 2010).

ESDM utilizes play therapy and positive reciprocal interactions to integrate a developmental curriculum designed for individuals based on current abilities and interests. Utilizing knowledge of typical development in infants, Rogers and Dawson created a model to accommodate this developmental trajectory in children at risk for ASD (Rogers and Dawson 2010). In practice, toddlers may be instructed in speech via nonverbal communication of smiles, gestures, and eye contact (i.e., skills that typically precede speech in typical children but which toddlers with ASD have not practiced). At the current time, ESDM is the only early intervention model validated in a randomized clinical trial for use with children with ASD as young as 18 months of age (Dawson et al. 2010). It has been found to be effective for children with ASD across an array of learning abilities. The ESDM couples the two modalities of autism intervention with the majority of research support. Results suggested that children possessing more significant learning challenges benefited from the model as much as children without great learning challenges (Rogers and Dawson 2010).

Origins

ESDM stems from the original Denver Model of 1981, Rogers and Pennington's 1991 model of interpersonal development, pivotal response training, and the model of social motivation of Dawson et al. 2010. Components of the original Denver Model have been implemented into the ESDM, including: (1) child's choice of activities, (2) positive affect toward the child, (3) turn taking and reciprocity, (4) empathic response toward the child, (5) fostering of communicative opportunities, (6) flexible variation in activities, (7) developmentally appropriate verbal and nonverbal language, and (8) scaffolding interests and behaviors through transitions (Rogers and Dawson 2010). The original Denver Model was deemed efficacious in peer-reviewed journals in 1989 as Rogers and Lewis reported gains in symbolic play and social communication (Rogers and Dawson 2010).

Those Serviced Under the ESDM

Unique to the ESDM, the model is an intensive intervention for toddlers with ASD coupling relationship-based approaches with ABA. ESDM is targeted at children aged 12–36 months with ASD. While the model targets toddlers, the programming continues through ages 48–60 months in refining skills. Originally, the program was developed with preschoolers aged 24–60 months in mind. However, recent changes in early identification of ASDs warranted a program to be utilized with recently screened and identified toddlers (Rogers and Dawson 2010). ESDM is not intended for children older than 60 months of age or younger than 9 months of age. Prerequisites for the development of programming include an interest in object use and combining two objects in play. Children that meet these prerequisites can receive interventions from the ESDM. For children that are functioning at the level of 48 months, interventionists may need to develop an advanced curriculum, as the ESDM curriculum may not capture deficits or appropriate interventions (Rogers and Dawson 2010).

Implementation

This model can be implemented by early childhood professionals in areas of psychology, education, speech/language, Occupational Therapy (OT), and ABA (Rogers and Dawson 2010). The model is delivered by supervised interventionists focusing on treatment fidelity, as incorporated into the program's philosophy. Notably, the program includes a Teaching Fidelity Rating System to assess the interventionist's mastery of the practices included in the manualized treatment model. Using a Likert Scale allows interventionists to be assessed for competence. The marker for competence here is defined as 85 % or higher in each activity (Rogers and Dawson 2010).

In addition to interventionists, family members can receive training to implement teaching strategies in the home environment. Parents are instructed on therapeutic techniques for 1–2 h per week and incorporate learning into the "natural" home environment (Rogers and Dawson 2010). It is anticipated that parents will gain greater expertise into their child's current functioning as well as their child's remaining needs for areas of further growth. Children can eventually be transitioned out of the ESDM with the availability of community support transition services (Rogers and Dawson 2010).

Getting Started

The first step in the ESDM program entails an assessment utilizing the "Curriculum Checklist" located in the Appendix of the manual. Two or three short-term objectives are created for the child in each developmental domain. Developmental domains include: receptive communication, expressive communication, social skills, and fine and gross motor skills (Rogers and Dawson 2010). Based on results of the Curriculum Checklist assessment, the team leader creates the quarterly objectives, the task analysis for each objective, data collection system, and ensuing activities (Rogers and Dawson 2010). The checklist provides a comprehensive set of targeted goals for each child. A 12-week individualized plan is devised including specific learning objectives. This process is repeated at the termination of the 12-week period, with new initiatives formulated (Rogers and Dawson 2010).

Short-Term Objectives

The Curriculum Checklist is organized into four skill levels which correspond with developmental age periods: (1) 12–18 months, (2) 18–24 months (3) 24–36 months, and (4) 36–48 months (Rogers and Dawson 2010). Skills focus more heavily on communication and social items, in comparison to typically developing peers (Rogers and Dawson 2010). The checklist is administered in a play-based interactive style, examining components of social and communication components. The assessment can be administered within one play session typically lasting 1–2 h. The conglomeration of the developmental curriculum, teaching strategies, and social interactions foster measurable treatment goals. The ESDM proposes the balancing of objectives from all domains rather than emphasizing one domain over all others. Placing too much emphasis on areas of weakness may lead to frustration for the child, whereas too much emphasis placed on strengths may yield uneven pattern of strength versus weaknesses—already present in many children with ASD (Rogers and Dawson 2010).

The authors recommend two to three objectives for each domain, developing 20 or more objectives per child. Typically, each goal includes four to six steps to be measured. In developing four to six steps, the interventionist may use a technique called "from the ends to the middle (Rogers and Dawson 2010, p. 81)." This entails beginning with the child's baseline performance in step one with the last step describing the general criterion of the objective (Rogers and Dawson 2010). If an interventionist is not confident whether the child will be able to pass an objective in 12 weeks, the interventionist can write fewer objectives in that particular domain or break an item into smaller components (Rogers and Dawson 2010). Criterion of mastery entails an appropriate level of difficulty that is dependent on the knowledge of the child's developmental rate.

Measuring Progress

ESDM achieves individuation of goals through incorporating family and child preferences/interests into teaching—a hallmark of the ESDM (Rogers and Dawson 2010). In cases where a child is struggling in progression of goals, a decision tree may be utilized in creating changes in teaching protocols if progress slows down or halts (Rogers and Dawson 2010). Under continual data review, the child's performance is evaluated in an effort to minimize child frustration resulting from activities that may prove to be too difficult.

Under the ESDM, progress is measured under rules of criterion. Criterion measurements may be measured by number of skills learned, latency of response, percent correct, or temporal duration (e.g., independent play in the absence of adult prompts) (Rogers and Dawson 2010). A word of caution is provided by the authors in the overutilization of percentage statements in dealing with criterion measurements. Percentages are most effective when the objective involves multiple behaviors over a period of time (Rogers and Dawson 2010). Well-written objectives allow for better operational definition of teaching effectiveness.

Tracking progress can be accomplished by examining the start date and the date passed for each objective. Employing a summary sheet for sessions 1 through 12, daily sheets summarize interval recordings of performance and cue the interventionist to skills and steps to be targeted (Rogers and Dawson 2010). At the end of a session, data should be acquired on performance of the maintenance and acquisition of each objective taught. If an objective is not covered in the current session, it can be the first to be covered in the following session (Rogers and Dawson 2010). Utilizing principles of ABA, ESDM promotes ongoing data collection and interpretation.

Topography of the ESDM

It is important while working with young children with ASD to appraise the physical environment since these children may be highly motivated to obtain favored objects. Materials that intrigue young children with ASD are, therefore, necessary in teaching sessions and eliciting positive responses (Rogers and Dawson 2010). The authors recommend an initial interaction in treatment as the imitation of the child by the interventionist. Through parallel play, young children may demonstrate positive responses to being imitated, while others may wish to control materials in the physical environment, allowing for interaction of the child and interventionist (Rogers and Dawson 2010). Once this interaction has materialized, the interventionist can become more active within the interaction. Depending on the child, the level of activity of the interventionist will vary in early sessions of intervention (Rogers and Dawson 2010).

Joint activities are an integral component of teaching within the ESDM. Joint activities encompass cooperative activity, playing together, and attending to the same stimulus (Rogers and Dawson 2010). At this point of implementation, social elements are being nurtured in the child. The joint activity allows teaching at three intervals: (1) adult response to child initiation, (2) prompts, and (3) delivery of positive consequences to child's response (Rogers and Dawson 2010). Teaching is then fostered when the child initiates an activity with the adult. A typical session involves a series of joint activities, lasting approximately 2–5 min each. With further success, activities increase in duration and may last up to 10 min (Rogers and Dawson 2010).

Outside of the intervals included in the ESDM, transitions are utilized as time periods in which learning may continue. The insertion of a cleanup routine allows children to shift from one activity to the next with a transition (Rogers and Dawson 2010). Ideally, children will learn to shift from one place to another independently. The interventionist needs to be cognizant of transitions and gauge whether the child is independently engaged in the transition or if the child is being physically prompted (Rogers and Dawson 2010). Similarly, if a child does not want to make a transition from one activity to the next due to increased repetition of a preferred activity, a transition should not be avoided unless there are further opportunities for learning and engagement in this repetitive activity. A child's acquisition of shifting attention, when asked, will be a vital skill for children with ASD to acquire (Rogers and Dawson 2010).

Problem Solving

During the course of any teaching objectives, children may become defiant, engaging in a myriad of unwanted behaviors. Within the model, unwanted behaviors are identified and frequency data are subsequently collected (Rogers and Dawson 2010). Functional behavioral assessments are utilized in this application and the focus may be placed on a positive behavior management plan as well as parent coaching to use in the home environment (Rogers and Dawson 2010).

What happens when children are not progressing in the program? The authors appreciate that not one teaching approach can be utilized for all children. Therefore, a decision making tree is offered in these situations to guide the interventionist in helping the child best (Rogers and Dawson 2010). Teaching approaches are modified to accommodate learning. Progress can typically be measured in 3–5 days for children receiving 20 h or more of individual teaching. The authors suggest that more than a few weeks should not pass without modifying a teaching plan for an objective that is not fruitful (Rogers and Dawson 2010). Instruction may be adjusted by modifying reinforcement strength, adding structure, or adding visual aids (Rogers and Dawson 2010). Furthermore, it may be necessary to identify highly motivating natural reinforcers to stimulate the child.

ESDM Within Group Settings

While one-on-one interactions with children have been described thus far, ESDM can also be implemented within group settings, including early childhood programs. Individual learning within the group setting entails the broad development of goals with individual instructional periods (Rogers and Dawson 2010). Interventions with peers predominantly target areas that provide strong social rewards from each other. The areas include imitating other children, observing others, sharing with another child, turn taking, and requesting objects (Rogers and Dawson 2010). Advantages of group settings include the allowance of further interaction with same age peers.

This group model requires precision in planning and communication between team members. Typically, daily group schedules will be posted in the classroom for all members to view and access (Rogers and Dawson 2010). For optimal results, the authors recommend individual learning interactions approximately every 30 s. Likewise, successful group experiences incorporate short (10 min) interactions with enjoyable activities in which all children are capable of being active members (Rogers and Dawson 2010). Notably, verbal scripts are utilized in these interactions to facilitate play interactions with other children. Here, the adult scaffolds the interactions between two children with basic skills called "play dates (Rogers and Dawson 2010, p. 203)." Although it is challenging to coordinate between teachers and children in a group setting, this modality can yield copious benefits.

Transitions to Kindergarten

As stated by ESDM authors, the optimal end result for children in the program is the transitioning to environments in which children can further succeed. When the child transitions from preschool to kindergarten, this provides an opportunity for a "real-life" transition. Along with this opportunity comes the fear that the transition may result in loss of the child's developed skills when joining the new environment (Rogers and Dawson 2010). The communication of information from one educator to the next should begin as soon as possible prior to the transition. Particular materials, such as picture schedules, may be adapted to the new setting prior to the transition occurring (Rogers and Dawson 2010).

Evidence of Effectiveness

In the last decade, ASD were rarely identified prior to age 3 or 4 years. With endorsements from the American Academy of Pediatrics, children are now identified as toddlers; yet little research exists on how to intervene effectively for toddlers (Vismara et al. 2010). Few randomized controlled trials (RCTs) of early intensive intervention in ASD have been recognized (Cook 2010). RCTs of early intervention typically begin with children aged 40 months, despite the fact that the American Pediatric Association recommends screening prior to 18 months (Dawson et al. 2010). According to some researchers, the ESDM has established itself through rigorous empirical support and developmental sensitivity (Warren et al. 2011). Disparate from other modalities, the ESDM authors disseminate data regarding efficacy prior to publishing the program (Paul 2011; Warren et al. 2011).

The ESDM has gained acceptance as an efficacious program through various studies. In the first review, 48 children diagnosed with ASD ages 18–30 months were randomly assigned to either: (1) 2 years of ESDM intervention or (2) referral to commonly available interventions in the community (Dawson et al. 2010). Children receiving the ESDM intervention demonstrated significant improvements in adaptive behavior, IQ, and diagnosis of autism, compared to community-intervention counterparts. Selected few children in the ESDM treatment group received a change in diagnosis from Autistic Disorder to Pervasive Developmental Disorder, Not Otherwise Specified (PDD-NOS), more so than the comparison group (Dawson et al. 2010). Relative to baseline scores, the 2-year study yielded an average improvement of 17.6 standard score points for those in the treatment group compared to just 7.0 points in the comparison group (Dawson et al. 2010). Similarly, the ESDM group maintained its rate of growth in the realm of adaptive behavior when compared with a normative sample of typically developing children (Cook 2010). While the ESDM group excelled over the 2-year period, the comparison group demonstrated delays in adaptive behavior (Dawson et al. 2010). According to Dawson et al. (2010) this is the first randomized controlled trial to demonstrate efficacy as a behavioral intervention for toddlers with ASD, improving cognitive and adaptive behavior coupled with reducing the severity of ASD diagnosis (Warren et al. 2011).

Cook (2010) reviewed the ESDM via use of the treatment manual and a trained university-based clinical research team. The ESDM team implemented 2-h sessions on weekdays for 24 months. Parents also implemented interventions at home for approximately 16 h per week (Dawson et al. 2010; Cook 2010). Improvements from mean standard Mullen Scales of Early Learning (MSEL) Early Learning Composite standard scores were reported: 61–79 for the ESDM group; 59–66 for the control group (Warren et al. 2011). On the Vineland Adaptive Behavior Scales (VABS) adaptive behavior composite: 70–69 in the ESDM group and 70–59 in the control group (Dawson et al. 2010). Changed diagnoses from Autistic Disorder to PDD-NOS were noted for treatment group members compared to controls (Dawson et al. 2010). While the children in the study were not "cured" of autism, improvements in ability to handle everyday tasks necessary for child functioning were observed (Cook 2010).

Further research including work by Rogers and Vismara (2008) lends support to the ESDM. A 9-month-old infant identified with a behavioral profile consistent with autistic disorder was provided with interventions from the ESDM. The infant received 12 weeks of individualized parent–child education (1.5 h per week). Results suggested that parents acquired numerous strategies related to the development of social communication behaviors within their infant (Vismara and Rogers 2010). Similarly, the severity of behavioral problems associated with ASD decreased.

Vismara et al. (2010) reviewed the efficacy of application of the ESDM. Vismara et al. (2010) focused on deficits in attention, communication, imitation, and play skills in young children with ASD as toddlers. Providing a 12-week program to eight newly diagnosed toddlers, this study allocated 1 h per week of individualized education to parents (Vismara et al. 2010). Parents employed "naturalistic therapeutic techniques" from ESDM with results suggestive of acquired parental strategies by the 6-week mark. At the midpoint of the 12 weeks, children exhibited sustained change in social communication (Vismara et al. 2010; Warren et al. 2011).

In the context of other early interventions for young children with ASD, Warren et al. (2011) systematically reviewed evidence of interventions for children aged 2 to 12. Studies between January 2000 and May 2010 were included in this review. Out of the 34 studies reviewed by these researchers, 1 study was rated as good quality, 10 as fair quality, and 23 as poor quality. Along with Lovaas–based interventions, the ESDM reported some improvements in cognitive performance, language skills, and adaptive behavior skills (Warren et al. 2011).

Suggested Weaknesses of ESDM

While specific studies comparing the ESDM to other approaches are not available at the current time, the authors of the ESDM point out that there is no "one best approach" for all children (Rogers and Dawson 2010, p. 33). Professionals working with children with ASD agree that early intervention is critical and they also agree on central aspects of this treatment (e.g., intensity, family involvement, and focus on generalization) (Corsello 2005). Difference in philosophy coupled with a lack of RCTs further exacerbates difficulties in comparing programs of early intervention for children with ASD (Rogers and Dawson 2010).

Although gains in cognition and language have been noted through utilization of the ESDM, it should be noted that these changes were not accompanied by improvements in social skills or repetitive behaviors (Dawson et al. 2010). One hypothesis suggests gains in social skills may take longer to develop than language or IQ (Warren et al. 2011). Warren et al. (2011) also add that it is difficult to parse out the effect of the total number of therapy hours on conclusions as control children received half the hours of intervention as treatment children received. As described by other researchers in the field of autism, significant variability exists as to how children will respond to interventions in general (Rogers and Vismara 2008). When averaging improvements in the treatment group, this average stems from a group of children making tremendous gains with others making little-to-no improvement (Corsello 2005; Warren et al. 2011).

The authors suggest that there are weaknesses within the model that are currently being addressed in replication studies (Dawson et al. 2010). One weakness lies within the delivery methodology of the program according to Vismara et al. (2010). As a clinic-based delivery method, the ESDM may limit access to parents. The addition of home delivery coupled with clinic delivery may enhance the program as natural and "artificial" settings would be accounted for (Vismara et al. 2010). In discussing the generalizability of skills learned in the clinical setting, training in the home setting would increase fidelity of skills learned in the natural setting (Vismara et al. 2010).

Regarding specific guidelines of the ESDM, critics argue that the manual is too prescribed or too technical for some audiences. For example, the manual proposes explicit arrangements for the therapy room (i.e., arranged to be empty with the exception of a table and chairs and a closed cabinet). While coined a "natural environment" by the authors of the ESDM manual, critics argue that this environment does not allow for natural, unmodified exploration of the environment by the child. Flexibility of the program comes into question by others when it is stated in the manual, "Our job is not to keep children happy; it is to teach them their objectives (Rogers and Dawson 2010)."

Some researchers have designated the ESDM as an "eclectic" intervention as it entails combining ABA- and non-ABA-based approaches. Strict behavior analysts claim that "eclectic" autism interventions are ineffective (Howard et al. 2005). The Association of Professional Behavior Analysts does not support eclectic approaches (Howard et al. 2005). Howard et al. (2005) compared intensive behavior analytic and eclectic treatments for young children with autism (prior to the publication of the ESDM). Fourteen months following treatment, the researchers examined cognitive, language, and adaptive skills in young children. Although three groups (intensive ABA group, eclectic group, and nonintensive community intervention group) were similar on key variables at intake, the follow-up yielded higher mean standard scores in all skill domains for the intensive ABA group versus groups 2 and 3. Statistically significant differences were not found between the eclectic group versus the nonintensive community interventions group (Howard et al. 2005). Although this study was completed prior to the publication of the ESDM, it lends assistance in comprehending the suggested scrutiny toward eclectic approaches in autism interventions. Further research will be necessary in comparing ESDM to other "eclectic" approaches in the future.

Although authors lend support to the program through the RCT study, the design of the ESDM RCT has come into question just as the design of other RCTs come into question (Warren et al. 2011). As with most interventions, exclusion criteria were applied in this trial. Children with severe or profound intellectual disability were excluded from review. Parents reported approximately 15 h per week of home interventions along with 5 h of non-ESDM interventions (Warren et al. 2011). Although the RCT includes more children than other trials of autism interventions, the trial sample size remains small. Additionally, the description of the control group does not allow for elaboration or understanding of the group makeup. Similarly, blinding is extremely difficult in RCTs. Although evaluators are purported to be naïve regarding the intervention status of a child, they are not described as being blind to the purpose of the study or of ESDM (Warren et al. 2011).

Conclusion and Future Directions

The ESDM has gained acceptance as an efficacious program through various studies for rigorous empirical support and developmental sensitivity (Rogers and Dawson 2010; Warren et al. 2011). This promising new model responds to the need for earlier interventions reflecting identification of children with ASD in the toddler years. At the current time, ESDM is the only early intervention model validated in a randomized clinical trial for use with children with ASD as young as 18 months of age (Dawson et al. 2010). Disparate from other modalities, the ESDM authors disseminate data regarding efficacy prior to publishing the program (Paul 2011).

According to the ESDM authors, the ESDM will allow for the provision of an individualized curriculum with a predictable routine for children and adults (Rogers and Dawson 2010). Coupling focused interactions with play-oriented and relationship-based approaches, a high level of structure can be provided with ongoing data collection and interpretation (Rogers and Dawson 2010). Similarly, the model maintains a focus on treatment fidelity to assess the application of the model and mastery of the practices included in the treatment manual. In application to various environments, "A classroom using the ESDM emphasizes children's development of independence, encouragement of social relationships and interactions, and the development of more and more sophisticated communication skills (Rogers and Dawson 2010, p. 207)."

As with all early behavioral interventions, longer term follow-up studies and replications will be required to demonstrate the consistency of evidence over time. The authors are confident that the benefit of their treatment approach is efficacious in posing an impact in improvements for children with early signs of ASD (Rogers and Dawson 2010). A variety of studies have indicated increases in language and cognitive abilities, adaptive skills, and social interaction with use of the ESDM.

While positive outcomes are reported in most cases of early intervention, the field does not yet possess treatment that meets the present criteria for well-established or probably efficacious treatment (Rogers and Vismara 2008). Most notably, will research findings translate to the community settings for any of these approaches? Further research requires evaluation, including age at start of treatment, treatment modality, intensity, and baseline language/IQ (Rogers and Dawson 2010). Recent preliminary data for intensive intervention in children younger than 2 years have been identified; however, these studies need to be replicated. Similarly, researchers need to identify which children are likely to benefit from which treatments and how well they will respond to interventions (Warren et al. 2011).

References

Baranek, G. T. (1999). Autism during infancy: A retrospective video analysis of sensory-motor and social behaviors at 9–12 months of age. *Journal of Autism and Developmental Disorders, 29*(3), 213–224. doi:10.1023/A:1023080005650.

Bourgondien, M., & Coonrod, E. (2012). TEACCH: An intervention approach for children and adults with autism spectrum disorders and their families. In S. Goldstein & J. Naglieri (Ed.), *Intervention for autism spectrum disorders*. New York: Springer Science.

Centers for Disease Control and Prevention. (2009). Autism and family history. Retrieved October 8, 2009 from http://www.cdc.gov/genomics/resources/diseases/autism.htm.

Cook, E. H., Jr. (2010). Reduction of increased repetitive self-grooming in ASD mouse model by metabotropic 5 glutamate receptor antagonism; randomized controlled trial of early start Denver model. *Autism Research, 3*(1), 40–42. doi:10.1002/aur.118.

Corsello, C. (2005). Early intervention in autism. *Infants and Young Children, 18*(2), 74–85. doi:10.1097/00001163-200504000-00002.

Dawson, G., Rogers, S., Muson, J., Smith, M., Winter, J., Greenson, J., Donaldson, A., & Varley, J. (2010). Randomized, controlled trial of an intervention for toddlers with autism: The Early Start Denver Model. *Pediatrics, 125*(1), e17–e23. doi:10.1542/peds.2009-0958.

Greenspan, S. I., & Wieder, S. (2005). Can children with autism master the core deficits and become empathetic, creative, and reflective? A ten to fifteen year follow up of a subgroup of children with autism spectrum disorders (asd) who received a comprehensive developmental, individual difference, relationship based (dir) approach. *The Journal of Developmental and Learning Disorders. 9,* 39–61.

Ghaziuddin, M. (2005). *Mental health aspects of autism and asperger syndrome*. London: Jessica Kingsley.

Ghuman, J. K., Peebles, C. D., & Ghuman, H. S. (1998). Review of social interaction measures in infants and preschool children. *Infants and Young Children, 11*(2), 21–44.

Gutstein, S. (2005). Relationship development intervention: Developing a treatment program to address the unique social and emotional deficits of autism spectrum disorders. *Autism Spectrum Quarterly* (Winter).

Howard, J., Sparkman, R., Cohen, H., Green, G., & Stanislaw, H. (2005). A comparison of intensive behavior analytic and eclectic treatments for young children with autism. *Research in Developmental Disabilities, 26*(4), 359–383. doi:10.1016/j.ridd.2004.09.005.

Howlin, P., Magiati, I., & Charman, T. (2009). Systematic review of early intensive behavioral interventions for children with autism. *American Journal on Intellectual and Developmental Disabilities, 114*(1), 23–41. doi:10.1352/2009.114;23-41.

Paul, R. (2011). Sally J. Rogers and Geraldine Dawson: Review of Early Start Denver Model for young children with autism: Promoting language, learning, and engagement. *Journal of Autism and Developmental Disorders, 41*(7), 978–980. doi:1007/s10803-010-1041-8.

Rogers, S. J., & Dawson, G. (2010). *The Early Start Denver Model: Promoting language, learning, and engagement*. New York: Guilford.

Rogers, S. J., & Vismara, L. A. (2008). Evidence-based comprehensive treatments for early autism. *Journal of Child Adolescent Psychology, 37*(1), 8–38. doi:10.1016/S0140-6736(10)60300-5.

Rubin, E., Prizant, B., Laurent, A., & Wetherby, A. (2012). Social Communication, Emotional Regulation and Transactional Support (SCERTS). In S. Goldstein & J. Naglieri (Eds.), *Intervention for autism spectrum disorders*. New York: Springer Science.

Stone, W. L., Coonrod, E. E., & Ousley, O. Y. (2000). Brief report: Screening tool for autism in two year olds (STAT): Development and preliminary data. *Journal of Autism and Developmental Disorders, 30*(6), 607–612. doi:10.1023/A:1005647629002.

Vismara, L. A., Colombi, C., & Rogers, S. J. (2009). Can one hour per week of therapy lead to lasting changes in young children with autism? *Autism, 13*(1), 93–115. doi:10.1177/1362361307098516.

Vismara, L. A., & Rogers, S. J. (2010). Behavioral treatments in autism spectrum disorder: What do we know? *Annual Review of Clinical Psychology, 6*, 447–468. doi:10.1146/annurev.clinpsy.121208.131151.

Vismara, L. A., Young, G. S., & Rogers, S. J. (2010). Community Dissemination of the Early Start Denver Model: Implications for Science and Practice. *Topics in Early Childhood Special Education*. doi:10.1177/0271121411409250.

Warren, Z., Veenstra-VanderWeele, J., Stone, W., Bruzek, J. L., Nahmias, A. S., Foss-Feig, J. H., Jerome, R. N., Krishnaswami, S., Sathe, N. A., Glasser, A. M., Surawicz, T., & McPheeters, M. L. (2011, April). Therapies for Children With Autism Spectrum Disorders. Comparative Effectiveness Review No. 26. (Prepared by the Vanderbilt Evidence-based Practice Center under Contract No. 290-2007-10065-I.) AHRQ Publication No. 11-EHC029-EF. Rockville, MD: Agency for Healthcare Research and Quality. www.effectivehealthcare.ahrq.gov/reports/final.cfm.

Warren, Z., McPheeters, M. L., Sathe, N., Foss-Feig, J. H., Glasser, A., & Veenstra-VanderWeele, J. (2011). A systematic review of early intensive intervention for autism spectrum disorders. *Pediatrics, 127*(5), e1303–e1311. doi:10.1542/peds.2011-0426.

Chapter 5
TEACCH: An Intervention Approach for Children and Adults with Autism Spectrum Disorders and their Families

Mary E. Van Bourgondien and Elaine Coonrod

Introduction and Overview

The TEACCH autism program is a clinical service and professional training program dedicated to serve individuals with autism spectrum disorder (ASD) of all ages and ability levels and their families. Established in the early 1970s by Dr. Eric Schopler and colleagues, the mission of TEACCH is to enable individuals with ASD to function as meaningfully and as independently as possible in their community by providing exemplary services to individuals, their families, and the professionals who serve and support them, and by generating and disseminating theory, practice, and research on autism nationally and internationally. TEACCH is based at the University of North Carolina at Chapel Hill and has a statewide presence, including regional service clinics across North Carolina, early intervention and supported employment programs, and a model adult residential community.

The primary intervention and educational strategy used in the TEACCH model is Structured Teaching, which is a set of teaching principles and intervention strategies based on an understanding of the learning style and unique needs of individuals with ASD (Mesibov et al. 2005). Because individuals with ASD will likely have some level of cognitive/learning differences throughout their lives, the end goal of Structured Teaching is not to cure autism but rather to help individuals with ASD live more productive, fulfilling, and independent lives. Structured Teaching emphasizes the use of visual and organizational supports and can be adapted for all ages and ability levels to address the many behavioral and educational challenges associated with autism. Individuals with ASD, their family members, and professionals from a variety of training backgrounds can be taught to implement Structured Teaching

M. E. Van Bourgondien (✉) · E. Coonrod
Chapel Hill TEACCH Center, The University of North Carolina,
Campus Box #6305, Chapel Hill, NC 27599-6305, USA
e-mail: mvan2@email.unc.edu

E. Coonrod
e-mail: Elaine_Coonrod@med.unc.edu

S. Goldstein, J. A. Naglieri (eds.), *Interventions for Autism Spectrum Disorders*,
DOI 10.1007/978-1-4614-5301-7_5,

strategies. The TEACCH model is in a constant state of evolution in response to the changing world of autism—such as increasing prevalence rates, identification of more intellectually capable and independent individuals on the autism spectrum, and diagnoses of autism occurring at younger, as well as much older, ages. Although the basic principles of Structured Teaching remain the same, as the face of autism has evolved and as more empirically supported treatments for autism become available, new approaches are continually being integrated into the TEACCH model and Structured Teaching methods.

The TEACCH model upholds best practices in interventions for individuals with ASD, and Structured Teaching provides an evidence-based approach to intervention. Mesibov and Shea (2010); Mesibov et al. (2005) describe in detail the evidence base for the TEACCH approach in terms of research findings in support of Structured Teaching and the TEACCH Program, the clinical expertise of TEACCH professionals, the focus on individualization of treatment strategies based on specific characteristics and needs of the individuals and families, positive findings from real life outcome measures, and generalizability of Structured Teaching strategies and the numerous home, school, and work environments in which they are applied, nationally and internationally. Professionals continue to discuss the best approach for validating the efficacy of a given treatment approach in the field of autism (Mesibov and Shea 2011; Odom et al. 2010; Reichow et al. 2008). In this review of the TEACCH method, we are taking two approaches to providing empirical support. First, empirical support for each of the essential components of the model is included within the description of each component. Second, the chapter concludes with a section summarizing the research which supports the overall TEACCH Program.

In this chapter, we begin by describing in more detail the theoretical and empirical underpinnings of the TEACCH psychoeducational model, focusing on evidence related to the patterns of neurobehavioral strengths and weaknesses in individuals with ASD, known at TEACCH as the "culture of autism", as well as the importance of family collaboration. From there, we discuss the role of assessment, formal and informal, in designing and implementing TEACCH interventions. Then, we discuss in detail the principles of Structured Teaching, including the basic elements of physical structure, visual schedules, work and activity systems, and visually structured activities, as well as the ways Structured Teaching continues to evolve, incorporating technological advances and other evidence-based intervention approaches. The final section summarizes the programmatic research to date utilizing the TEACCH method.

TEACCH and the Culture of Autism

The TEACCH approach and Structured Teaching are grounded in a philosophy of respect for and understanding of the "culture of autism". Just as culture in the traditional sense refers to shared patterns of human behavior, the culture of autism refers to the shared patterns of neurobehavioral strengths and weaknesses in individuals with ASD (Mesibov and Shea 2010). There is tremendous heterogeneity across the phenotypic presentation of ASD—individuals vary significantly in terms of their overall intellectual ability, their temperament, their interests, and the specific level of impairment in their social communication and adaptive skills. However, just as all individuals possess diagnostically identifiable impairments in their social-communication skills and repetitive behaviors, they also demonstrate a characteristic set of strengths and weaknesses in their learning style and information processing abilities. Because there is currently no intervention that completely reverses the neurologically based impairments associated with ASD, the TEACCH model focuses on mutual accommodation—both teaching new skills and providing environmental supports. This is done best by appreciating the differences in learning and understanding associated with ASD, and then teaching the skills needed to function in our neurotypical culture (Mesibov and Shea 2010). Thus, the TEACCH Structured Teaching method focuses on designing interventions and supports around the specific learning style and neuropsychological strengths and weaknesses of the individual.

Below is a review of the learning style and information processing characteristics that make up the culture of autism. Identification of these characteristics is grounded in the observations and reports of TEACCH clinicians, first-hand accounts of individuals with ASD and their family members, as well as empirical support from years of studies examining the performance of individuals with ASD on tests of neuropsychological functioning.

Strong Visual Learning

Individuals with ASD are visual learners, and many demonstrate relative strengths and preserved abilities in visual processing as compared to auditory or verbal processing (Grandin 1996; Mesibov and Shea 2010; Mesibov et al. 2005; Quill 1997; Tsatsanis 2005). Clinically, this means that individuals may struggle to process and learn information presented in a verbal format (i.e., language) that could be more easily understood if it were presented in a visual format, such as pictures or written words.

Impairment in Generating Meaning, Narrowly Focused Attention and Weak Central Coherence

Individuals with ASD demonstrate a relative strength in detail-focused attention and information processing as compared to integrating multiple details or sources of information for higher conceptual meaning (Frith 1989; Happé 2005; Mesibov and Shea 2010; Mesibov et al. 2005; Tsatsanis 2005). This pattern of attention is sometimes described like the narrow beam of a flashlight; the individual can only attend to one small, circumscribed aspect of the environment at a time. Similarly, although multiple pieces of information may be observed, the individual has difficulty understanding how those details fit together or how to prioritize their relevance.

Clinically, this means that individuals with ASD need assistance in understanding what parts of the environment or what pieces of information are the most important. They also need explicit information about big picture concepts that others might be able to correctly infer by integrating individual pieces of information.

Concrete vs. Abstract Thinking

Individuals with ASD show strengths in processing and learning rote, concrete information and difficulty with abstraction and generalization (Mesibov et al. 2005; Ropar and Peebles 2007). Clinically, this means that teaching strategies should focus on making concepts and instructions as concrete and literal as possible.

Executive Function

Executive function is a broad construct that refers to the cognitive processes related to complex, goal-directed behavior (Duncan 1986; Ozonoff and Griffith 2000). Under this umbrella of skills, individuals with ASD have deficits in their ability to sequence, plan, and organize (Bramham et al. 2009; Lopez et al. 2005; Ozonoff et al. 1991; Zalla et al. 2006), as well as difficulties with cognitive flexibility and set shifting (Ambery et al. 2006; Lopez et al. 2005; Ozonoff et al. 2005b). Deficits in executive function have also been linked to the presence of repetitive behaviors and restricted interests (Boyd et al. 2009; Lopez et al. 2005). Clinically, this means that when presented with complex or multistep tasks, individuals may carry out activities in an illogical or inefficient order, or miss important steps along the way. They also have difficulty shifting attention and transitioning between ideas and activities, and can become overly focused on rigidly completing established routines or favorite activities.

Sensory Perception and Responses

Individuals with ASD often experience and respond to sensory input (e.g., visual, auditory, tactile) in a disordered fashion (Baranek et al. 2005; Rogers and Ozonoff 2005; Tsatsanis 2005). Atypical sensory responses and overstimulation are associated with repetitive behavior (Gabriels et al. 2008) and other behavior problems (Grandin 1996; Schopler 1995). In planning interventions for behavior and learning, it is important to consider each individual's subjective experience of the sensory environment so that environmental modifications or appropriate supports can be made as necessary.

Individually, these characteristics identified as the culture of autism are not specific to individuals with ASD, as individuals with a variety of neurodevelopmental or psychiatric disorders, such as intellectual disability, ADHD, anxiety, or psychosis, often show one or more of these characteristics. For example, unusual sensory responses occur commonly in individuals with ASD, though not more commonly than in individuals with other disabilities (Baranek et al. 2005; Rogers and Ozonoff 2005). What is unique to individuals with ASD is the number, frequency, and intensity with which these characteristics occur (Mesibov et al. 2005). By understanding the culture of autism, we have more information about how individuals with ASD learn best, and the ways in which interventions might be most effectively designed.

Family Collaboration

Working together with parents as co-therapists or collaborators in the assessment and treatment of their children is one of the most fundamental principles in the TEACCH approach (Marcus et al. 2005; Mesibov et al. 2005; Schopler et al. 1984; Schopler and Reichler 1971).

From the first encounter, the parents are viewed as experts on their children who know their own child better than anyone else. Information gathered from parent's observations in both the assessment and intervention stages provides a more comprehensive understanding of the child which enhances our ability as professionals to better diagnose and design intervention strategies. At the same time, parents are eager for information from professionals about the nature of their child's problems and what it means to them to have a diagnosis of an Autism Spectrum Disorder (ASD; Midence and O'Neill 1999). Parents benefit from the understanding that autism is a developmental disorder and that the behavioral difficulties the children demonstrate are the result of neurological differences that affect their communication, socialization, cognitive and learning processes. Understanding that autism is a pervasive problem that to some degree pervades all aspects of a child's life gives the parents the information they need to develop a strategy for improving their child's behavior and skills as well as coping with the stresses created by the disorder.

At the time that Schopler and Reichler (1971) were developing the TEACCH model, the idea that the most effective treatment approach for children with autism was one that involved working collaboratively with families was a novel approach. Today, parent training has been demonstrated to be a component of all successful early intervention programs (Dawson and Osterling 1997) and is among the empirically based intervention strategies for autism cited by the National Professional Development Center on Autism Spectrum Disorders (NPDC on ASD; http://autismpdc.fpg.unc.edu/). Within the TEACCH Program, parents have been shown to be effective teachers of their children (Marcus et al. 1978; Schopler et al. 1982; Short 1984). Parent training can contribute to reducing mothers' depressive symptoms (Bristol et al. 1993) and increasing positive family interactions (Koegel et al. 1996; Moes 1995). As a program that works with individuals with ASD of all ages throughout their lifespan, the involvement of family members goes beyond parents at times to include spouses, siblings, and other concerned family members.

The parent training and family teaching sessions at the TEACCH model are individualized based on the particular concerns and needs of each family. Parental concerns and needs often reflect the child's age and current developmental level (Marcus et al. 2005). A common concern across all age groups is learning how to decrease negative behaviors which is addressed by utilizing the individual's visual strengths to address the underlying cognitive issues. Increasing the individual's positive engagement, communication, social and adaptive skills are also areas of focus. As the child ages, the family's advocacy efforts change from thinking about early intervention to school and eventually to vocational, residential and recreational issues. As professionals, our job is to help the parents learn to articulate their child's learning style so that throughout their child's life they can best advocate for the services he/she needs at each stage of life.

At all ages of development, one of the most sought after service is where parents and other family members come together with other families to share information and provide a true understanding and support for each other. The nature of family support groups continues to evolve to reflect the changes in the field and the aging of the population being served. Mothers groups, fathers groups, and siblings groups now have expanded to include support groups for parents of adults with ASD. As the population of individuals with high functioning ASD has grown and aged, there is an increasing need for support groups for adults with ASD themselves and for siblings.

Assessment

Along with family collaboration, another guiding principle of the TEACCH approach is assessment. There are several goals of assessment—first is to determine diagnostically whether or not an individual shares the established diagnostic features of ASD. The second goal of an assessment process is to determine what is unique about this individual's learning style which then enables us to design an individualized intervention plan. Other important aspects of assessment are functional behavioral assessments (Thomas and Williams 2004) and taking data during intervention times in order to determine the progress of the individual and to help determine how to improve the intervention.

Diagnostic Evaluation

The TEACCH diagnostic procedure is consistent with the best practices of evidence-based assessment outlined by Ozonoff et al. (2005a). The evaluation is conducted from a developmental perspective with information gathered from multiple sources and contexts. Regardless of whether the person being evaluated is a child or an adult, information from family members who know the person's early history as well as from spouses or others who know their current functioning is essential.

Table 5.1 CARS2 Standard Version items and CARS2 High Functioning Version items

	CARS-ST	CARS-HF
1	Relating to people	Social–emotional understanding
2	Imitation	Emotional expression and regulation
3	Emotional response	Relating to people
4	Body use	Body use
5	Object use	Object use in play
6	Adaptation to change	Adaptation to change/restricted interests
7	Visual response	Visual response
8	Listening response	Listening response
9	Taste, smell and touch response	Taste, smell and touch response
10	Fear or nervousness	Fear or anxiety
11	Verbal communication	Verbal communication
12	Nonverbal communication	Nonverbal communication
13	Activity level	Thinking/cognitive integration skills
14	Consistency of intellectual response	Level and consistency of intellectual response
15	General impressions	General impressions

The first step in the diagnostic process involves gathering both developmental and current information from the parents and others about the individual's communication, social, and behavioral development. Information is gathered both through parent and teacher questionnaires (e.g., PEP-3 and CARS2; Schopler et al. 2005; Schopler et al. 2010), as well as through direct interviews with parents and other informants. The interview is roughly based on the clinical, brief version of the ADI-R (LeCouteur et al. 2003). To differentiate between other possible diagnoses, it is essential to have information about the individual's early development before they started in school, as well as their developmental progression.

In accordance with professional practice standards (Filipek et al. 2000), an equally important part of the process is directly interacting and observing the child or adult suspected of having an ASD. The diagnostic assessment tools utilized within the TEACCH program include the recently revised Childhood Autism Rating Scale–2nd Edition (CARS2; Schopler et al. 2010) as well as the Autism Diagnostic Observation Scales-2 (ADOS-2; Lord et al. 2012). The CARS2 comprises of two different scales, the Childhood Autism Rating Scale 2nd Edition–Standard version (CARS2-ST; Schopler et al. 2010) and the Childhood Autism Rating Scale 2nd Edition–High Functioning version (CARS2-HF; Schopler et al. 2010). Both scales are comprised of 15 items rated on a 7-point scale (1 through 4 with mid points). See Table 5.1 for a description of items.

The CARS2-ST is appropriate for children under 6 or older individuals whose IQ score is less than 80 and/or those who do not have fluent language. It contains the same items as the original version of the CARS (Schopler et al. 1988). The CARS is a well researched screening tool which has been shown to be a reliable and valid measure for rating the behaviors related to autism (Lord and Corsello 2005; Magyar and Pandolfi 2007). In the CARS2 (Schopler et al. 2010), the reliability and validity were re-verified and t-scores added with an updated sample ($N = 1{,}034$). The CARS-ST has a sensitivity of .88 and a specificity of .86 in identifying individuals with autism as compared to individuals without autism. Ratings can be made based on direct observation during a clinic visit, during a school observation, or based on a parent interview (Schopler et al. 2010).

To complement the CARS2-ST, the CARS2-High Functioning (HF) version was developed at TEACCH to assess individuals older than 6 years with IQ scores 80 or above and fluent language. The items reflect current research on the diagnostic features of individuals with high functioning autism. The reliability and validity of the CARS2-HF is quite good with a sensitivity of .81 and specificity of .87 (Schopler et al. 2010). The CARS2-HF requires information from multiple sources including at least a direct observation and a caregiver interview in order to determine the pervasiveness of the difficulties over time and over settings.

To complete the diagnostic process, information about the individual's current level of cognitive, academic, language, and adaptive functioning are also essential elements of the evaluation.

Assessment and Individualization

Assessment is part of the child or adult's initial evaluation, and also continues beyond that point. The purpose of assessment is to identify the person's strengths, weaknesses, interests, learning style, and emerging skills from a variety of perspectives. Our ultimate goal is to use the assessment information to develop appropriate individualized goals and intervention strategies and to continue to evaluate their effectiveness over time.

Utilizing information from parents, teachers, and the individual with ASD, individualized teaching goals are developed based on the perceived needs and weaknesses in different settings. Respect for the individual with ASD necessitates choosing goals and objectives based on recognition of the child or adult's specific wants and interests. Emerging skills identified through the assessment process are used to form developmentally appropriate and achievable goals. Emerging skills are those skills that the child or adult is showing a beginning or partial understanding of but has not yet mastered the concept. For a young child, he/she may be starting to sort by color recognizing one or two colors but not consistently putting like colors together. For an adolescent learning to care for his/her own needs, he/she may be able to hold a broom correctly and make the sweeping motion, but does not yet have the concept of how to sweep an entire area. Part of the assessment process includes assessing the parent's interests, needs, and skills as they are essential collaborators in this process. Carefully listening to parents is perhaps the most valuable assessment skill one can have (Morrell and Palmer 2006). Taking the time early on and throughout one's relationship with a family to hear their story and to recognize their greatest concerns and needs creates a foundation that is essential to the ongoing collaboration.

A second aim of the assessment process is to identify the person's learning style in order to individualize the teaching strategies and behavioral interventions. Knowing the person's strengths—whether he/she is good at matching or decoding objects, pictures, letters, numbers or words—is the beginning step to Structured Teaching.

The TEACCH approach has always been to utilize the strengths of the individual to help compensate for areas he/she is not yet ready to learn. Along with identifying strengths, defining the unique interests of the client is a very important aspect of the assessment process. Motivating individuals on the autism spectrum can be challenging especially if we make the erroneous assumption that what is meaningful to us is meaningful to them. Intense and atypical interests are defining features of autism spectrum disorders. As will be discussed shortly, Structured Teaching utilizes the clients' special interests to increase their engagement, appropriate attention, and motivation to complete tasks.

Ongoing assessment is an important aspect of any intervention or educational program. Taking data on either the acquisition of a skill or the frequency of occurrence of a negative behavior helps us to determine whether or not the goal is being achieved. When targeting high frequency or high intensity negative behaviors one may actually have a successful behavior plan but subjectively not recognize progress without objective data that is regularly analyzed and charted. Data on teaching goals helps us determine when the intervention plan is working or not working and may provide information on how to refine the teaching method.

Formal developmental and functional assessment tools The two most widely used formal assessment tools developed at TEACCH are the Psychoeducational Profile–3rd Edition (PEP-3; Schopler et al. 2005) and the TEACCH Transition Assessment Profile (TTAP; Mesibov et al. 2007).

The Psychoeducational Profile (PEP 1971) was originally developed at a time when children with autism were often thought to be "untestable" (Alpern 1967; Marcus and Baker 1986). Standardized tests often require an inflexible, language based administration that does not fully reflect the uneven profile of children with autism. A developmental measure, the Psychoeducational Profile (PEP) was designed to assess the functioning of children whose communication deficits may impair their ability to understand what is being asked of them on a more language based standardized test.

The PEP-3 (Schopler et al. 2005), the most recent update of this measure, includes both a direct assessment of the child's skills and behaviors as well as a caregiver questionnaire. The direct assessment scale is comprised of six developmental subtests and four maladaptive scales. Developmental items range from 7 to 81 months. In general, the test is best utilized with children whose cognitive ability is younger than 6 years of age. The six developmental subtests include cognitive verbal/preverbal, expressive language, receptive language, fine motor, gross motor, and visual motor imitation. Each item is scored as a 2, 1, or 0 with 2 being a passing skill that the child can do without extra demonstration or teaching; 1 is an emerging skill where the child demonstrates some ability to perform the skill or needs extra demonstration or teaching to be successful; or 0 is a failure indicating an inability to complete any aspect of the task. These scores are totaled to yield developmental ages and percentile ranks for each area.

The Maladaptive Behavior subtests include items related to Affective Expression; Social Reciprocity, Characteristics Motor Behaviors, and Characteristic Verbal Behaviors. Lower scores represent atypical or autistic behaviors.

The Caregiver Report provides information about the parents' perceptions of their child's current developmental level, diagnostic categories, problem behavior, personal self-care, and adaptive behavior. Parent estimates of current child functioning in communication, motor, social, self help, thinking, and overall skills are generally accurate and broadly sensitive to developmental difficulties (Glascoe and Sandler 1995). They are also an excellent gauge of likely parent reactions to the feedback from the assessment.

Overall, analysis of reliability and validity indicate that the PEP-3 demonstrates sound psychometric properties (Schopler et al. 2005). It was developed using data collected during 2002 through 2003 in a normative sample comprised of 407 children and adolescents with ASDs and 148 children with typical development from across the United States. Both groups were similar to the general U.S. population as measured by 2001 Census data on the characteristics of race, family income, and parent educational attainment. The gender of the typically developing sample was also similar to the general population, while the gender of the sample with ASD (4:1 males to females) was similar to reported prevalence rates for autism. Coefficient alphas were calculated for all subtests and composites from the sample of individuals with ASDs at 11 age intervals (ages 2 through 12 years); average coefficients indicated high reliability and for the Developmental subtests ranged from .92 to .97, for the Maladaptive Behavior subtests ranged from .90 to .93, for the Caregiver Report subtests ranged from .84 to .90, and for the Composites ranged from .97 to .99. Test-retest reliability was assessed over a period of two weeks in a subsample of 33 children with ASDs. Raw scores were used to calculate correlation coefficients for each subtest and all indicate high reliability: Developmental subtest correlation coefficients ranged from .97 to .99, Maladaptive Behavior subtest correlation coefficients ranged from .94 to .98, and Caregiver Report subtest correlation coefficients ranged from .98 to .99.

Validity was evaluated in a series of studies correlating scores from the PEP-3 with scores from other developmental and behavioral assessments used to measure similar constructs, including the Vineland Adaptive Behavior Scales, the Childhood Autism Rating Scales, and the Autism Behavior Checklist–Second Edition. Overall, the vast majority of correlations were large (.50 and above) and in the expected direction, thus supporting the validity of the PEP-3 as a measure of development and autism characteristics (Schopler et al. 2005).

The PEP-3 can be used to identify a starting point for designing both teaching goals and Structured Teaching intervention strategies for a preschool child with autism. For developing teaching goals for home or a school IEP, the emerging skills in each development area combined with the information about parents' greatest area of concerns typically provides an ideal starting point. The observations of the child's strengths, and responses to the different teaching strategies utilized within the test administration, give valuable insights into the child's learning style and where to start in developing the visual strategies discussed later in this chapter.

TEACCH Transition Assessment Profile–Second Edition (TTAP; Mesibov et al. 2007) is a criterion referenced assessment tool developed to assist in the assessment of skills and development of goals for older children and adolescents as they transition to adulthood. It is also useful for assessing and developing goals for many adults on the autism spectrum. Originally developed as the Adolescent and Adult Psychoeducational Profile (AAPEP; Mesibov et al. 1988), this second edition has been expanded to include more high functioning skills in recognition of the increasing incidence of high functioning autism diagnoses. The interrater reliability for the total score of the original APPEP was .865, and the validity of the AAPEP was established by comparing the recommendations generated by the AAPEP with those already in the client's IEPs or IHPs. Ratings by independent, blind observers rated the recommendations based on the AAPEP as superior to those on the current IEP (Van Bourgondien and Mesibov 1989b). The reliability and validity studies for the new edition, TTAP, are currently in progress. Also added to the TTAP is an informal community-based assessment to assist in the transition to adult life by evaluating the individual in a variety of vocational and living situations. The Individuals with Disabilities Education Act (IDEA) of 1997 and the reauthorization of IDEA in 2004 require that an evaluation be made and a transition plan be put into place by age 16 years at the latest.

The formal assessment aspect of the TTAP assesses six functional areas across three different contexts. The six areas assessed are vocational skills, vocational behaviors, independent functioning, leisure skills, functional communication, and interpersonal behaviors. The Direct Observation Scale provides a skill based observation and evaluation of the client by the examiner. The Home scale and the School/Work scale each complement the information gathered in the direct assessment with information from the caregiver and from either the teacher or a work supervisor. The information from these interview scales provide valuable information about a larger range of strengths and weaknesses, the generalization of skills across different contexts, and the individual's ability to flexibly use his/her skills.

The scoring system is the same as used in the PEP-3 with a pass, emerge, or fail. In addition to the scores in each functional area across the three contexts, the TTAP formal assessment section also includes a Structure Checklist that helps to identify the environmental accommodations the individual needs to be most successful. The TTAP directly assesses the individual's ability to benefit from the different types of schedules, work systems, and visual instructions described later in this chapter.

An added feature of the TTAP is its informal assessment components. Best practices indicate that effective transitions are facilitated by a combination of both formal and informal assessment tools (Mesibov et al. 2007). The Cumulative Record of Skills (CRS) and additional TTAP forms provide information on a greater variety of skill sets that can be assessed, taught, and re-evaluated within the job site. With its comprehensive list of skills, it goes beyond an assessment tool to become both a curriculum of skills needed in community environments and a potential record/resume of skills acquired during multiple community interventions.

The assessment process Formal assessment is an ideal place to start working with any child, student, or adult. This formal assessment provides us with a useful developmental perspective and helps identify the general teaching goals not only in the areas of greatest concern—communication and socialization—but also in all areas of cognitive, academic, and adaptive development. However, often the goals

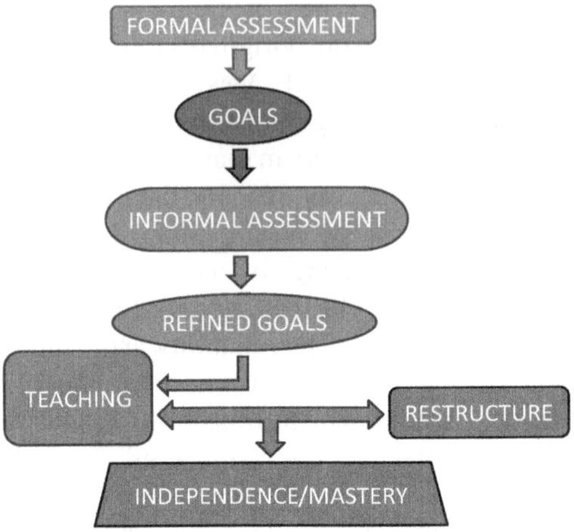

Fig. 5.1 The assessment and teaching process: from formal assessment to independence

from the standardized or formal assessment are very broad or vague, e.g. improve individual's reading comprehension skills. The next step in the process is to take the general goal and to assess that skill area more informally and more in-depth in the actual setting the teaching will occur. For example, for the reading comprehension goal, one might assess the individual's ability to comprehend nouns versus verbs versus adjectives. By looking more in-depth at the original goal and trying out different ways of increasing the student understanding, one develops more refined goals and teaching strategies that can translate into immediate teaching objectives in the classroom, home, or vocational setting.

The next step in this process is to implement the teaching activity and to observe the success of this effort. Every teaching opportunity is also a chance to reassess not just the individual's skill, but also the learning style and what teaching strategy works best. Restructuring our teaching activities is a fundamental aspect of the Structured Teaching philosophy. By carefully observing the child or adult's response to our teaching efforts, we learn what works best for him or her. Ultimately, through this dynamic process of teaching and restructuring, the individual achieves mastery of the concept and independence in performing the skill (see Fig. 5.1).

Structured Teaching

TEACCH's predominant intervention methodology is Structured Teaching, a set of teaching principles and intervention strategies based on our understanding of the culture of autism as well as the unique needs, skills, interests, and preferences of each individual with ASD (Mesibov et al. 2005). Given the neurological basis of the culture of autism, Structured Teaching emphasizes both teaching new skills as well as developing compensatory strategies and environmental supports, much as a cognitive remediation program seeks to improve and/or compensate for cognitive deficits arising from brain dysfunction (Ozonoff et al. 2005b). Structured Teaching emphasizes the use of visual and organizational supports and can be applied in flexible ways in a variety of settings for individuals of all ages and all abilities levels. Structured Teaching can be used to develop or improve skills in communication, social interaction, academic achievement, daily living and self-help, leisure, and vocation. It can also be used to help prevent behavior problems (Van Bourgondien et al. 2003) and adapt interventions focusing on mental health issues (DeRamus and Naftel 2008). Although Structured Teaching draws heavily from behavioral and cognitive behavioral principles, it is most closely aligned with cognitive–social learning theory in that it emphasizes the importance of recognizing the client's thoughts, expectations, and understanding when designing interventions to change behavior and teach new skills (Mesibov et al. 2005). The effectiveness of visual systems as an intervention technique has been documented in numerous studies with children and adults in a variety of settings (Bryan and Gast 2000; Dettmer et al. 2000; Francke and Geist 2003; Hume and Odom 2007; Mesibov 1997; Mesibov et al. 2002; Mesibov and Shea 2010; Mesibov et al. 2005; Panerai et al. 1998; Panerai et al. 2002; Panerai et al. 2009; Persson 2000; Probst et al. 2010; Probst and Leppert 2008; Quill 1997; Short 1984; Van Bourgondien et al. 2003; Vaughn and Horner 1995).

The primary goals of Structured Teaching are to (1) create an organized and predictable environment that enables individuals with ASD to move beyond fragmented details and begin to understanding meaningful connections in the world around them, and (2) teach skills that are functional and help promote personal independence at whatever level the individual is capable of (Mesibov et al. 2005). The basic elements of Structured Teaching include (1) organization of the environment and physical space, (2) visual schedules, (3) structured work and activity systems, and (4) visually structured activities. Each is discussed in the following section.

Physical Structure

Physical structure refers to the way the environment and physical space is organized to give it clearer context and meaning and to accommodate the specific needs of the individual with ASD. Physical structure can be applied in many environments, including homes, classrooms, leisure settings, and work sites. In designing physical structure, one adds clear visual and physical cues and boundaries to visually answer the question "What happens here?" as well as organizing the environment to minimize distractions and irrelevant information. Clear physical boundaries can be achieved by rearranging furniture to enclose larger spaces, adding visual cues such as wide strips of tape or carpet mats to clearly outline the area where the activity will be happening, or doing something as simple as closing a door. Visual and physical cues give further information about the function of the space, such as using pictures or signs to label the area, having the appropriate activity materials be out and visible, and removing all irrelevant information and materials from the activity area. Thoughtful physical structure can also reduce visual and auditory distractions in ways such as creating work spaces away from doors and windows, TVs, and areas where other students, family members, or coworkers congregate. Further, it is important to consider the traffic pattern of the overall layout to minimize the need for others to intrude unnecessarily in the area (e.g., not placing a work area near a bathroom frequently used by others) and minimize transitions for the individual (e.g., having all materials necessary for the work in the work area, having direct paths from one work area to another).

Visual Schedule

A visual schedule is a visual cue or set of cues that indicate to the individual with ASD what activities will occur and in what sequence. Visual schedules help keep the individuals organized and focused, and allow them to predict what they will be doing next and understand when certain activities will happen in the future, thus reducing stress and anxiety about the unknown. A visual schedule provides a concrete, visual way for understanding what is expected and what is happening, rather than the individual having to rely on verbal communications that are difficult to process, or having to rely on his or her own memory or desires for a specific routine. Teaching a client to use a visual schedule to guide his or her activities, rather than teaching him or her to always follow a specific routine, helps the client be more flexible about necessary changes in routine. Schedules also promote independence, because the individuals are guided through their daily routine by the schedule, as opposed to having to rely on another person to prompt them through every activity change (Krantz et al. 1993; MacDuff et al. 1993).

Visual schedules take many forms, but overall their purpose is to help the client understand "Where am I supposed to be now?" and "When will I get to _______?" Within the schedule, there are a variety of ways to individualize the schedule including the type of visual cue, the way it is organized, the length of the schedule, how the student manipulates or interacts with the schedule.

Visual cue The type of visual cue chosen for the schedule depends on the needs and abilities of each individual client. Because the purpose of the schedule is to provide meaning and structure to the day, and not to teach language or reading, it is important that the specific cue chosen be clear and meaningful. Possible visual cues, in order from most concrete to most abstract, include objects, photographs, drawings or icons, and written words. The client should be able to understand and use the schedule independently, so it is counterproductive to choose a visual cue that is too abstract. For young children and individuals with an intellectual disability, using objects that represent the upcoming activity is often the clearest and most meaningful visual cue. For older children, or individuals with a milder intellectual disability, using photographs or drawing/icons that the individual clearly understands to represent activities may be most appropriate. Once a child or individual is reading, often written words are a good choice for a schedule, because they are meaningful and easy for everyone in the environment to create.

Organization and length Typically, the visual cues are organized in either a left to right or top to bottom sequence, because those are the ways individuals are taught to read and scan for information in our Western culture. In other cultures, a right to left or bottom to top sequence may be more intuitive. The length of the schedule also depends on the needs and abilities of the individual. Young children or older individuals with significant intellectual disability may need to see only one or two objects or pictures at a time, helping them to understand a simple sequence of "First ______, then ______." Older children and individuals with mild intellectual disability may be best served by having the day's schedule broken down into parts, and seeing only a few hours or half a day's worth of activities at a time. For older and higher functioning individuals, having the entire day's schedule presented at once may be the most useful.

Although age of the individual and overall intellectual ability can provide a useful starting point for deciding on the specific visual cue and length of the schedule, each client's array of strengths and weaknesses need to be taken into account. Some individuals with significant intellectual impairment can learn to read and comprehend single words quite well, and thus a schedule with words may be most appropriate. Some individuals with intellectual impairment become anxious when they do not have enough information about their day, and thus a full-day schedule may be the most appropriate to use with them. Conversely, some very intelligent adults with ASD become easily overwhelmed and distracted by having too much information at once, and thus would do better with a half-day schedule.

Manipulation No matter the type of schedule used, individuals should actively manipulate the schedule, such as by carrying the object or picture to the next activity or crossing or checking off the activity when finished. Individuals with ASD are less likely to reference and be engaged with a schedule when they are not able to manipulate and interact with it in some way. It also is more difficult for them to track what activities they have completed and what activities are upcoming if they are not able to remove or cross off schedule cues after completion.

Finally, as the individual with ASD ages and develops, it is important to remember that the long term goal is not to fade or remove the schedule from his or her environment. The same way students and adults without disabilities need schedules and calendars to effectively organize their time and activities, the individual with ASD will benefit from using some sort of schedule support throughout his or her life. However, it is very appropriate to change the cue, length, content, and organization of the schedule to reflect developmental changes in the individual's needs and skills. Thus, a client who uses a first–then schedule as a young child may progress to a half-day picture schedule as a kindergartener, and then a full-day written schedule by the time he or she is in middle school. As the child ages, the goal is to make the schedule more portable and more blended with the natural environment. Although written lists and calendars work well for many clients, more options are becoming available through widely available technologies. For example, smartphones, tablet computers, and other PDA devices provide a relatively affordable, user-friendly, and age-appropriate platform in which to incorporate schedules and other forms of visual supports for older children, adolescents, and adults. Advantages of these devices include their portability, their flexibility (e.g., schedules can be presented using words, photographs, or pictures), and their popularity, which allows the individual to use them in a more discrete fashion than a paper schedule. Research is needed to investigate the utility of electronic schedules. The preliminary research, however, indicated that adolescents who used visual checklists on handheld computers to self-monitor behaviors and feelings were rated higher than the wait list controls by adult supervisors on dimensions of initiative and self-regulation (Levine et al. 2010).

Work and Activity Systems

Physical structure and visual schedules communicate to the individual with ASD the day's activities and where to go for each activity. Once the individual is in the specified area, the work system, sometimes called the activity system, provides information about what is to be done. The goal of the work system is to give the individual a systematic strategy to approach the work or activity that needs to be completed. This learned strategy helps the person understand what to do and stay focused, while also building independence and enabling the individual to generalize skills into other environments (Hume and Odom 2007). The systems are designed to answer visually the four questions: (1) What is the task or activity?, (2) How much work and/or how many activities are there, or how long will the activity last?, (3) How will I know that progress is being made and when I am finished with the work or activity, and (4) What happens next after the work or activity is finished?

Similar to visual schedules, work systems are individualized to the client's developmental level and strengths and weaknesses. Some individuals use a Left to Right work system, in which materials for work and activities are presented in an organized fashion on the left of where the individual is seated. Activities are taken and worked on one at a time, and then placed in a finished area as they are each completed. The four questions are answered by visually observing the work to be done and then the work gradually disappearing into the finished area or basket. The last item in the line of work activities is a cue which indicates what the individual will do next. For a higher functioning individual, the work system might be a written list of tasks. The list of tasks tells the individual what and how much work to do. As the individual completes each activity, he or she would cross it off the list, thus showing the progress being made. When all activities were crossed off, the individual would know that the work was finished and that it was time to do whatever was written next on the system.

The work system in many ways addresses the issues and strengths presented by the culture of autism—described earlier as the shared characteristics and predictable patterns of thinking and behavior of individuals with ASD. First, no matter the ability level of the individual, the work system is presented visually. The system clarifies what aspects of the environment the individual needs to be attending to, and provides an organizational structure to complete the activities that the individual may not be able to generate independently or internally. The system adds predictability and a clear end or finished point, which reduces anxiety and can give the individual with ASD a naturally motivating feeling of satisfaction and closure at completion. Similar to schedules, the work system helps develop a multitude of skills. Once the work system is learned, it can be transferred to a variety of settings and contain a variety of tasks, including academic work, self care and daily living activities, and vocational activities. Ultimately, the individual can have a variety of work systems located throughout their classroom, home or job setting. The system also provides an ideal way to organize leisure activities. While leisure time can be rewarding and relaxing to individuals with typical development, open-ended, unstructured time is often confusing and anxiety-provoking for individuals with ASD. Using the work system to structure leisure activities has been shown to increase independence on task behavior and the variety of play materials utilized in play situations (Hume and Odom 2007). Also like the schedule, the work system should not be faded over time. Rather, as the individual develops, the work system—and the activities within it—should change to reflect the individual's current developmental level and needs.

Visually Structured Activities

Finally, it is important to consider the visual structure of the activities within the work system. Even with an appropriate schedule and work system, a person with an ASD will struggle with the tasks if they are not appropriately visually structured.

Visual instructions First, providing visual instructions will enable the individual to know where to begin the task and what sequence of steps to follow. Visual instructions enable the individual to know exactly what to do, but also allow for the flexibility of changing the instructions when a new approach may be necessary. Again, the type of visual instructions depends on the individual client. Younger or more intellectually impaired individuals may do best with instructions in the form of matching jigs, product samples, or photo or picture series. For older or less cognitively impaired individuals, written directions may be appropriate.

Visual organization The organization of the work materials, by limiting, organizing, and stabilizing them, helps the individual maintain attention and focus on the task at hand, rather than becoming distracted by too many or poorly contained materials or approaching the task in a disorderly or inefficient fashion. Using separate containers for materials, whether they are folders for school work or baskets of materials to sort, is often helpful. Although individuals with ASD are typically quite poor at generating organizational strategies themselves, some can be taught to organize materials for themselves with practice, such as the student who learns to file every homework handout in the appropriate folder to complete later.

Visual clarity Techniques to provide visual clarity and draw attention to the most important pieces of information in a task include color coding, highlighting, or labeling. Reducing or reorganizing written academic information so that there is more space on each page is a simple but effective way to add visual clarity.

Beginning Steps of Structured Teaching

The beginning step of the Structured Teaching process is to use the information about an individual's unique strengths, interests, needs and learning style to design interventions that address the most pressing needs of the individual and the family. Goals for the home are individualized based on the person's immediate needs and parental or family priorities. Typically, increasing the person's social engagement, communication skills, and self care skills are priorities along with decreasing behavior problems. Individualized goals for a classroom setting should reflect a thorough curriculum to address both the deficits of autism as well as the skills needed for success of an adult. The goal in teaching all skills is to make the activity meaningful at the appropriate developmental level, use teaching strategies that recognize the person's ability to utilize symbols, and individualize the approach utilizing the person's strengths and interests.

Communication Problems with communication is one of the defining features of autism. The communication problems of individuals with ASD affect both their expressive communication as well as their receptive ability to understand others' communication to them (Lord 1985; Lord and Paul 1997). Difficulties in communication interfere with the ability to express basic needs and wants, to engage in social–communication interactions such as conversations, and can be a major reason behind the behavioral difficulties seen in individuals with ASD. Confusion over what is happening, others' expectations, or frustrations over not being able to convey needs and wishes are often linked to the occurrence of behavioral problems.

The TEACCH approach to developing communication skills emphasizes the development of both receptive and expressive communication skills. The previously described visual systems of Structured Teaching provide both a receptive communication system, a way for others to communicate expectations to the person with ASD, as well as meaningful, preverbal foundations and context within which to build expressive communication skills. Having an orderly, predictable world enables the person to develop the understanding, routines and expectations that are necessary to the communication process (Mesibov et al. 2005).

Spontaneous expressive communication skills are taught utilizing an individualized approach based on the information from the assessment process. Segmenting and teaching each new communication concept individually—then building on these components—avoids introducing too many new concepts at a time. Watson et al. (1989) identify five basic elements of communication. First, the word or phrase used (if not verbal than the meaning of the communication); the form (e.g. gesture, object, photo, drawing, written, spoken); the function (getting attention, requesting, rejecting, commenting, giving information, seeking information, social routines emotional expression); the context (with whom, in what setting); and the semantic category (such as object wanted; action being done; location of a person). The ultimate goal is for the person with ASD to be able to flexibly and spontaneously communicate a variety of types of information across many contexts. A common component of the teaching approach for all levels of communications is to use visual cues at the appropriate level of abstraction to provide the individual with concrete information about what, how, and to whom to communicate. Research has shown that utilizing visual systems to teach communication enhances both nonverbal and verbal communication skills (Frost and Bondy 1994; Konstantareas 1996; Magiati and Howlin 2003; Yoder and Layton 1988). For more details about the TEACCH Communication Curriculum, see Mesibov et al. 2005 and Watson et al. 1989.

For beginning learners, this use of visuals may involve an exchange of an object, picture, or word that helps make the communication process more obvious and meaningful. Exchange communication systems have been listed among the empirically validated interventions cited by the NPDC on ASD (Frost and Bondy 1994) (http://autismpdc.fpg.unc.edu/). For more verbal individuals, the focus is on standard speech and language therapy goals, e.g. expanding vocabulary, length of sentences, use of verbs, nouns, plurals. Some areas frequently targeted for more able individuals with ASD include the conversational skills of choosing topics, taking turns and staying on topic (Mesibov et al. 2005). Again, even for more able individuals, visual support or written directions that make abstract concepts more concrete can be very helpful (Faherty 2000, 2010).

Social skills and engagement Socialization difficulties are perhaps the most pervasive of all the characteristics of people with ASD (Reichow and Volkmar 2010), and the feature that most differentiates children with autism from those with other developmental disorders (Klin et al. 2007). The TEACCH priority in the area of engagement and social skill development is to make play and socializing enjoyable (Mesibov et al. 2005). Neurotypical people without autism ultimately pursue social and recreational activities with others because we find these experiences enjoyable. For people on the autism spectrum, creating and practicing individually meaningful experiences in social contexts also serves as the foundation for the development of social skills.

The starting point regardless of the age or level of severity is to build interactions based on the individual's interests. For example, engagement in individual play activities in a 2 year old with autism may be facilitated by the use of her interest in "Dora the Explorer" while the adults in a support group may initiate getting together outside the group based on their interests in classic cars. Eckenrode et al. (2009) provide lots of vivid examples of how the TEACCH approach builds social engagement and joint attention utilizing the child's interests, predictable routines, our own reactions and visual cues.

There are numerous studies that have demonstrated the effectiveness of a variety of interventions in increasing the social behavior in individuals with autism (Reichow and Volkmar 2010). Structured social groups have been a longstanding intervention strategy employed at TEACCH (Mesibov 1984, 1986). These social groups vary in size based on the age and ability level of the participants. For 2 or 3 year olds, a three-person group may be considered while a high school group for teens in regular education settings may have 10 to 15 peers. Typically developing peer group members, as well as actively participating staff or teachers, can provide enthusiasm, persistence, and appropriate social skill models. Using visual aids within these groups helps the participants with ASD feel comfortable knowing what to expect and enhances each person's ability to participate.

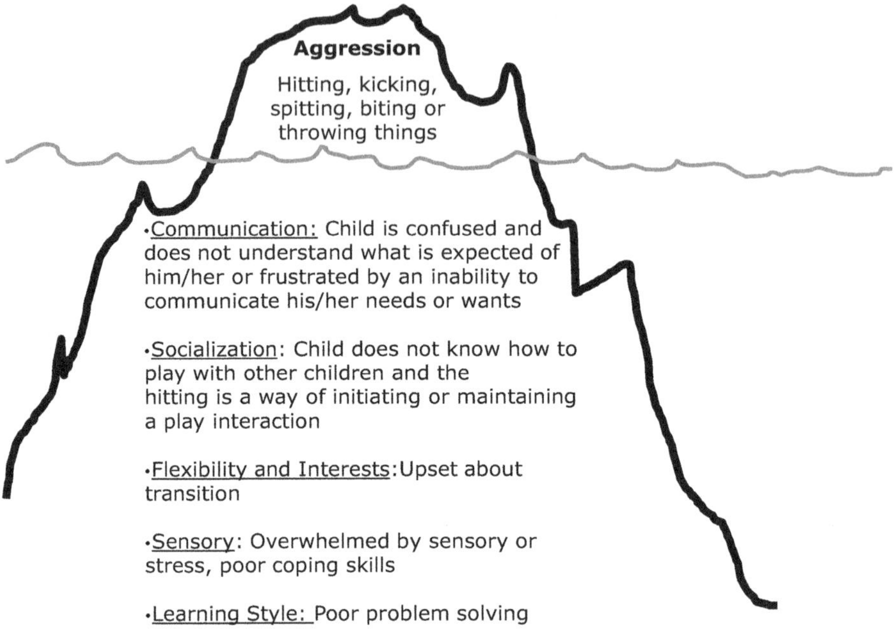

Fig. 5.2 Iceberg analogy for understanding the behavior problems of autism: Aggression and the underlying deficits of autism

Challenging behavior In addition to concerns about lack of communication or poor social skills, parents' initial concerns often center around a variety of behavioral problems. For parents of preschool children, these concerns may include aggression, lack of response to discipline, eating problems, sleeping problems, toileting problems, lack of initiative, poor play skills, or temper tantrums (Van Bourgondien 1993). As children approach adolescence, concerns may include issues related to the onset of puberty and sexuality (Gabriels and Van Bourgondien 2007). These behavioral deficits or excesses have been conceptualized as being the result of underlying deficits related to autism (Schopler 1989, 1995; Van Bourgondien 1993). The concept of an iceberg has been used at TEACCH to illustrate that the observable behavior is above the surface of the water, but the cause or function of the behavior is related to a core deficit of autism which is below the surface of the water. Figure 5.2 illustrates this concept with aggressive behavior. Above the surface one may observe hitting, kicking, spitting, biting, or throwing things, but below the surface underlying these behaviors could be difficulty with communication either because the child is confused and does not understand what is expected of him/her or frustrated by an inability to communicate his/her needs or wants. Another hypothesis is that the child does not know how to play with other children and that the hitting is a way of initiating or maintaining a play interaction. Through the assessment and data collection process, the most likely explanations can be identified and used to develop an appropriate intervention strategy. The intervention may involve teaching the child a new skill to initiate a play activity appropriately, or it may involve restructuring the situation to decrease confusion or unneeded sensory input. An individualized schedule may be utilized to show the child what will come next and when he/she will get time to do a desired activity again. Some children need to be taught coping strategies so they have a way of calming themselves when things do not go as planned, e.g. learning to take slow breaths, using a counting system with pictures of a special interest. Once the individual has an effective stress reduction activity, this activity can be built into the schedule preventatively to keep stress from building throughout the day.

Schopler (1995) collaborated with TEACCH staff members and parents to compile a list of the most common parental concerns and strategies for addressing these concerns utilizing the Iceberg model. In a review of the literature Machalicek et al. (2007) found that preventative approaches, such as those used by TEACCH, that are based on antecedent manipulations and changes in instructional contexts are effective methods for reducing challenging behavior. In a study of adults in residential programs, Van Bourgondien et al. (2003) found that use of Structured Teaching over time was associated with a decrease in behavior difficulties.

Teaching other skills TEACCH intervention strategies go beyond the communication, social and behavioral concerns to also address the teaching of a wide variety of skills. Learning fine motor and writing skills, basic concepts, language art skills, math and other academic skills can be taught utilizing the Structured Teaching approach (Boswell et al. 2005; Eckenrode et al. 2003). Self care skills, domestic, life skills and vocational skills are important not just for success at home, but also for success in the community and on the job (Eckenrode et al. 2004; Van Bourgondien and Chapman 2005). Many skills need to be taught in a one-to-one teaching context by the teacher, parent, caretaker, or job coach. More able individuals can also be taught skills in small group settings. As always, an individualized approach to teaching each skill utilizing the individual's visual strengths and interests (Boyd et al. 2007) will be the most effective.

Long Term Goals of Intervention Strategies

Ultimately, the long term goal of the Structured Teaching approach is to help the individual with an ASD enjoy a meaningful life in the greater community. To maximize the individual's quality of life and their ability to function as independently as possible, one needs to go beyond teaching just the basic skills. Five of the most important concepts for long term success are independence, flexibility, self-advocacy, generalization, and well-being.

Independence Difficulty with being able to use one's skills independently is one of the greatest challenges faced by individuals with ASD (Hume et al. 2009). If individuals need to rely on the presence of adult to remain engaged, then they are not truly independent, and their ultimate outcome as an adult is negatively affected by this lack of independence (Hume et al. 2009). Therefore, the goal is to teach each person with ASD to understand what is expected and to meet these expectations as independently as possible to promote both a sense of individual well being as well as to help them succeed in the adult world (Mesibov et al. 2005). Work systems (Hume and Odom 2007) and visual schedules (Anderson et al. 1997; Krantz et al. 1993; Pierce and Schreibman 1994) increase independence in performing tasks. As time goes on, the goal is to continually increase the amount of time and the number of sequential tasks that the student can perform independently thus increasing his or her potential as a future employee, as well as their overall self-efficacy.

Flexibility Rigidity, repetitive behaviors and difficulty breaking routines are defining features of ASD that interfere with the individual's ability to be more flexible. As we prepare the person for success in adult life, our goal is to use the visual systems to help the person cope better with change and to be more flexible in how they do a given task. For example, each time one goes to the grocery store, we do not buy exactly the same thing or when working in a bookstore or a library, the books we shelve will vary day to day. So when teaching students or adults, we need to make sure to use the visual systems to teach the concepts of change, surprise and flexibility. The order and occurrence of specific events on the schedule and work systems will change each day to mirror the changes in life's activities. The visual instructions in tasks will change to reflect that the menu changes each day or the number of servings of coffee will change, etc.

Generalization Problems with generalization have been a long recognized problem in children and adults on the spectrum (Fein et al. 1979; Hume et al. 2009; Mesibov et al. 2005). Individuals with autism have trouble generalizing what they learn from one setting to another, to new people and to a new set of materials. A child who learns to sort and identify colored blocks may not recognize that a red ball is also red. A boy who learns to go to the toilet independently at home may not automatically generalize this skill to a bathroom at school. We need to systematically teach individuals with ASD how to use their skills in new contexts, with a variety of people, and with differing materials. Again, the use of visual cues such as work systems and visual instructions help the individual not only be less dependent on an adult prompt, but also recognize how and when to use learned skills in new settings with new materials (Hume et al. 2009; Mesibov et al. 2005). Our ultimate goal is for the person with ASD to be able to utilize his/her skills to be able to work, live and recreate in the community.

Self-advocacy With diagnostically defined deficits in social–communication, it is not surprising that individuals at all levels of severity have difficulty communicating with others about their needs and preferences. Even if someone has been taught a communication strategy in one setting, they need to be taught strategies and given visual systems that enable them to use these skills with new people, in new places. For the more concrete learners with autism, we work toward having portable communication systems that allow them to express a variety of communicative functions in different settings including letting someone know when they are hurt or do not like something. For more able individuals with high functioning autism or Asperger

Syndrome, self advocacy also means learning to recognize their own learning style and being able to advocate for the supports they need at school, on the job, or at college (Faherty 2000, 2010; Palmer 2006; Shore 2004).

Well-being All intervention programs share the ultimate goal of providing a high quality of life for a person with ASD. While skill enhancement enriches the life of a person with autism, quality of life is also influenced by the same factors that affect neurotypical individuals—being healthy, experiencing less stress, and being able to pursue activities or topics of interest.

Structured Teaching principles are also used to address these aspects of life. Helping the individual make healthy food choices can be promoted by the use of visuals. Including exercise on the schedule along with counting systems to help define when an exercise activity is complete promotes a healthier lifestyle. Stress reduction activities can be taught using visual systems. In addition, an individual's circumscribed interests can be used within an activity (Boyd et al. 2007) or after an activity to promote motivation and learning (Mesibov and Shea 2010).

Compatibility with Other Evidence-Based Methods

The overall Structured Teaching approach includes assessment of each person's unique learning style, utilizing the strengths of the individual to teach new skills while structuring the environment to increase independence and decrease behavioral problem. Parent collaboration is an integral part of all aspects of this process. Within this context, there are many other empirically based intervention techniques (NPDC on ASD; http://autismpdc.fpg.unc.edu/) that can be integrated in this framework. Some recent clinical examples include joint attention interventions (Kasari et al. 2008), Social Stories™ (Gray 2000), cognitive behavioral interventions (Lyubomirsky 2008; Turner-Brown et al. 2008), relaxation techniques (Cautela and Groden 1978), and video modeling (Bellini and Akullian 2007).

Research Support

Fidelity Measures

To determine whether a classroom, residential program, or vocational setting is representative of the TEACCH approach, one must look at all aspects of the setting. The two empirically validated measures of fidelity are the TEACCH Fidelity Form for classrooms (Hume et al. 2011) and the Environmental Rating Scale (ERS; Van Bourgondien and Mesibov 1989; Van Bourgondien et al. 1998). Hume et al. (2011) demonstrated that the TEACCH classroom fidelity measure has interrater agreement of 95.3 %, test–retest reliability utilizing interclass correlations of .805 for the total score and internal consistency of .932. As a measure of validity, they found that the measure significantly discriminated between TEACCH preschool classrooms, LEAP preschool programs (Hoyson et al. 1984), and preschool classrooms using a nonspecific eclectic approach. Van Bourgondien et al. (1998) found that the ERS had good reliability with an internal consistency alpha coefficient of .96, test–retest reliability with a mean kappa of .55, and an intraclass correlation of .81 for the total score. As a measure of validity, the ERS significantly differentiated residential programs designed for individuals with autism utilizing the TEACCH principles from generic developmental disability group homes as well as individual family homes.

Both measures evaluate the degree to which the setting has the following characteristics:

1. Structured approach to learning that is individualized in the use of physical structure, schedules, work systems and visual systems.
2. Assessment, teaching goals, and strategies that show recognition and individualization based on an appreciation of the culture of autism and the individual's strengths, needs and developmental level. Focus on independence and generalization of skills.
3. Supports to enhance receptive language, appropriate functional expressive communication goals, actively teaching and stimulation of communication throughout the day.
4. Individualized social leisure goals and interventions to increase leisure activities and social interactions.
5. Behavior management strategies that emphasize an understanding of autism, and a proactive approach and data collection.
6. Family collaboration.

Empirical Evidence

As described above, each of the major components of the TEACCH approach—culture of autism, parent collaboration and training, assessment, use of structure, visual supports and individual interests, communication, and social skills training have been supported through more focused studies. The direct support for the overall TEACCH program which is reviewed by Mesibov and Shea (2010) and Odom et al. (2010) is summarized below.

Historically, research conducted within the TEACCH program using quasi experimental designs demonstrated that structure increased relatedness, appropriate affect, meaningful engagement in activities, while reducing repetitive self stimulating behaviors, in individuals with ASD (Schopler et al. 1971), and parent training increased mothers' teaching skills and children's cooperation and engagement in tasks (Marcus et al. 1978). Parents who participated in the TEACCH Program reported high overall satisfaction with the program and markedly improved child behaviors (Schopler et al. 1982). Short (1984) described significant improvement in child communication and engagement with materials and parent involvement with and guidance of their children's behavior. Bristol et al. (1993) found that mothers of 2 to 6 year olds who received TEACCH intervention in the form of clinic based parent training in Structured Teaching reported a significant decrease in depressive symptoms compared to those in the no treatment comparison group whose symptoms did not decrease.

More recently, Van Bourgondien et al. (2003) in a part random, part clinical assignment admission procedure compared adults who participated in a TEACCH based residential and vocational program to comparison groups of adults who were either receiving other community services or lived at home with their parents. While there was no significant difference in skill acquisition between the groups, individuals who were receiving TEACCH based interventions showed a decrease in negative behaviors over time and parents were significantly more satisfied with their adult child's lifestyle, living and work environments.

Welterlin (2009) evaluated the TEACCH 12 session in home early intervention program using a random assignment to treatment or waitlist control condition. Preliminary results showed significant increases in fine motor skills, decreased maladaptive behavior, and increased independence for children in the treatment condition as compared to children not yet receiving intervention.

Researchers outside of the TEACCH Program (Ozonoff and Cathcart 1998) compared pre and post treatment developmental skills of a group of preschoolers receiving the TEACCH home based parent teaching program with a matched comparison group of children who received other community interventions. Results indicated that children receiving the TEACCH home based program showed significantly greater improvements in overall development, imitation, fine motor, gross motor, and cognitive performance skills than did children in the comparison group. Panerai et al. (2002) demonstrated that children and adults with autism and severe intellectual disabilities in TEACCH based interventions in an Italian residential program made significantly more progress in a year in developing skills than a matched comparison group who lived at home and attended regular Italian public school classrooms with a support teacher. In a later study, Panerai et al. (2009) compared a sample of children with autism and severe disabilities who were participating in a TEACCH based residential program to children living at home who were attending the regular Italian public special education classroom option and to children living at home who were attending regular Italian mainstream classes whose parents also received training in the TEACCH method. Results indicated no significant differences in children receiving the two TEACCH approaches, but children in both TEACCH conditions showed significant improvement over three years compared to the non-TEACCH comparison group in imitation, gross motor, cognitive performance, daily living skills, socialization skills, and maladaptive behaviors. All three of these studies have the limitation on using consecutive admissions and not random assignment.

Tsang et al. (2007) conducted a longitudinal study in China with 34 children with autism. In a full-time center based TEACCH program 18 children were enrolled, while 16 children in the comparison group received different types of individualized or group training, but not training based on the TEACCH method. After six months, the TEACCH group demonstrated significantly greater improvements in perception, fine motor, and gross motor skills. The comparison group children, who also had significantly greater IQ scores at baseline, showed significantly greater improvement in their daily living skills.

Each of the components of the TEACCH program have strong empirical support (Hume and Odom 2007; Mesibov and Shea 2010), more research that evaluates TEACCH as a comprehensive program is needed and is currently underway (Odom et al. 2010).

Summary

The TEACCH model and general principles continues to be a valued intervention approach because both are based on an understanding of the culture of autism, and because the Structured Teaching techniques continue to evolve based on the changing world of autism and current research findings. The guiding principles include respect for the learning style of individuals with autism and utilizing assessment information to create a strength-based and individualized intervention to promote independence in the community (Marcus and Corsello 1997). Because we work with children and adults of all ages and ability levels, the collaboration that started out with parents and their children has expanded to include teachers, employers, residential providers, spouses, siblings and the adult with ASD. These multiple perspectives help us to continually refine and expand the ways in which we support individuals with ASD in our community and throughout the world.

References

Alpern, G. D. (1967). Measurement of "untestable" autistic children. *Journal of Abnormal Psychology, 72*(6), 478–486.

Ambery, F. Z., Russell, A. J., Perry, K., Morris, R., & Murphy, D. G. M. (2006). Neuropsychological functioning in adults with Asperger syndrome. *Autism, 10*(6), 551–564.

Anderson, M. D., Sherman, J. A., Sheldon, J. B., & McAdam, D. (1997). Picture activity schedules and engagement of adults with mental retardation in a group home. *Research in Developmental Disabilities, 18*(4), 231–250.

Baranek, G. T., Parham, L. D., & Bodfish, J. W. (2005). Sensory and motor features in autism: assessment and intervention. In F. R. Volkmar, R. Paul, A. Klin & D. Cohen (Eds.), *Handbook of autism and pervasive developmental disorders, Vol. 2: assessment, interventions, and policy* (3rd ed.). (pp. 831–857). New Jersey: Wiley.

Bellini, S., & Akullian, J. (2007). A meta-analysis of video modeling and video self-monitoring interventions for children and adolescents with autism spectrum disorders. *Exceptional Children, 73*, 264–287.

Boswell, S., Reynolds, B., Faukner, R., & Benson, M. (2005). *Let's get started.* North Carolina: Lulu.

Boyd, B. A., Conroy, M. A., Mancil, G. R., Nakao, T., & Alter, P. J. (2007). Effects of circumscribed interests on the social behaviors of children with autism spectrum disorders. *Journal of Autism and Developmental Disorders, 37*(8), 1550–1561.

Boyd, B. A., McBee, M., Holtzclaw, T., Baranek, G. T., & Bodfish, J. W. (2009). Relationships among repetitive behaviors, sensory features, and executive functions in high functioning autism. *Research in Autism Spectrum Disorders, 3*(4), 959–966.

Bramham, J., Ambery, F., Young, S., Morris, R., Russell, A., Xenitidis, K., et al. (2009). Executive functioning differences between adults with attention deficit hyperactivity disorder and autistic spectrum disorder in initiation, planning and strategy formation. *Autism, 13*(3), 245–264.

Bristol, M. M., Gallagher, J. J., & Holt, K. D. (1993). Maternal depressive symptoms in autism: response to psychoeducational intervention. *Rehabilitation Psychology, 38*(1), 3–10.

Bryan, L. C., & Gast, D. L. (2000). Teaching on-task and on-schedule behaviors to high-functioning children with autism via picture activity schedules. *Journal of Autism and Developmental Disorders, 30*(6), 553–567.

Cautela, J. R., & Groden, J. (1978). *Relaxation: a comprehensive manual for adults, children, and children with special needs*. Champaign: Research Press Co.

Dawson, G., & Osterling, J. (1997). Early intervention in autism. In M. J. Guralnick (Ed.), *The effectiveness of early intervention* (pp. 307–326). Baltimore: Brookes.

DeRamus, M., & Naftel, S. (2008). *Counseling adolescents and adults with high-functioning autism*. Paper presented at the TEACCH Winter Inservice Conference.

Dettmer, S., Simpson, R. L., Myles, B. S., & Ganz, J. B. (2000). The use of visual supports to facilitate transitions of students with autism. *Focus on Autism and Other Developmental Disabilities, 15*(3), 163–169.

Duncan, J. (1986). Disorganization of behavior after frontal lobe damage. *Cognitive Neuropsychology, 3*, 271–290.

Eckenrode, L., Fennell, P., & Hearsey, K. (2003). *Tasks galore*. North Carolina: Tasks Galore.

Eckenrode, L., Fennell, P., & Hearsey, K. (2004). *Tasks galore for the real world*. North Carolina: Tasks Galore.

Eckenrode, L., Fennell, P., Hearsey, K., & Reynolds, B. (2009). *Tasks galore: let's play: structured steps to social engagement and symbolic play*. North Carolina: Tasks Galore.

Faherty, C. (2000). *What does it mean to me?* Texas: Future Horizons, Inc.

Faherty, C. (2010). *Communication: what does it mean to me?* Texas: Future Horizons.

Fein, D., Tinder, P., & Waterhouse, L. (1979). Stimulus generalization in autistic and normal children. *Journal of Child Psychology and Psychiatry, 20*(4), 325–335.

Filipek, P. A., Accardo, P. J., Ashwal, S., Baranek, G. T., Cook Jr., E. H., Dawson, G., et al. (2000). Practice parameter: screening and diagnosis of autism: report of the Quality Standards Subcommittee of the American Academy of Neurology and the Child Neurology Society. *Neurology, 55*(4), 468–479.

Francke, J., & Geist, E. A. (2003). The effects of teaching play strategies on social interaction for a child with autism: a case study. *Journal of Research in Childhood Education, 18*(2), 125–140.

Frith, U. (1989). *Autism: explaining the enigma*. Oxford: Blackwell.

Frost, L. A., & Bondy, A. S. (1994). *PECS: the picture exchange communication system training manual*. New Jersey: Pyramid Educational Consultants.

Gabriels, R. L., & Van Bourgondien, M. E. (2007). Sexuality and autism. In R. L. G. D. E. Hill (Ed.), *Growing up with autism* (pp. 58–72). New York: Guilford Press.

Gabriels, R. L., Agnew, J. A., Miller, L. J., Gralla, J., Pan, Z., Goldson, E., et al. (2008). Is there a relationship between restricted, repetitive, stereotyped behaviors and interests and abnormal sensory response in children with autism spectrum disorders? *Research in Autism Spectrum Disorders, 2*(4), 660–670.

Glascoe, F. P., & Sandler, H. (1995). Value of parents' estimates of children's developmental ages. *Journal of Pediatrics, 127*, 831–835.

Grandin, T. (1996). *Thinking in pictures*. New York: Vintage Books.

Gray, C. (2000). *The new social story book*. Texas: Future Horizons.

Happé, F. (2005). The weak central coherence account of autism. In F. R. Volkmar, R. Paul, A. Klin & D. Cohen (Eds.), *Handbook of autism and pervasive developmental disorders, Vol. 1: diagnosis, development, neurobiology, and behavior* (3rd ed., pp. 640–649). New Jersey: Wiley.

Hoyson, M., Jamieson, B., & Strain, P. S. (1984). Individualized group instruction of normally developing and autistic-like children: The LEAP curriculuam model. *Journal of the Division for Early Childhood, 8,* 157–172.

Hume, K., & Odom, S. (2007). Effects of an individual work system on the independent functioning of students with autism. *Journal of Autism and Developmental Disorders, 37*(6), 1166–1180.

Hume, K., Loftin, R., & Lantz, J. (2009). Increasing independence in autism spectrum disorders: a review of three focused interventions. *Journal of Autism and Developmental Disorders, 39*(9), 1329–1338.

Hume, K., Boyd, B., McBee, M., Coman, D., Gutierrez, A., Shaw, E., Sperry, L., Allessandri, M., & Odom, S. (2011). Assessing implementation of comprehensive treatment models for young children with ASD: reliability and validity of two measures. *Research in Autism Spectrum Disorders, 5,* 1430–1440.

Kasari, C., Paparella, T., Freeman, S., & Jahromi, L. B. (2008). Language outcome in autism: randomized comparison of joint attention and play interventions. *Journal of Consulting and Clinical Psychology, 76*(1), 125–137.

Klin, A., Saulnier, C.A., Sparrow, S.S., Cicchetti, D.V., Volkmar, F. R., & Lord, C. (2007). Social and communication abilities and disabilities in higher functioning individuals with autism spectrum disorders. The Vineland and the ADOS. *Journal of Autism and Developmental Disorders, 37,* 748–759.

Koegel, R. L., Bimbela, A., & Schreibman, L. (1996). Collateral effects of parent training on family interactions. *Journal of Autism and Developmental Disorders, 26*(3), 347–359.

Konstantareas, M. M. (1996). Communication training approaches in autistic disorder. In J. H. Beitchman, N. J. Cohen, M. M. Konstantareas & R. Tannock (Eds.), *Language, learning, and behavior disorders: developmental, biological, and clinical perspectives* (pp. 467–488). New York: Cambridge University Press.

Krantz, P. J., MacDuff, M. T., & McClannahan, L. E. (1993). Programming participation in family activities for children with autism: parents' use of photographic activity schedules. *Journal of Applied Behavior Analysis, 26*(1), 137–138.

LeCouteur, A., Lord, C., & Rutter, M. (2003). *The Autism Diagnostic Interview (ADI-R).* Los Angeles: Western Psychological Services.

Levine, M., Hearsey, K., Mesibov, G., Calvanio, R. (2010). Self-monitoring with handheld computers by teens with high functioning autism/Asperger's syndrome in mainstream settings. Poster presented at the International Meeting for Autism Research.

Lopez, B. R., Lincoln, A. J., Ozonoff, S., & Lai, Z. (2005). Examining the relationship between executive functions and restricted, repetitive symptoms of autistic disorder. *Journal of Autism and Developmental Disorders, 35*(4), 445–460.

Lord, C. (1985). Autism and the comprehension of language. In E. Schopler & G. B. Mesibov (Eds.), *Communication Problems in Autism* (Vol. 257–281). New York: Plenum.

Lord, C., & Corsello, C. (2005). Diagnostic instruments in autistic spectrum disorders. In F. R. Volkmar, R. Paul, A. Klin & D. Cohen (Eds.), *Handbook of autism and pervasive developmental disorders, Vol. 2: assessment, interventions, and policy* (3rd ed., pp. 730–771). New Jersey: Wiley.

Lord, C., & Paul, R. (1997). Language and communication in autism. In J. Cohen & F. R. Volkmar (Eds.), *Handbook of autism and pervasive developmental disorders* (2nd ed.). New York: Wiley.

Lord, C., Rutter, M., DiLavore, P. C., Risi, S., Gotham, K., & Bishop, S. L. (2012). *Autism Diagnostic Observation Schedule (ADOS): Manual* (2nd ed.). Los Angeles Western Psychological Services.

Lyubomirsky, S. (2008). *The how of happiness: a scientific approach to getting the life you want.* New York: Penguin Press.

MacDuff, G.S., Krantz, P.J., & McClannahan, L. E. (1993). Teaching children with autism to use photographic activity schedules: maintenance and generalizations of complex response chains. *Journal of Applied Behavior Analysis, 26,* 89–97.

Machalicek, W., O'Reilly, M. F., Beretvas, N., Sigafoos, J., & Lancioni, G. E. (2007). A review of interventions to reduce challenging behavior in school settings for students with autism spectrum disorders. *Research in Autism Spectrum Disorders, 1*(3), 229–246.

Magiati, I., & Howlin, P. (2003). A pilot evaluation study of the Picture Exchange Communication System (PECS) for children with autistic spectrum disorders. *Autism, 7*(3), 297–320.

Magyar, C.I., & Pandolfi, V. (2007). Factor structure evaluation of the childhood autism rating scale. *Journal of Autism and Developmental Disorders, 37*, 1787–1794.

Marcus, L. M., & Baker, A. (1986). Assessment of autistic children. In R. J. Simeonsson (Ed.), *Psychological assessment of special children* (pp. 279–304). Boston: Allyn & Bacon.

Marcus, L. M., & Corsello, C. (1997). Clinical principals and practices. Unpublished manuscript. Division TEACCH; UNC Chapel Hill.

Marcus, L. M., Kunce, L. J., & Schopler, E. (2005). Working with families. In F. R. Volkmar, R. Paul, A. Klin, & D. Cohen (Eds.), *Handbook of autism and pervasive developmental disorders, vol. 2: assessment, interventions, and policy* (3rd ed., pp. 1055–1086). New Jersey: Wiley.

Marcus, L. M., Lansing, M., Andrews, C. E., & Schopler, E. (1978). Improvement of teaching effectiveness in parents of autistic children. *Journal of the American Academy of Child Psychiatry, 17*(4), 625–639.

Mesibov, G. B. (1984). Social skills training with verbal autistic adolescents and adults: a program model. *Journal of Autism and Developmental Disorders, 14*(4), 395–404.

Mesibov, G. B. (1986). A cognitive program for teaching social behaviors to verbal autistic adolescents and adults. In E. Schopler & G. B. Mesibov (Eds.), *Social behavior in autism* (pp. 265–283). New York: Plenum.

Mesibov, G. B. (1997). Formal and informal measures on the effectiveness of the TEACCH programme. *Autism, 1*(1), 25–35.

Mesibov, G. B., Browder, D. M., & Kirkland, C. (2002). Using individualized schedules as a component of positive behavioral support for students with developmental disabilities. *Journal of Positive Behavior Interventions, 4*(2), 73–79.

Mesibov, G. B., Schopler, E., Schaffer, B., & Landrus, R. (1988). *Adolescent and adult psychoeducational profile (AAPEP)*. Texas: Pro-Ed.

Mesibov, G. B., & Shea, V. (2010). The TEACCH program in the era of evidence-based practice. *Journal of Autism and Developmental Disorders, 40*(5), 570–579.

Mesibov, G. B., Shea, V. (2011). Evidence-based practices and autism. *Autism, 15*(1), 114–133.

Mesibov, G. B., Shea, V., & Schopler, E. (2005). *The TEACCH approach to autism spectrum disorders*. New York: Springer.

Mesibov, G. B., Thomas, J. B., Chapman, S. M., & Schopler, E. (2007). *TEACCH Transition Assessment Profile (TTAP) Second Edition: Manual*. Texas: Pro-Ed.

Midence, K., & O'Neill, M. (1999). The experience of parents in the diagnosis of autism: a pilot study. *Autism, 3*(3), 273–285.

Moes, D. R. (1995). Parent education and parent stress. In R. L. Koegel & K. L. Koegel (Eds.), *Teaching children with autism: strategies for initiating positive interactions and improving learning opportunities* (pp. 79–93). Baltimore: Brookes.

Morrell, M. F., & Palmer, A. (2006). *Parenting across the autism spectrum: unexpected lessons we have learned*. Philadelphia: Kingsley.

Odom, S. L., Boyd, B. A., Hall, L. J., Hume, K. (2010) Evaluation of comprehensive treatment models for individuals with autism spectrum disorders. *Journal of Autism and Developmental Disorders, 40*, 425–436.

Ozonoff, S., & Cathcart, K. (1998). Effectiveness of a home program intervention for young children with autism. *Journal of Autism and Developmental Disorders, 28*, 25–32.

Ozonoff, S., & Griffith, E. M. (2000). Neuropsychological function and the external validity of Asperger Syndrome. In A. Klin, F. Volkmar & S. Sparrow (Eds.), *Asperger Syndrome* (pp. 72–96). New York: Guilford.

Ozonoff, S., Pennington, B., & Rogers, S. (1991). Executive function deficits in high-functioning autistic individuals: relationship to theory of mind. *Journal of Child Psychology and Psychiatry, 32*(7), 1081–1105.

Ozonoff, S., Goodlin-Jones, B. L., & Solomon, M. (2005a). Evidence-based assessment of autism spectrum disorders in children and adolescents. *Journal of Clinical Child and Adolescent Psychology, 34*(3), 523–540.

Ozonoff, S., South, M., & Provencal, S. (2005b). Executive functions. In F. R. Volkmar, R. Paul, A. Klin & D. Cohen (Eds.), *Handbook of autism and pervasive developmental disorders, Vol. 1: diagnosis, development, neurobiology, and behavior* (3rd ed., pp. 606–627). New Jersey: Wiley.

Palmer, A. (2006). *Realizing the college dream with autism or Asperger syndrome: a parent's guide to student success*. Philadelphia: Kingsley.

Panerai, S., Ferrante, L., Caputo, V., & Impellizzeri, C. (1998). Use of structured teaching for treatment of children with autism and severe and profound mental retardation. *Education and Training in Mental Retardation and Developmental Disabilities, 33*, 367–374.

Panerai, S., Ferrante, L., & Zingale, M. (2002). Benefits of the Treatment and Education of Autistic and Communication Handicapped Children (TEACCH) programme as compared with a non-specific approach. *Journal of Intellectual Disability Research, 46*(4), 318–327.

Panerai, S., Zingale, M., Trubia, G., Finocchiaro, M., Zuccarello, R., Ferri, R., et al. (2009). Special education versus inclusive education: the role of the TEACCH program. *Journal of Autism and Developmental Disorders, 39*(6), 874–882.

Persson, B. (2000). Brief report: a longitudinal study of quality of life and independence among adult men with autism. *Journal of Autism and Developmental Disorders, 30*(1), 61–66.

Pierce, K. L., & Schreibman, L. (1994). Teaching daily living skills to children with autism in unsupervised settings through pictorial self-management. *Journal of Applied Behavior Analysis, 27*(3), 471–481.

Probst, P., & Leppert, T. (2008). Brief report: outcomes of a Teacher Training Program for Autism Spectrum Disorders. *Journal of Autism and Developmental Disorders, 38*(9), 1791–1796.

Probst, P., Jung, F., Micheel, J., & Glen, I. (2010). Tertiary-preventive interventions for autism spectrum disorders (ASD) in children and adults: an evaluative synthesis of two TEACCH based outcome studies. *Life Span and Disability, 13*(2), 129–167.

Quill, K. A. (1997). Instructional considerations for young children with autism: the rationale for visually cued instruction. *Journal of Autism and Developmental Disorders, 27*(6), 697–714.

Reichow, B., & Volkmar, F. R. (2010). Best-evidence synthesis of social skills interventions for individuals with autism spectrum disorders. *Journal of Autism and Developmental Disorders, 40*(2), 149–166.

Reichow, B., Volkmar, F. R. & Cicchetti, D.V. (2008). Development of an evaluative method for evaluating and determining evidence-based practices in autism. *Journal of Autism and Developmental Disorders, 38(7)*, 1311–1319.

Rogers, S. J., & Ozonoff, S. (2005). Annotation: what do we know about sensory dysfunction in autism? A critical review of the empirical evidence. *Journal of Child Psychology and Psychiatry, 46*(12), 1255–1268.

Ropar, D., & Peebles, D. (2007). Sorting preference in children with autism: the dominance of concrete features. *Journal of Autism and Developmental Disorders, 37*(2), 270–280.

Schopler, E. (1989). Principles for directing both education, treatment and research. In C. Gillberg (Ed.), *Diagnosis and treatment of autism* (pp. 167–183). New York: Plenum Press.

Schopler, E. (1995). *Parent survival manual*. New York: Plenum.

Schopler, E., & Reichler, R. (1971). Parents as cotherapists in the treatment of psychotic children. *Journal of Autism and Childhood Schizophrenia, 1*(1), 87–102.

Schopler, E., Brehm, S. S., Kinsbourne, M., & Reichler, R. J. (1971). Effect of treatment structure on development in autistic children. *Archives of General Psychiatry, 24*, 415–421.

Schopler, E., Mesibov, G. B., & Baker, A. (1982). Evaluation of treatment for autistic children and their parents. *Journal of the American Academy of Child Psychiatry, 21*(3), 262–267.

Schopler, E., Mesibov, G. B., Shigley, R. H., & Bashford, A. (1984). Helping autistic children through their parents: The TEACCH model. In E. Schopler & G. B. Mesibov (Eds.), *The effects of autism on the family* (pp. 65–68 l). New York: Plenum.

Schopler, E., Reichler, R., & Renner, B. (1988). *Childhood Autism Rating Scale (CARS)*. Los Angeles: Western Psychological Services.

Schopler, E., Lansing, M., Reichler, R., & Marcus, L. (2005). *Psychoeducational profile: Third edition (PEP-3)*. Texas: Pro-Ed.

Schopler, E., Van Bourgondien, M., Wellman, J., & Love, S. (2010). *Childhood Autism Rating Scale—Second edition (CARS2): Manual*. Los Angeles: Western Psychological Services.

Shore, S. (2004). *Ask and tell: self advocacy and disclosure for people on the autism spectrum*. Shawnee Mission, KS: Autism Asperger Publishing.

Short, A. B. (1984). Short term treatment outcome using parents as co-therapists for their own autistic children. *Journal of Child Psychology and Psychiatry, 25*(3), 443–458.

Thomas, J. B., & Williams, G. A. (2004). Functional behavior assessment for individuals with autism. Unpublished manuscript. Division TEACCH, University of North Carolina at Chapel Hill.

Tsang, S., Shek, D., Lam, L., Tang, F., & Cheung, P. (2007). Brief report: application of the TEACCH Program on Chinese pre-school children with autism—does culture make a difference? *Journal of Autism and Developmental Disorders, 37*(2), 390–396.

Tsatsanis, K. D. (2005). Neuropsychological characteristics in autism and related conditions. In F. R. Volkmar, R. Paul, A. Klin & D. Cohen (Eds.), *Handbook of autism and pervasive developmental disorders, vol. 1: Diagnosis, development, neurobiology, and behavior* (3rd ed., pp. 365–381). New Jersey: Wiley.

Turner-Brown, L. M., Perry, T. D., Dichter, G. S., Bodfish, J. W., & Penn, D. L. (2008). Brief report: feasibility of social cognition and interaction training for adults with high functioning autism. *Journal of Autism and Developmental Disorders, 38*(9), 1777–1784.

Van Bourgondien, M. E. (1993). Behavior management in the preschool years. In E. Schopler, M. E. Van Bourgondien & M. M. Bristol (Eds.), *Preschool issues in autism.* (pp. 129–145). New York: Plenum.

Van Bourgondien, M. E., & Chapman, S. M. (2005). Adult services. In G. B. Mesibov, V. Shea & E. Schopler (Eds.), *The TEACCH approach to autism spectrum disorders* (pp. 155–188). New York: Springer.

Van Bourgondien, M. E., & Mesibov, G. B. (1989a). Environmental rating scale. Division TEACCH, UNC Chapel Hill.

Van Bourgondien, M.E., & Mesibov, G.B. (1989b). Diagnosis and treatment of adolescents and adults with autism. In G. Dawson (ED.), *Autism* (pp. 367–385). New York: Guilford.

Van Bourgondien, M. E., Reichle, N. C., Campbell, D. G., & Mesibov, G. B. (1998). The Environmental Rating Scale (ERS): a measure of the quality of the residential environment for adults with autism. *Research in Developmental Disabilities, 19*(5), 381–394.

Van Bourgondien, M. E., Reichle, N. C., & Schopler, E. (2003). Effects of a model treatment approach on adults with autism. *Journal of Autism and Developmental Disorders, 33*(2), 131–140.

Vaughn, B., & Horner, R. H. (1995). Effects of concrete versus verbal choice systems on problem behavior. *Augmentative and Alternative Communication, 11*(2), 89–92.

Watson, L. R., Lord, C., Schaffer, B., & Schopler, E. (1989). *Teaching spontaneous communication to autistic and developmentally handicapped children*. Texas: Pro-Ed.

Welterlin, A. (2009). The Home TEACCHing Program: a study of the efficacy of a parent training early intervention model. Unpublished doctoral dissertation, Rutgers University.

Yoder, P. J., & Layton, T. L. (1988). Speech following sign language training in autistic children with minimal verbal language. *Journal of Autism and Developmental Disorders, 18*(2), 217–229.

Zalla, T., Labruyere, N., & Georgieff, N. (2006). Goal-directed action representation in autism. *Journal of Autism and Developmental Disorders, 36*(4), 527–540.

Chapter 6
Social Communication, Emotional Regulation, and Transactional Support (SCERTS)

Emily Rubin, Barry M. Prizant, Amy C. Laurent and Amy M. Wetherby

Comprehensive Versus Focused Approaches in Educational Programs

Educational programming for individuals with Autism Spectrum Disorders (ASD) can be described at two different levels: focused approaches and comprehensive approaches. Focused approaches utilize evidence-based strategies directed at particular symptoms. Examples include, but are not limited to, focused interventions aimed at reducing behaviors which interfere with learning (Horner et al. 2002; Odom et al. 2003), improving speech and expressive language skills (Garrison-Harrell et al. 1997; Light et al. 1998; Mirenda 2003; Schlosser and Lee 2000), improving play skills (Thorp et al. 1995), and fostering interactions with peers (Kalyva and Avramidis 2005; Thiemann and Goldstein 2004). These evidence-based strategies are indeed essential for supporting individuals with ASD in relation to particular areas of need.

In contrast, a comprehensive approach provides a framework that is broad in scope and is designed to improve overall functioning and to produce positive long-term outcomes in adulthood. The SCERTS® Model is a comprehensive, multidisciplinary educational approach that was developed to maximize long-term positive outcomes

E. Rubin (✉)
Communication Crossroads, 931 Monroe Dr., Suite 102, Box 110,
Atlanta, GA 30308, USA
e-mail: Emily@CommXroads.com

B. M. Prizant
Childhood Communication Services, Center for the Study of Human Development,
Brown University, 35 Kent Place, Cranston, RI 02905, USA
e-mail: bprizant@gmail.com

A. C. Laurent
University of Rhode Island, Kingston, RI, USA

A. M. Wetherby
Department of Clinical Sciences, College of Medicine, Florida State University,
Tallahassee, FL, USA

S. Goldstein, J. A. Naglieri (eds.), *Interventions for Autism Spectrum Disorders*,
DOI 10.1007/978-1-4614-5301-7_6, © Springer Science+Business Media New York 2013

Table 6.1 SCERTS® Model core values and guiding principles (Adapted from Prizant et al. 2006)

1	The development of spontaneous, functional communication abilities and emotional regulatory capacities, which support development and independence, are the highest educational priorities.
2	Principles and research on child development frame assessment and educational efforts. Goals and activities are developmentally appropriate and relevant to a child's life.
3	All domains of child development are viewed as interrelated and interdependent. Assessment and intervention must address these relationships.
4	All behavior is viewed as purposeful. For children who display unconventional and/or problem behaviors, there is an emphasis on determining the functions of the behaviors and supporting the development of more appropriate ways to accomplish those functions.
5	A child's unique learning profile of strengths and weaknesses is used to determine appropriate transactional supports for facilitating the development of social communicative and emotional regulatory competence.
6	Natural routines across home, school, and community environments provide educational and treatment contexts for learning and the development of relationships. Progress is measured in relation to increasing competence and independence across these natural routines.
7	Professionals bear the primary responsibility for establishing and maintaining positive relationships with children and family members. All are treated with dignity and respect.
8	Family members are considered experts about their child. Assessment and educational efforts are collaborative processes.

for individuals with ASD and their families while embracing a wide range of more focused evidence-based interventions (Prizant et al. 2006). The acronym "SCERTS" refers to the model's focus on the following three domains: (1) social communication (SC), which refers to the development of spontaneous, initiated, functional communication, the development of secure and trusting relationships with children and adults, and an understanding of the conventions of different social situations; (2) emotional regulation (ER), which refers to the development of the ability to utilize specific strategies to cope with everyday stressors and to be most available for learning and interacting; and (3) transactional support (TS), which refers to the development and implementation of supports to help partners to be highly responsive to an individual's needs and interests, modify and adapt the environment, and provide tools to enhance learning. Specific plans are also developed to provide educational and emotional support to families and to foster collaboration across service providers and family members.

The comprehensive nature of the SCERTS Model ensures that a range of meaningful goals and objectives are addressed by utilizing evidence-based strategies. Furthermore, practices in the SCERTS Model are consistent with explicitly stated core values and guiding principles, which are critical in supporting fidelity of programming and allow for broad application of practice across a wide range of abilities and chronological ages. These core values and guiding principles of the SCERTS Model are summarized in Table 6.1.

As a comprehensive approach, the SCERTS Model is designed to be implemented over longer periods of time and across a wider variety of settings and partners than many focused approaches. In fact, the core domains of the model are applicable throughout the lifespan, across settings (e.g., home, school, and community), and across partners (e.g., teachers, family members, peers, coworkers). The overarching goal is to provide a systematic framework for assessment and selection of the most critical and developmentally appropriate goals, namely those goals that are predictive of long-term positive outcomes in social communication and emotional regulation. At the same time, the model integrates focused approaches or strategies from a range of evidence-based methodologies into the daily routines of an individual with ASD. Focused approaches or strategies include those from the fields of behavioral psychology, developmental psychology, speech-language pathology, occupational therapy, mental health, and others.

In the SCERTS Model, specific guidelines are provided for helping educational teams and families to support an individual with ASD to (1) become a competent and confident SC and (2) become more available for learning and engaging with others by developing greater capacity for ER. These goals are realized by training teams and families to implement developmentally appropriate TS, such as evidence-based interpersonal supports and learning supports, and by developing plans to support families and to engender collaboration and support among service providers. Effective programming using the SCERTS framework results in active participation in daily activities in home, school, and community contexts while preventing problem behaviors that interfere with learning and the development of relationships. SCERTS is designed to help families, educators, and therapists work cooperatively as a team, in a carefully coordinated manner, to maximize progress in supporting an individual.

Prioritizing Social Communicative Competence

The rationale for selecting social communication, emotional regulation, and transactional support as the most critical domains within the SCERTS Model is derived from the literature base defining the core challenges of ASD that affect social-adaptive functioning (ASHA 2006; NRC 2001). It is also derived from the strong correlations that have been found between social communication and emotional regulation and long-term positive outcomes for all human beings (Prizant et al. 2006; NRC 2000). These developmental domains contribute to everyone's ability to form relationships and to adapt to the demands of everyday social situations. The choice of these domains as the highest level priorities in educational programming is supported by both large group studies of individuals with ASD as well as large group studies of typically developing individuals over time in the areas of social, communicative, cognitive, emotional, and sensory-motor development (Prizant et al. 2006).

Challenges in Social Communication

While the population of ASD presents with tremendous heterogeneity, there are common characteristics and challenges that compromise the development of critical social communication skills and interfere with social communicative competence (ASHA 2006). Regardless of an individual's cognitive abilities or learning style differences, individuals with ASD face core challenges with establishing shared attention (i.e., joint attention) and therefore predicting the actions of social partners (Volkmar et al. 2004). When an individual has difficulty predicting the actions of one's social partners, the development of social communication can be compromised. Core challenges in social communication have been noted with respect to joint attention, including difficulties with social orienting, establishing shared attention, monitoring emotional states, and considering another's intentions. In addition, limitations in social reciprocity have been noted, including difficulties with initiating bids for interaction, maintaining interactions by taking turns, and providing contingent responses to bids for interaction initiated by others. If one has difficulty predicting the actions of another, predicting that others can be a source of engagement, assistance, and comfort may be compromised, reducing the individual's overall rate of spontaneous bids for communication. Challenges in social communication have also been noted with respect to an individual's symbol use or language and related cognitive skills (e.g., understanding and using nonverbal and verbal communication, symbolic play, and the conventions and "rules" of social conversations in different situations). In typically developing children, a high rate of spontaneous communication is correlated with the acquisition of more symbolic and sophisticated forms of communication. Thus, individuals with ASD are at a significant disadvantage with learning more conventional forms of communication when their rate of communication is infrequent and the intervention is focused on their response to others versus their initiation (Prizant et al. 2006; NRC 2001).

These challenges are relevant across the entire developmental range in ASD, including those identified with Asperger syndrome (AS). Although individuals with AS demonstrate higher-level abilities on standardized measures of cognitive and language ability, outcome studies with this population highlight that cognitive, academic, and even strong expressive language abilities do not necessarily ensure an individual's ability to establish and maintain satisfying relationships that contribute to success at school, at home, and in the community (Saulnier and Klin 2007; Tsatsanis et al. 2004). Challenges in social communication significantly compromise social adaptive functioning and the ability to achieve longer-term vocational goals even in those with strong intellectual abilities (Gilchrist et al. 2001; Little 2001; Saulnier and Klin 2007; Tantam 2000; see also Tsatsanis 2003). Such vulnerabilities also place the individual at risk for mental health conditions such as anxiety and depression (Tsatsanis et al. 2004). Therefore, when developing a comprehensive educational program for individuals with ASD, addressing social communication is a critical priority across all levels of functioning.

In the SCERTS Model manuals (Prizant et al. 2006), a curriculum-based assessment tool is provided so that an individualized educational plan can be developed based on an individual's profile, rather than using the same prescribed curriculum for all individuals (Prizant et al. 2006). The *SCERTS Assessment Process* assesses individual differences in the domain of social communication from preverbal to more advanced language stages, covering a wide developmental and chronological age span. A carefully laid out scope and sequence of goals and objectives is provided to provide a means to select developmentally appropriate and meaningful goals in the components of the social communication domain, i.e., joint attention and symbol use, to address an individual's specific needs, and to monitor progress over time (Prizant et al. 2006). This ensures that multidisciplinary teams have a means to select targets and measure progress over time with a sustainable tool beginning in early intervention and carrying on through the school-age years, possibly into adulthood.

The core challenges in social communication as experienced by individuals with ASD are assessed using a three-stage developmental continuum divided into the Social Partner, Language Partner, and Conversational Partner stages. Within each stage, potential goals and objectives are delineated to allow teams to select the most appropriate targets based on three criteria. (1) Functional: will achievement of this objective make a meaningful difference for this individual, (2) Family Priority: is this objective consistent with family priorities, and (3) Developmental: is this objective consistent with the individual's developmental abilities as measured on the *SCERTS Assessment Process*. The Social Partner stage in the SCERTS Model encompasses two transitions that typically develop during the first few years of life, namely the ability to communicate with intent with others and the acquisition and use of conventional gestures and vocalizations. The Language Partner stage encompasses the transition to the intentional and meaningful use of single symbols (e.g., words, signs, photos, icons) as well as the creative combinations of symbols, which typically occurs between 2 to 4 years of age. This stage is particularly challenging for individuals with ASD, as limited social orientation, unconventional verbal behavior (e.g., echolalia), and limited understanding of the intentions of others makes the acquisition of early word combinations such as agent + action (e.g., "mommy hug" or "daddy tickle") a particular challenge. As this skill is predictive of creative language acquisition in all children, this is a strong emphasis of the Language Partner Stage. Lastly, the Conversational Partner stage includes the acquisition of sentence grammar and conversational discourse and represents a stage where individuals with ASD are challenged with learning how to be a true conversational partner by adapting their language and conversational style based upon the social expectations and perspectives of those around them. This stage is particularly relevant through the school-aged years and beyond.

Challenges in Emotional Regulation

Core challenges have also been documented with respect to emotional regulation, a developmental capacity that plays a significant role in fostering social communicative competence (NRC 2000). In individuals with ASD, challenges have been noted with respect to effectively regulating one's emotional state and behavior, focusing attention to salient aspects of the environment, and engaging in executive functioning, which refers to an ability to solve problem, plan, and self-monitor goal-directed behavior. Difficulties with emotional expression, interpretation of nonverbal social cues, and mood regulation are widely discussed in the ASD literature (Klin and Volkmar 2003). For individuals with ASD, there is often a mismatch between (1) a child's ability to remain actively engaged, adapt to novel stimuli, and inhibit impulsive reactions and (2) the expectations for that child regarding appropriate and socially conventional behavior in a given context (Laurent and Rubin 2004; Miller et al. 2004). Limitations in emotional regulation abilities also contribute to the development of a variety of challenging behaviors. Such behaviors can have a significant impact on an individual's access to educational and social opportunities (Koegel et al. 1996; Prizant and Laurent 2011; Walker et al. 2004).

At the core of the disability, individuals with ASD have difficulty predicting the actions of their social partners (Klin and Volkmar 2003). While these challenges clearly compromise the development of social communication skills, as described above, they also contribute to challenges in emotional regulation. An individual needs to accurately predict the behavior or intent of others in order to maintain active engagement in social situations, to feel comfortable, and to initiate engagement with others. Difficulty in these areas leads to increased frustration and anxiety and may contribute to withdrawal and depression (Little 2001; Tantam 2000). Emotional regulation challenges can, in fact, provide a significant obstacle toward the achievement of social communicative competence if left unaddressed or if considered a lesser priority than academic skills (NRC 2000).

In the SCERTS Model, two components of emotional regulation are of primary interest: (1) mutual regulation and (2) self-regulation. Mutual regulation refers to the ability to respond to or solicit assistance in regulating one's emotional state. As individuals with ASD frequently misinterpret social cues, they often fail to recognize assistance that is offered by partners (e.g., parents, service providers, peers; Laurent and Rubin 2004) and may avoid opportunities to request support from others because of increased anxiety and/or social withdrawal. Likewise, partners of individuals with ASD often miss opportunities to provide support because of the subtle and atypical signals of emotional distress in this population. Specific challenges in this capacity include, but are not limited to (1) expressing emotion, (2) responding to assistance, (3) responding to feedback and guidance regarding behavior, (4) requesting assistance, and (5) recovering from distress with the support of partners (Prizant et al. 2006). A carefully laid out scope and sequence of goals and objectives is provided in the SCERTS assessment process to provide a means to select developmentally appropriate and meaningful goals in mutual regulation, to address an individual's specific needs, and to monitor progress over time (Prizant et al. 2006).

The capacity for self-regulation is also a component of emotional regulation that is of interest (Laurent and Rubin 2004). As the development of conventional or socially acceptable strategies for self-regulation requires an ability to imitate others, follow instructions, and consider the perspective of others, regulatory behaviors modeled by social partners are often missed. As a result, an individual with ASD may use behaviors that are atypical, unconventional, or simply not based on an understanding of the perspective of others. These behaviors have been described in the literature as "odd," "disruptive," or "deviant." In fact, many sensory-motor patterns of behavior that may be attempts at self-regulation are often referred to as "autistic behaviors" because of their repetitive and unconventional nature (e.g., rocking, spinning, staring at fingers, gaze aversion). Specific challenges in this capacity include (1) demonstrating availability for engaging, (2) using conventional behaviors to regulate arousal during familiar activities, (3) using conventional language strategies to regulate arousal during familiar activities, (4) using metacognitive strategies (i.e., the ability to reflect and plan) to regulate arousal during familiar activities, (5) regulating emotion during new and changing situations, and (6) recovering from extreme distress by oneself (Prizant et al. 2006).

Individuals with ASD often continue to use early developing and/or atypical strategies to regulate their emotions and arousal beyond early childhood. Behaviors such as insisting on specific routines, hoarding preferred items, and averting gaze may persist in older individuals with ASD, but are actually quite common in typically developing young children. In addition, when an individual is not tuned into models provided by others, the use of language for self-regulation may follow more idiosyncratic or atypical patterns. Individuals with ASD may recite the lines of a favorite movie or book or repetitively talk about areas of special interest when faced with distressful social circumstances (Prizant and Laurent 2011; Rydell and Prizant 1995). Unusual patterns in self-regulation can lead to social isolation, as the negative perception of these behaviors can create barriers to building relationships and contribute to an increased risk for depression (Little 2001; Tantam 2000).

As emotional regulation is a critical developmental process that is correlated with the development of social relationships, behavioral adjustment, and academic success (Martinez-Pons 1996; Rydell et al. 2003), this is considered an essential domain in the SCERTS Model. A carefully laid out scope and sequence of goals and objectives provided in the *SCERTS Assessment Process* provide a means to select developmentally appropriate and meaningful goals in self-regulation, to address an individual's specific needs, and to monitor progress over time (Prizant et al. 2006).

Challenges in Transactional Support

Addressing social communication and emotional regulation cannot be achieved solely in isolated teaching contexts such as one-on-one therapy or a social skills group. Rather, these developmental achievements need to be supported across social activities, social partners, and social contexts (e.g., home, school, and community). A comprehensive educational program will ensure that supports are embedded throughout an individual's daily routines. In addition, the importance of partner training is evident, as setting targets for the individual with ASD does not always ensure that partners will modify their communicative style and the environment to accommodate the individual's unique learning style, address family priorities, and facilitate generalization across situations and contexts (Simpson et al. 2003). Family support, personnel preparation, and peer training are characteristics of an effective comprehensive model as a means to ensure individualized supports are embedded across contexts and activities (Prizant et al. 2006; Wetherby and Woods 2006).

The *SCERTS Assessment Process* was not only designed to identify goals and objectives that have been shown to address the core challenges that compromise social communicative competence, but was also designed to provide a tool for measuring program fidelity across partners, contexts, and activities (Prizant et al. 2006). In other words, progress is documented not only in an individual with ASD but also in how consistently partners use interactive styles and environmental arrangements that are evidence-based to foster more successful engagement across daily routines. In the SCERTS Model, this domain is referred to as transactional support. Essentially, this domain emphasizes that when partners are responsive to the individual with ASD, individuals with ASD are more competent social communicators.

A partners' ability to provide these supports is often compromised by the transactional nature of the social disability (Prizant et al. 2003). The atypical style of individuals with ASD compromises the ability of a communicative partner to provide these supports. In more focused approaches, which often have a sole target on enhancing the skills of the individual with the disability, supports are not necessarily being implemented across all partners; thus, the consistency of partner behavior is less of a challenge. However, when implementing a comprehensive educational approach, the emphasis shifts toward those who interact with the individual throughout the day. Those who interact with the individual, as a result, often require direct coaching and support to ensure competent communicative exchanges (Prizant et al. 2006).

Intervention research has demonstrated a strong correlation with how communicative partners adapt their communicative styles and modify the environment with learning supports and the social communicative competence of an individual with ASD (ASHA 2006; NRC 2001). An individual with ASD must experience successful social interactions with partners across a range of social contexts in order to develop skills in both social communication and emotional regulation. Unfortunately, partners do not have an easy task in providing these accommodations, as subtle and unconventional bids for communication and emotional distress can lead to frequent misinterpretations. For example, an individual with ASD might initiate a request for comfort by seeking physical proximity, but if such an attempt is sudden or unconventional, and therefore is perceived as potentially harmful, the attempt might be rejected or responded to negatively by staff. While the teacher might perceive this behavior as inappropriate or even threatening, the individual's difficulty in inhibiting impulsive reactions, considering another's perspective, and using more appropriate communication (e.g., speech or conventional gestures) masks the true intent of the behavior (i.e., requesting comfort). While an intervention approach can certainly address this using more appropriate communicative forms with the individual with ASD, empowering the partners with the knowledge of why these behaviors are occurring and how to alter their own communicative style to foster success can have a more efficient impact on social exchanges (e.g., provide visual models for communicative forms, responding to bids for interaction). Partners, in these circumstances, might be encouraged to not only acknowledge the bids from the individual with ASD (e.g., "It looks like you need a hug . . . need a break") but also explicitly model and encourage imitation of a more appropriate communicative act (e.g., using a sign for hug, asking to go for a walk).

In a similar manner, unconventional coping strategies such as reciting lines from a movie during a boisterous group activity in the classroom might be perceived as avoidant, disruptive, and disrespectful to the group. Yet, this may also be a result of that individual's increased anxiety with the task demands and the lack of a clear and predictable endpoint to the task. As such, while a plan might be developed to support the use of more socially conventional coping strategies (e.g., asking for help or a break), partners would also be encouraged to recognize signals of distress and to provide support. Service providers, for example, might be encouraged to label the individual's emotions (e.g., "It looks like you might be frustrated...") while modeling coping strategies (e.g., "Let's write down the steps we need to complete this task").

Prioritizing Transactional Supports

While a range of focused strategies are available that hone in on the individual's acquisition of targeted skills, the SCERTS Model has been designed to ensure that partners provide appropriate interpersonal and learning supports and are accountable for implementing supports across the natural routines and social contexts of that individual's life (Prizant et al. 2006). In the SCERTS curriculum-based assessment, the domain of TS provides an ongoing assessment of how team members are implementing both interpersonal supports and learning supports across partners and contexts (i.e., school, home, and community). Interpersonal supports refer to the adjustments made by social partners with respect to their interactive style. These include the ability to (1) respond to the individual's needs, (2) ensure opportunities for the individual with ASD to initiate, (3) respect independence and intentions, (4) engage the individual, (5) provide developmental support, (6) adjust language input to be developmentally appropriate, and (7) model appropriate behaviors. Learning supports refer to the modifications that are made to support learning, including visual and organizational supports that foster the ability to establish shared attention and attend to relevant social stimuli in the environment, and curriculum modifications. Sample goals and objectives adapted from the transactional support domain of the *SCERTS Assessment Process* (Prizant et al. 2006) are outlined in Table 6.2 under the components of interpersonal support and learning support.

When partners embed learning supports across natural activities, these accommodations will take on different forms based on the unique circumstances and demands of the social setting. Likewise, how these partners adapt their interactive style for an individual (i.e., interpersonal supports) should differ based on that individual's unique learning style differences and preferences for modes of instruction (Tsatsanis 2004). While many partners may be adapting their interaction style unconsciously, this SCERTS process brings these adaptations to a more conscious level. Furthermore, it is important to note that addressing the development of social communication and emotional regulation in individuals with ASD should not take the form of overly

Table 6.2 SCERTS® curriculum-based assessment: sample transactional support goals and objectives (Adapted from Prizant et al. 2006)

Transactional support
Interpersonal support
1) Partners will be responsive to the individual
a. attuning to the emotion and pace of the individual
b. responding to subtle communicative signals
c. recognizing signs of dysregulation and offers support
d. providing information or assistance to regulate state
2) Partners will foster initiation
a. offering choices
b. waiting for and encouraging initiation
c. providing a balance between initiated and respondent turns
3) Partners will respect the independence of the individual
a. allowing the individual to take breaks to move about as needed
b. providing time for the individual to solve problems or complete activities at own pace
c. interpreting problem behaviors as communicative and/or regulatory
d. honoring protests, rejections, or refusals when appropriate
4) Partners will set the stage for engagement
a. securing individual's attention prior to communicating
b. using appropriate proximity and nonverbal behavior to encourage interaction
c. sharing emotions and internal states and mental plans
5) Partners will provide developmental support
a. providing guidance for success in interacting with peers
b. attempting to repair breakdowns in communication
c. providing guidance on expressing emotions and understanding the cause of emotion
d. providing guidance on interpreting others' feelings and opinions
6) Partners will adjust language input
a. using nonverbal cues to support understanding
b. adjusting complexity of language input to individual's developmental level
c. adjusting complexity of language input to individual's arousal level
7) Partners will model appropriate behavior
a. modeling appropriate nonverbal communication and emotional expressions
b. modeling a range of communicative functions
c. modeling appropriate behavior when individual using inappropriate behavior
d. modeling the use of self-talk
Learning support
1) Partners will structure activities for active participation
a. defining a clear beginning and ending to activity
b. providing a predictable sequence to activity
c. offering repeated learning opportunities
2) Partners will use augmentative communication support to foster development
a. using visual or written support to enhance communication and expressive language
b. using visual or written support to enhance understanding of language and social behavior
c. using visual or written support to enhance emotional expression
d. using visual or written support to enhance emotional regulation
3) Partners will use visual and organizational support
a. using support to define steps within a task
b. using visual support to enhance smooth transitions between activities
c. using visual support to enhance active involvement in group activities

Table 6.2 (continued)

4) Partners will modify the goals, activities, and learning environment
   a. adjusting the social complexity to support organization and interaction
   b. adjusting task difficulty
   c. modifying the sensory properties of the environment
   d. arranging the environment to promote initiation
   e. infusing motivating and meaningful materials and topics in activities
   f. alternating between movement and sedentary activities as needed

simplified methodologies that suggest a one-to-one correspondence between a specific interpersonal support or learning support and specific social communication and emotional regulation goals. Rather, it is more likely that the partner will need to make a number of conscious changes in these areas in order to make a significant impact on a specific aspect of an individual's social communication or emotional regulation profile. As a result, it will be important to continually monitor the effectiveness of specific interpersonal and learning supports in different social situations. For example, when encouraging an individual with ASD to spontaneously initiate bids for communication at the Language Partner stage, partners would not simply be implementing one learning support, such as the use of augmentative communication (e.g., picture symbols), but will also likely be encouraged to offer choices of desired items, provide a balance between initiated and respondent turns, and ensure that the individual is motivated to engage by modifying the environment to provide developmentally appropriate activities.

The following transactional supports are offered to provide essential priorities to illustrate the influence of partner behavior and transactional support goals on the achievement of social communication and emotional regulation skills. They are not intended to provide specific instructions or guidelines, merely examples of the variables, which might be considered when developing a comprehensive educational plan based upon the SCERTS Model.

Interpersonal Supports

There are seven partner goals, each with underlying objectives, included within the interpersonal support component of the transactional support domain, as illustrated in Table 6.2. In the *SCERTS Assessment Process*, these goals and objectives are provided in order to ensure that progress is tracked with respect to how consistently evidence-based interpersonal supports are provided across social partners and whether these more focused supports are available across social contexts and natural activities. In the sections that follow, partner goals and objectives are discussed in detail with respect to how they may address the need for accommodating the primary challenges in ASD, namely those that fall in the domains of social communication and emotional regulation, as summarized above.

Partner is Responsive As individuals with ASD have significant challenges predicting the intentions of others, partners must have coaching that enables them to be extremely responsive to even the most subtle communicative acts. This is particularly essential at the Social Partner stage when shifting toward the use of spontaneous bids for communicative intent is the transition that is being addressed. For example, when an individual with ASD is not yet using gestures paired with gaze to share intent for assistance with opening a container, partners may need to be taught to respond to subtle signals such as that individual's gaze toward the container. This responsiveness will help facilitate the development of expressing communicative intent based on a developing awareness that others can be a source of assistance. Over time, this developmental achievement leads to the ability to repair communicative breakdowns by using more directed behaviors such as taking another's hand and pulling it toward an object and, ultimately, looking toward their partner to be sure that their message was received. The expression of communicative intent, even at this early presymbolic level, requires that partners are consistently responsive (McDuffie and Yoder 2010). This interpersonal support remains critical throughout development, as even the most able individuals with ASD at the Language and Conversational Partner stages may not predict that their partners will provide emotional support when they are distressed. In the SCERTS Model, partners are explicitly taught to recognize signals of distress and offer support in order to help individuals with ASD recognize others as predictable sources of comfort and engagement.

Partner Fosters Initiation An individual with ASD needs to be able to predict that others are a source of assistance, a source of pleasure or engagement, and a source of comfort in order to initiate bids for communication. By teaching partners to offer choices and balance their bids for communication with frequent opportunities for the individual with ASD to initiate, a focus is placed on the most critical variables that predict positive long-term outcomes, i.e., functional, spontaneous communication (NRC 2001). A range of focused intervention strategies for fostering initiation are embraced within the SCERTS Model including offering choices and providing a balance between initiated and respondent turns (ASHA 2006). For children at the Social Partner stage, choices of preferred toys (e.g., cars for a wooden race track or puppets representing social/song routines) could be offered in see-through containers so that the child is aware of the options and might then have an opportunity to request assistance by either looking toward the containers or giving them to a partner and looking toward that partner's face. Similarly, at the Language Partner stage, a strip with photo/picture symbols could be placed on the see-through container reminding the individual with ASD to look toward another and use agent + action + object word combination (e.g., "Nancy open cars").

At the Conversational Partner stage, the need for offering choices and balancing initiated and respondent turns remains quite essential. For example, educational teams often question whether to encourage an individual's initiation of conversations about special interests. It is not uncommon to observe educational goals written for discouraging "movie talk" or special interest discussions at all. Such an unwillingness to respond to functional communicative attempts may result in an individual learning that others have little interest in that individual's "passions" and therefore are not a source of engagement and pleasure. As many adolescents with higher functioning autism and Asperger syndrome are at risk for mental health conditions such as extreme social anxiety and depression, this is a legitimate concern. By fostering initiation and modeling a balance of respondent and initiated opportunities, we are modeling mature and socially conventional conversational skills.

Partner Respects Individual's Independence One of the most essential goals of partner training in the SCERTS Model is the notion of creating an interpersonal environment that enables the individual with ASD to establish trusting relationships with others. This is a particular challenge for individuals who have difficulty predicting the intentions of others, requesting assistance from others, and initiating bids for social engagement and pleasure. Without trusting relationships, however, an individual with ASD will likely not only demonstrate decreased initiations but also exhibit anxiety, lack of responsiveness, and decreased motivation to engage in activities initiated by others (Prizant 2009). Thus, particularly in educational programs that are required to address academic content standards and other curricula, it is essential that partners are taught to respect the independence of individuals with ASD as a means to build trusting relationships (Prizant and Carley 2009). This can be accomplished by allowing individuals to take breaks to move about as needed, to provide time to solve a problem at their own pace, and to honor protests and refusals when appropriate. For example, a third-grade teacher supporting a child at the Conversational Partner stage to write words in cursive was observed to offer a break following that child's behavior of putting his head down on the table and indicating that he did not know why he was being asked to write a list of words. As he left the table, she modified the task so that he could better predict the intent of writing a list, i.e., writing cursive could be a useful tool for completing a silly word puzzle. She showed him that after the list was finished, she would place each word into a fill-in-the-blank story and that it would come out as quite humorous. His break from the task was short-lived, he was observed to return to his work with greater motivation, and, most importantly, his trust and motivation to engage with his teacher was only enhanced by this respect. An individual with ASD needs to learn to trust others in order to feel safe and resilient.

Partner Sets the Stage for Engagement Individuals with ASD often attend to less relevant stimuli in the environment (e.g., the alphabet letters posted on the classroom wall, the fire evacuation route sign, or an interesting shirt that a classmate might be wearing). An inability to attend to relevant social stimuli is one of the core challenges of ASD and cannot simply be attributed to inattentiveness (Klin and Volkmar 2003). One of the most effective strategies for securing the attention of those with ASD is to ensure that partners receive support as to how one might set the stage for engagement. This might entail providing guidance as to the most effective strategies for securing attention prior to communicating (e.g., getting down at the child's level, coming face-to-face in close proximity, using visual supports) and using appropriate words and intonation to support optimal arousal and engagement (e.g., using a high-pitched excited tone versus a quiet flat tone depending upon the preferences of the individual).

Partner Provides Developmentally Appropriate Support For individuals with ASD, it is not uncommon for repeated failures in social interactions with peers and/or in academic activities to lead to negative emotional memories. These failures are often not solely related to challenges in the individual with ASD but also due to partners providing developmentally inappropriate support. Thus, this is an area of partner training that is crucial for ensuring individuals with ASD gain more positive emotional experiences at school and when engaging with their peers. For example, one educational team sought support for a student at the Social Partner stage, a stage representative of presymbolic children who are still learning about intentional communication and conventional gestures, but most importantly that others are a predictable source of engagement and support. This little girl was hoarding her toys during free play opportunities in the classroom. When peers approached her to request a turn or to simply take one of these toys, she would screech and, occasionally, lash out at the peers. The problem was being perceived as her lack of willingness to share. When her team was taught to recognize her developmental level and provide developmentally appropriate support, challenges were reduced significantly. For a child at the Social Partner stage, sharing toys and taking turns is not consistent with expectations for that stage and skills are more consistent with higher-level Language Partner stage children who already have established trusting relationships and predict others as sources of engagement. The team, as a result, worked on duplicating some of the key toys that this child preferred so that other children would have access and also taught her peers how to follow her lead and imitate her actions in a more parallel play manner. This little girl soon began to realize that her peers were sources of pleasure and not distress and, as her language develops, will likely learn to share and take turns once these skills are in her zone of proximal development (Prizant et al. 2006).

Partners Adjust Language Input As individuals progress through developmental stages of language acquisition, it has been well documented that the language modeling of communicative partners provides scaffolding for next steps in semantic relationships, grammar, syntax, and functional use of language (Prizant et al. 2006). In the SCERTS Model, appropriate support is provided so that that partners are able to adjust their language input to enhance both comprehension (e.g., providing nonverbal cues to support understanding) and expression along a developmental continuum. For individuals at the Social Partner stage, partners would be encouraged to model a range of more conventional gestures (e.g., giving an object to another, pointing toward items, pushing away, a head nod, a head shake) before targeting single words, signs, and/or picture symbols, a range of single words, and a range of word combinations. Likewise, for individuals at the Conversational Partner stage, partners would be encouraged to adjust language input to model more complex sentences representing clauses to clarify background information for a listener who may not have been present at an event (e.g., "Mark, *who I played with on the playground yesterday*, was wearing a dinosaur shirt"). Adjusting language input might also require simplifying language models and input when an individual is highly aroused or distressed, as emotional dysregulation compromises language expression and comprehension.

Partner Models Appropriate Behavior Replacement of challenging or unconventional behavior with functional equivalents is now a well-documented focused approach for individuals with ASD (Horner et al. 2002; NRC 2001). Thus, this focused strategy is embraced within the comprehensive approach of the SCERTS Model. Partners are taught to provide models for appropriate nonverbal communication, emotional expression, appropriate play skills, and the use of self-talk for self-regulation so that individuals with ASD can predict how to regulate their emotions in a manner sensitive to others. This is particularly relevant when partners are called upon to model appropriate behavior when an individual with ASD uses inappropriate behavior. The developmental framework of SCERTS allows this guidance to be fine-tuned to that of individual's developmental level. For example, if an individual at the Social Partner stage uses hoarding as a means to self-regulate when making transitions, partners may be taught to replace that behavior with another sensory-motor strategy to serve the same function (e.g., providing objects to represent the upcoming activity with interesting sensory properties). If this individual were at the Language Partner stage, the replacement might include the use of self-talk for self-regulation paired with visuals to enhance smooth transitions (e.g., a picture schedule to represent upcoming transitions). Lastly, if an individual at the Conversational Partner stage was hoarding during transitions, the replacement might be more cognitive-based. For example, one might be able to talk through the possible sources of anxiety in upcoming activities and alternative strategies for coping with that anxiety (e.g., writing out a schedule for the day, storing one's precious items in a secure spot, and using more socially acceptable coping strategies like drawing in one's journal at one's desk). In addition, the use of visual supports might be planned out with the individual to serve as a reminder for coping strategies that are socially acceptable (e.g., "when I am feeling . . . , I can . . . .").

Learning Supports

There are four primary partner goals and accompanying objectives included within the learning support component of the transactional support domain, as illustrated in Table 6.2. These are provided to ensure that progress is tracked with respect to how consistently evidence-based learning supports are provided across social partners and whether these supports are available across social contexts and natural activities. In the sections that follow, these partner goals and objectives are discussed in detail with respect to how they may address the need for accommodating one of the primary challenges in ASD, namely those that fall in the domains of social communication and emotional regulation as summarized above.

Partner Structures Activities for Active Participation Activity accommodations, such as visual supports that illustrate a clear beginning and endpoint, and predictable sequence to an activity are well-documented, evidence-based focused strategies for individuals with ASD (MacDuff et al. 1993; Bryan and Gast 2000). These focused strategies are embraced within the SCERTS Model and are seen as essential transactional support for fostering social communication and emotional regulation skills. Partners are taught to provide clear expectations for activities whether they are social routines with caregivers, academic tasks with teachers, or vocational tasks in a transition to adult programming. When a clear beginning and ending is not defined, the individual with ASD must rely on his ability to predict the intentions of another; thus, the stage may be set for confusion, emotional distress, and/or disengagement. In contrast, partners may be encouraged to use predictable carrier phrases to indicate a routine, such as "ready, set... go" and "1, 2, 3, ... stop" paired with visual supports to indicate the length of the activity. Such a strategy is relevant when coaching a parent on how to initiate or terminate a preferred activity, such as pushing a child on the swing or finishing an activity on a computer, so that the child can anticipate the steps within the activity and the predictable endpoint. Similarly, having materials clearly laid out from left to right paired with a visual model of a completed sample may help a student in a classroom complete an art project in the classroom and, lastly, an adolescent with Asperger syndrome might benefit from a written checklist of hygiene routines prior to leaving for school each morning.

Partner Uses Augmentative Communication Support For individuals with ASD at all stages of development, ensuring that partners provide augmentative communication support to foster expressive language, understanding of language, and emotional regulation is an essential part of the comprehensive approach within the SCERTS Model (Rubin et al. 2008). With respect to fostering expressive communication, in particular, the use of augmentative communication support is considered an essential focused approach. Partners are assessed as to their knowledge and consistent use of these tools across contexts and settings using the *SCERTS Assessment Process*.

At the Social Partner stage, the provision of augmentative communication supports to enhance communication and expressive language might involve the use of objects to foster an individual's ability to initiate bids for interaction and use conventional gestures to share intentions. For example, partners might be encouraged to pair objects with preferred social routines to support a child's ability to represent and request a social game across contexts. A specific scarf might be used for a Ring-Around-the-Rosie song or a toy rocket ship might be paired with a "3, 2, 1,... blast off" routine. Eventually, a see-through tub of these objects can be presented by the partner to allow the child with ASD to make a choice. Within feeding routines, a communication board might be created with several of the individual's preferred snack items sealed in see-through containers and attached with Velcro. Eventually, this support can be used to facilitate the use of a conventional gesture such as a touch paired with communicative gaze or a giving gesture. By providing a successful means of communication, augmentative communication has also been shown to be an effective support for preventing or replacing challenging behaviors (Frea et al. 2001; Mirenda 1997).

At the Language Partner stage, partners are taught to use a range of augmentative communication methods depending upon the unique learning style of the individual with ASD as well as the unique requirements of specific social contexts (e.g., sign language, photographs or graphic symbols, or Speech Generating Devices (SGDs)). These supports can foster a range of word types, early word combinations, and creative simple sentence structures. For example, the use of color coding paired with photographs and graphics can be incorporated across social partners and natural routines to foster agent + action + object word combinations. For example, during a snack routine at school, a placemat menu might be created with photographic representations of a student's teachers (e.g., "Emily" and "Amy") enhanced with a thick red border; graphic representations of different actions (e.g., "open," "help," "cut," "eat") enhanced with a thick green border; and graphic representations of different objects in that activity (e.g., "yogurt," "juice," and "pizza") enhanced with a thick yellow border. The student could then be provided with a sentence template that includes a blank white box with a red border, a blank white box with a green border, and blank white box with a yellow border to elicit an agent + action + object word combination. These augmentative supports have shown promise for fostering initiation of early sentences and creative word combinations (Binger et al. 2010).

At the Conversational Partner stage, the provision of augmentative communication to foster expressive communication and language might be used to help an individual follow the conventions for initiating and taking turns in conversation (ASHA 2006; Charlop-Christy and Kelso 2003; Johnston et al. 2003; Krantz and McClannahan 1993). For example, at recess, a student might be provided with a small notebook with the names or photographs of each of his or her classmates included on separate pages. Written conversation starters related to the classmate's preferred topics might then be provided on each page.

Partner Uses Visual and Organizational Support As part of the comprehensive approach of the SCERTS Model, focused intervention strategies such as the use of visual supports for enhancing smooth transitions, defining steps within a task, and organizing segments of time across the day are embraced (Pierce and Schreibman 1994; Prizant et al. 2006). Visual supports are also seen as essential for enhancing attention and active engagement in group activities (ASHA 2006; Barry and Burlew 2004; Goldstein and Cisar 1992). These types of supports are viewed as lifespan transactional supports within the SCERTS Model. Partners are taught to implement concrete visual tools for those at the Social Partner stage (e.g., using actual objects to represent upcoming transitions), using photographs or graphic symbols for the Language Partner stage, and the written word for the Conversational Partner stage. Rather than fading these supports, the support is modified to reflect the current developmental stage, and particularly, for those making the transition to more advanced stages and/or into adulthood, the responsibility of creating the supports is shifted to the individual with ASD (Watanabe and Sturmey 2003).

Partner Modifies Goals, Activities, and the Learning Environment For individuals with ASD, challenges in predicting the intentions of others, social monitoring, and initiating bids for mutual regulation can create significant hurdles in educational programs, particularly when the learning environment is focused on adult-directed tasks, which may or may not have a clear intent that is visually apparent. Thus, an individual with ASD may not be able to predict why they are being asked to engage in a specific task and may, in turn, not cooperate or may disengage secondary to limitations in the ability to seek assistance and comfort in a conventional manner. In the SCERTS Model, partners are provided guidance so that they can make conscious and proactive modifications such as adjusting task difficulty to ensure success, ensuring tasks are developmentally appropriate and ensuring that motivating and meaningful endpoints are embedded in activities. These modifications are essential tools for differentiated instruction for individuals with ASD. For example, at the Social Partner stage, teachers are provided with coaching to ensure that academic activities are suited to the neurodevelopmental level of the individual usually requiring the introduction of materials that enable sensory-motor exploration (e.g., cause-effect, music, rhythm, and multisensory stimulation). At the Conversational Partner stage, the emphasis shifts toward project-based instruction as a means to ensure that the individual with ASD is able to predict why they are engaged in a task. For example, one kindergarten teacher modified a daily handwriting practice by changing it from simply writing the three words of the day on the paper as a rote practice strategy to embedding those words in a fill-in-the-blank letter of the day (e.g., a birthday card to a student in the class, a letter to the school principal, or an invitation for an upcoming class event). Embedding handwriting and sight word practice into this meaningful project served as a key strategy that fostered active engagement and participation in her student with ASD and was also quite beneficial for her typically developing students as well.

Future Research

While efficacy research on focused approaches and intervention strategies provides an invaluable contribution to the field of ASD, these strategies are typically aimed at training specific skills or improving specific areas of need in individuals with ASD. Comprehensive approaches, such as the SCERTS Model, shift this focus toward a broader goal of improving overall quality of life and improving outcome over time by establishing educational goals most predictive of long-term positive outcomes and ensuring that more focused interventions for these goals are embedded in natural activities, across partners and settings, and over time. The SCERTS Model and its curriculum-based assessment have been derived from descriptive group research studies indicating that developmental achievements in the domains of social communication and emotional regulation are predictive of longer-term gains in language acquisition, social adaptive functioning, self-determination, and academic achievement, areas which foster social competence into adulthood (Prizant et al. 2006). In addition, the SCERTS Model is most focused on acquisition of meaningful abilities in social communication and emotional regulation that can be applied across natural activities, settings, and across many partners. Thus, the transactional support domain has been developed to support a high level of awareness of the critical impact of partner behavior and ensures that all team members are "on the same page" by providing essential elements for monitoring treatment fidelity and progress across partners and contexts.

There is a critical need to operationalize more comprehensive approaches and evaluate their effectiveness in the contexts where they will be most relevant. To date, few randomized controlled trials of a comprehensive approaches for school-aged children with ASD, in particular, have been conducted in public school settings, which is the most ecologically valid and sustainable context for the delivery of services. The SCERTS Model manuals (Prizant et al. 2006) were written to provide an impetus for this type of intervention research and were designed to address many of the acknowledged inadequacies of available research. When a comprehensive approach is "manualized," i.e., guided by a detailed comprehensive manual, it ensures for greater fidelity of practice, thereby improving the quality of the research in question. We are confident that ongoing and future research in the SCERTS Model will contribute to the body of literature on how to most effectively support individuals with ASD and their families.

References

American Speech-Language-Hearing Association (ASHA) (2006). Guidelines for speech-language pathologists in diagnosis, assessment, and treatment of autism spectrum disorders across the life span. http://www.asha.org/docs/html/gl2006-00049.html. Accessed 28 December 2011.

Barry, L. M., & Burlew, S. B. (2004). Using social stories to teach choice and play skills to children with autism. *Focus on Autism and Other Developmental Disabilities, 19,* 45–51.

Binger, C., Kent-Walsh, J., Ewing, C., & Taylor, S. (2010). Teaching educational assistants to facilitate the multisymbol message productions of young students who require augmentative and alternative communication. *American Journal of Speech-Language Pathology, 19,* 108–120.

Bryan, L. C., & Gast, D. L. (2000). Teaching on-task and on-schedule behaviors to higher functioning children with autism via picture activity schedules. *Journal of Autism and Developmental Disorders, 30,* 553–567.

Charlop-Christy, M. H., & Kelso, S. E. (2003). Teaching children with autism conversational speech using a cue card/written script program. *Education and Treatment of Children, 26,* 103–127.

Frea, W. D., Arnold, C., & Vittimberga, G. L. (2001). A demonstration of the effects of augmentative communication on the extreme aggressive behavior of a child with autism within an integrated preschool setting. *Journal of Positive Behavior Interventions, 3,* 194–198.

Garrison-Harrell, L., Kamps, D., & Kravits, T. (1997). The effects of peer networks on social-communicative behaviors for students with autism. *Focus on Autism and Other Developmental Disabilities, 12,* 241–254.

Gilchrist, A., Green, J., Cox, A., Burton, D., Rutter, M., & Le Couteur, A. (2001). Development and current functioning in adolescents with Asperger syndrome: A comparative study. *Journal of Child Psychology and Psychiatry, 42*(2), 227–240.

Goldstein, H., & Cisar, C. L. (1992). Promoting interaction during sociodramatic play. Teaching scripts to typical preschoolers and classmates with disabilities. *Journal of Applied Behavior Analysis, 25,* 265–280.

Horner, R. H., Carr, E. G., Strain, P. S., Todd, A. W., & Reed, H. K. (2002). Problem behavior interventions for young children with autism: A research synthesis. *Journal of Autism and Developmental Disorders, 32,* 423–446.

Johnston, S., Nelson, C., Evans, J., & Palazolo, K. (2003). The use of visual supports in teaching young children with autism spectrum disorder to initiate interactions. *Augmentative and Alternative Communication, 19,* 86–103.

Kalyva, E., & Avramidis, E. (2005). Improving communication between children with autism and their peers through the 'circle of friends': A small-scale intervention study. *Journal of Applied Research in Intellectual Disabilities, 18,* 253–261.

Koegel, R. L., Koegel, L. K., & Dunlap, G. (Eds.). (1996). *Positive Behavioral Support: Including people with difficult behavior in the community.* Baltimore: Paul H. Brookes.

Klin, A., & Volkmar, F. R. (2003). Asperger syndrome: Diagnosis and external validity. *Child and Adolescent Psychiatric Clinics of North America, 12,* 1–13.

Krantz, P.J., & McClannahan, L. E. (1993). Teaching children with autism to initiate to peers: Effects of a script-fading procedure. *Journal of Applied Behavior Analysis, 26,* 121–132.

Laurent, A. C., & Rubin, E. (2004). Challenges in emotional regulation in Asperger syndrome and high-functioning autism. *Topics in Language Disorders, 24*(4), 286–297.

Light, J., Roberts, B., Dimarco, R., & Greiner, N. (1998). Augmentative and alternative communication to support receptive and expressive language for people with autism. *Journal of Communication Disorders, 31,* 153–180.

Little, L. (2001). Peer victimization of children with Asperger spectrum disorders. *Journal of the American Academy of Child and Adolescent Psychiatry, 40*(9), 995–996.

MacDuff, G. S., Krantz, P. J., & McClannahan, L. E. (1993). Teaching children with autism to use photographic activity schedules: Maintenance and generalization of complex response chains. *Journal of Applied Behavior Analysis, 26,* 89–97.

Martinez-Pons, M. (1996). Test of a model of parental inducement of academic self-regulation. *The Journal of Experimental Education, 64,* 213–227.

McDuffie, A., & Yoder, P. (2010). Types of parent verbal responsiveness that predict language in young children with autism spectrum disorders. *Journal of Speech, Language, and Hearing Research, 53,* 1026–1039.

Miller, L. J., Robinson, J., & Moulton, D. (2004). Sensory modulation dysfunction: Identification in early childhood. In R. Del-Carmen-Wiggins, & A. Carter (Eds.), *Handbook of infant, toddler, and preschool mental health assessment* (pp. 247–270). New York: Oxford University Press.

Mirenda, P. (1997). Functional communication training and augmentative communication: A research review. *Augmentative and Alternative Communication, 13,* 207–225.

Mirenda, P. (2003). Toward functional augmentative and alternative communication for students with autism: Manual signs, graphic symbols, and voice output communication aids. *Language, Speech, and Hearing Services in Schools, 34,* 202–215.

National Research Council (NRC). (2000). *From neurons to neighborhoods.* Washington: National Academy Press.

National Research Council (NRC). Committee on Educational Interventions for Children with Autism, Division of Behavioral and Social Sciences and Education. (2001). *Educating children with autism.* Washington: National Academy Press.

Odom, S. L., Brown, W. H., Frey, T., Karasu, N., Smith-Canter, L. L., & Strain, P. S. (2003). Evidence-based practices for young children with autism: Contributions from single-subject design research. *Focus on Autism and Other Developmental Disabilities, 18,* 166–175.

Pierce, K., & Schreibman, L. (1994). Teaching daily living skills to children with autism in unsupervised settings through pictorial self-management. *Journal of Applied Behavior Analysis, 27,* 471–482.

Prizant, B. M. (2009). The primacy of trust. Part I. *Autism Spectrum Quarterly, Fall,* 32–34.

Prizant, B. M., & Carley, M. J. (2009). The primacy of trust. Part II. *Autism Spectrum Quarterly, Winter,* 29–32.

Prizant, B. M., & Laurent, A. C. (2011). Behavior is not the issue: An emotional regulation perspective on problem behavior. Part I. *Autism Spectrum Quarterly, Spring,* 28–30. (Part II, Winter, 34–37).

Prizant, B. M., Wetherby, A. M., Rubin, E., & Laurent, A. C. (2003). The SCERTS® model: A transactional, family-centered approach to enhancing communication and socioemotional abilities of children with autism spectrum disorder. *Infants and Young Children, 16*(4), 296–316.

Prizant, B., Wetherby, A., Rubin, E., Laurent, A., & Rydell, P. (2006). *The SCERTS® model: A comprehensive educational approach for children with autism spectrum disorders* (Vols. 1 and 2). Baltimore: Paul H. Brookes.

Rubin, E., Laurent, A. C., Prizant, B. M., & Wetherby, A. M. (2008). AAC and the SCERTS® Model; incorporating AAC within a comprehensive, multidisciplinary educational program. In P. Mirenda, & T. Iacono (Eds.), *Autism and Augmentative and Alternative Communication (AAC)* (pp. 195–218). Baltimore: Paul H. Brookes.

Rydell, A., Berlin, L., & Bohlin, G. (2003). Emotionality, emotion regulation, and adaptation among 5- to 8-year-old children. *Emotion, 3,* 30–47.

Rydell, P., & Prizant, B. (1995). Assessment and intervention strategies for children who use echolalia. In K. Quill (Ed.), *Teaching children with autism: Strategies to enhance communication and socialization* (pp. 105–129). Albany: Delmar.

Saulnier, C. A., & Klin, A. (2007). Brief report: Social and communication abilities and disabilities in higher functioning individuals with autism and Asperger syndrome. *Journal of Autism and Developmental Disorders, 37*(4), 788–793.

Schlosser, R. W., & Lee, D. (2000). Promoting generalization and maintenance in augmentative and alternative communication: A meta-analysis of 20 years of effectiveness research. *Augmentative and Alternative Communication, 16,* 208–227.

Simpson, R. L., de Boer-Ott, S. R., & Myles, B. S. (2003). Inclusion of learners with autism spectrum disorders in general education settings. *Topics in Language Disorders, 23*(2), 116–133.

Tantam, D. (2000). Adolescence and adulthood of individuals with Asperger syndrome. In A. Klin, F. R. Volkmar, S. S. Sparrow (Eds.), *Asperger syndrome* (pp. 367–399). New York: The Guilford Press.

Thiemann, K., & Goldstein, H. (2004). Effects of peer training and written-text cueing on social communication of school-age children with pervasive developmental disorder. *Journal of Speech, Language, and Hearing Research, 47,* 126–144.

Thorp, D. M., Stahmer, A. C., & Schreibman, L. (1995). The effects of sociodramatic play training on children with autism. *Journal of Autism and Developmental Disorders, 25,* 265–282.

Tsatsanis, K. D. (2003). Outcome research in Asperger syndrome and autism. *Child and Adolescent Psychiatric Clinics of North America, 12,* 45–63.

Tsatsanis, K. D. (2004). Heterogeneity in learning style in Asperger syndrome and high-functioning autism. *Topics in Language Disorders, 24*(4), 260–270.

Tsatsanis, K. D., Foley, C., & Donehower, C. (2004). Contemporary outcome research and programming guidelines for Asperger syndrome and high-functioning autism. *Topics in Language Disorders, 24*(4), 249–259.

Volkmar, F. R., Lord, C., Bailey, A., Schultz, R. T., & Klin, A. (2004). Autism and pervasive developmental disorders. *Journal of Child Psychology and Psychiatry, 45,* 145–170.

Walker, H. M., Ramsay, E., & Gresham, F. M. (2004). *Antisocial behavior in school: Evidence-based practices.* Belmont: Thomson/Wadsworth Learning Publishing.

Watanabe, M., & Sturmey, P. (2003). The effect of choice-making opportunities during activity schedules on task engagement of adults with autism. *Journal of Autism and Developmental Disorders, 33,* 535–538.

Wetherby, A., & Woods, J. (2006). Effectiveness of early intervention for children with autism spectrum disorders beginning in the second year of life. *Topics in Early Childhood Special Education, 26,* 67–68.

Chapter 7
Maximizing Global Access to Effective Treatment: Center for Autism and Related Disorders (CARD), CARD eLearning™, and Skills™

Doreen Granpeesheh, Adel C. Najdowski and Evelyn R. Gould

The Center for Autism and Related Disorders (CARD) was founded in 1990 by Dr. Doreen Granpeesheh. CARD provides services to approximately 1,200 children around the globe ranging in age from less than 1 year up to 21 years old, with a diagnosis of Autistic Disorder, Asperger's Disorder, Pervasive Developmental Disorder-Not Otherwise Specified (PDD-NOS), or any other developmental delays typical of an autism spectrum disorder (ASD), including children at-risk for a diagnosis of autism.

CARD offers a range of different services, including behavioral, diagnostic, and psychometric assessments; specialized outpatient services, such as feeding and challenging behavior interventions; early intensive behavioral intervention (EIBI) to children (0–8 years) in the child's home, school, and community; and programs for older clients (9–21 years) focusing on increasing independent living, leisure, social, and communication skills. CARD also provides training to parents and other professionals through the provision of continuing education classes and online trainings.

There are currently 21 CARD offices in the USA (across seven states) and two international offices, with one in New Zealand and the other in Australia. CARD also has affiliate sites in the United Arab Emirates and South Africa and provides services through a consultative workshop model to families all over the world. It is CARD's mission to provide global access to the highest quality of behavioral intervention to children with autism. In an effort to achieve this mission and to extend the dissemination of the CARD model both to families and to other treatment providers, CARD has developed two web-based programs: CARD eLearning™ and Skills™. CARD eLearning™ is a web-based program for training individuals to deliver behavioral intervention to children with autism, and Skills™ is a web-based tool that provides three basic resources for individuals designing behavioral intervention programs: (1) a comprehensive assessment, (2) lesson plans within a set of curricula linked directly from items flagged in the assessment, and

D. Granpeesheh (✉) · A. C. Najdowski · E. R. Gould
Center for Autism and Related Disorders, 19019 Ventura Blvd Suite 300, Tarzana, CA 91356, USA
e-mail: doreen@centerforautism.com

S. Goldstein, J. A. Naglieri (eds.), *Interventions for Autism Spectrum Disorders*,
DOI 10.1007/978-1-4614-5301-7_7,

(3) a tracking system which graphically depicts the child's progress during behavioral intervention.

This chapter will describe the CARD model and the development of its dissemination tools: CARD eLearning™ and Skills™. We will begin with a description of the core assumptions at the heart of the CARD treatment model and the key features of typical CARD early intervention programs. Finally, we will provide overviews of CARD eLearning™ and Skills™ and outline how these web solutions further CARD's mission to extend the CARD treatment model and high-quality applied behavior analysis (ABA)-based services globally to as many families and children as possible.

Assumptions at the Heart of the CARD Treatment Model

CARD treatment programs are based on core behavior principles of ABA and a philosophy that providing a holistic approach to treat the child within their home, school, and community is essential to best outcome. With the right treatment, we believe that recovery from autism is possible (see Granpeesheh 2008 and Granpeesheh et al. 2009c for discussions of recovery). In treating thousands of children over the course of over 20 years, we have seen many children recover from autism (Granpeesheh et al. 2009c). That is, with the right treatment, some children with autism reach the point where they no longer display clinically significant impairments related to autism; are indistinguishable from typical peers on standardized tests of intelligence, language, socialization, and daily living skills; are earning passing grades in a regular classroom without support; and no longer qualify for an autism spectrum diagnosis as evaluated by a qualified professional. Although this is one goal of intervention for this population, it is the outcome for a group of children with particular characteristics and is not the single most important goal for each child. Rather, the goal for each child is always to help him or her reach the maximum potential possible in order to live life to the fullest.

The CARD approach to intervention is rooted in ABA, which is the application of scientifically supported principles of learning and motivation to socially significant behavior change (i.e., to increase adaptive behaviors and decrease problematic ones), while experimentally demonstrating that the procedures employed are responsible for that behavior change. The scientific evidence supporting the use of ABA for children with autism has led several independent bodies to acknowledge and endorse its use for children with autism, including the US Surgeon General (US Department of Health and Human Services 1999), the New York State Department of Health (New York State Department of Health, Early Intervention Program 1999), the National Academy of Sciences (National Research Council 2001), and the American Academy of Pediatrics (Myers and Plauché Johnson 2007). In 2010, Vismara and Rogers of the MIND Institute stated, "ABA is an educational-behavioral intervention for children with ASD that has generated the most extensive research and thus has been identified as the treatment of choice to address learning deficits" (Vismara and Rogers 2010, p. 460). The impact of such endorsements is evidenced by public policy changes, such as state-level legislative decisions mandating insurance coverage for ABA treatment (e.g., Steven's Law 2008). Taking an ABA approach to intervention reflects several core assumptions at the heart of the CARD treatment model. Firstly, a person's behavior is a result of complex interactions between that person and his or her environment, thus people are not just "slaves to their genes," and behavior is not "fixed."

Secondly, everything that a person says or does is considered behavior, including covert behaviors, such as thoughts, feelings, beliefs, and desires. These two assumptions suggest that both overt and covert behaviors are amenable to change through the manipulation of environmental variables.

Thus, our third assumption is that all individuals, with and without autism or other disabilities, are capable of learning (though not everyone will learn at the same rate or in the same way). A person's disability or "label" cannot be used to explain why a behavior or skill is occurring or not occurring or why a teaching procedure or intervention plan fails.

The importance of environment in shaping a person's behavior leads to a fourth assumption: continuous learning opportunities (helpful and problematic) are presented in the environment throughout our waking hours as we interact with people and objects and engage in everyday activities. Typically, developing children appear to learn effortlessly from their environment continuously, whereas children with autism spectrum disorders do not. Thus, CARD treatment programs maximize both structured and unstructured teaching opportunities during therapy sessions and train individuals primarily interacting with the child outside of sessions (family members, teachers, classroom aides, etc.) to continue to capture and contrive learning opportunities at other times of the day. In addition, all efforts are made to identify and remove any barriers that may be hindering the child's ability to attend to and benefit from environmental teaching opportunities. This may include the implementation of dietary, medical, or other interventions that may improve the child's ability to sleep, attend, and learn.

Our fifth assumption is that, in order to track progress and ensure that intervention is effective and individualized, ABA-based interventions require ongoing data collection and data monitoring. At CARD, accountability and reliable demonstration that treatment procedures are effective are essential. Detailed data collection and data monitoring allow CARD clinicians to make any needed changes to treatment procedures so that every child reaches his or her full potential and achieves the best quality of life possible.

The final assumption at the heart of the CARD treatment model is that family members should always participate in treatment. The family is generally the child's primary environment and thus plays an essential role in shaping and maintaining the child's skills. There must also be a good contextual fit between every child's individualized treatment plan and his or her personal, social, and educational environments. Parent training and participation are thus a vital part of the CARD treatment process. Family participation helps to identify skills which may be most functional for their child and to identify which behaviors are most problematic. It is also essential for the reduction of challenging behavior and the maintenance and generalization of skills throughout the child's daily life (Moes and Frea 2000, 2002).

CARD Model of ABA Treatment

CARD treatment programs share key components of programs oftentimes referred to as "EIBI" or "Intensive Behavioral Treatment" (Howard et al. 2005; Love et al. 2009; Sallows and Graupner 2005; Tarbox and Granpeesheh 2011). These key components are as follows:

1. Intervention begins as early as possible;
2. Intervention is intensive;
3. Intervention is supervised by qualified and experienced individuals;
4. Treatment plans are comprehensive and individualized;
5. Treatment procedures are rooted in ABA; and
6. The ultimate goal is integration into a mainstream classroom setting.

In addition, CARD programs are built on an overall holistic approach and emphasize the importance of treating the whole child by considering his or her health, sleep patterns, and sensory issues. Let us now examine each of these components of the CARD Model in more detail.

Intervention Begins as Early as Possible

CARD therapy programs are initiated as early as possible (typically around age 2–3 years). Research has shown that children who begin ABA treatment between the ages of 20 and 59 months have an increased likelihood of an optimal outcome (Fenske et al. 1985; Granpeesheh et al. 2009a).

Intervention is Intensive

At CARD, the intensity of services is based on each child's educational, social, and behavioral needs, and duration of treatment is determined by how fast a child progresses through curricula, with the optimal outcome being recovery. Typically, CARD early intervention programs involve between 30–40 h per week of 1:1 intervention provided by trained CARD therapists for at least 2 years. This level of treatment intensity is consistent with research suggesting that high intensity programs (i.e., 30–40 h per week) are associated with significant child progress (e.g., Cohen et al. 2006; Granpeesheh et al. 2009b; Green 1996; Lovaas 1987; Reed et al. 2007; Sallows and Graupner 2005) and that optimal progress is seen when intervention is provided consistently for at least 2 years (Granpeesheh et al. 2009b; Green 1996; Lovaas 1987; Sallows and Graupner 2005).

Granpeesheh et al. (2009a) note that, while some children have achieved an optimal outcome in less than 2 years, it is more common for children to continue ABA treatment for approximately 4 years. Treatment intensity is generally decreased as the child's functional skills develop and skill deficits diminish, allowing the child to integrate into typical educational and social settings.

Intervention is Supervised by Qualified and Experienced Individuals

Effective EIBI programs are supervised by experienced and suitably qualified individuals (Love et al. 2009). At CARD, we refer to these individuals as "clinical supervisors." Their role is to direct the course of each child's treatment and to train therapists and family members to implement treatment protocols and collaborate with other service providers (e.g., speech language pathologists, occupational therapists, classroom teachers). Doing so involves regularly meeting with the rest of the treatment team and parents of each child.

Every CARD supervisor possesses a master's degree or is actively seeking a master's degree. Each supervisor also has advanced training and experience in the provision of EIBI to children with ASDs. Each CARD supervisor is also strongly encouraged to become a Board Certified Behavior Analyst (BCBA), and at the time of this writing, 45 supervisors at CARD are board certified, making CARD perhaps the largest employer of board certified individuals providing behavioral treatment for autism spectrum disorders today.

All CARD treatment team members, from the parent right up to the highest-level clinicians, are required to partake in comprehensive training designed to teach them how to provide the best quality ABA-based treatment possible. Training procedures at CARD are intensive, ongoing, and based on published research on staff training (e.g., Bolton and Mayer 2008; Leblanc et al. 2005; Sarokoff and Sturmey 2004; Schepis et al. 2001; Sturmey 2008; Thomson et al. 2009).

Treatment Plans are Comprehensive and Individualized

The primary goal of treatment at CARD is to maximize the child's strengths and remediate the child's deficits by developing a unique and individualized program based on each child's specific needs. Skills taught must be functional, age appropriate, and consistent with overall program goals. Over the past 20 years, doctoral and master's-level clinicians and researchers at CARD developed a fully comprehensive internal assessment and set of curricula that allow CARD supervisors to design the most effective treatment program for each child. CARD's assessments and curricula cover all areas of the child development, including: social, motor, language, adaptive, play, executive functions, cognition, and academic skills, as well as a focus on higher level complex behavior, such as perspective taking (Theory of Mind), complex social language, and executive functions.

In order to formulate an individualized program, all children are fully assessed across all areas of functioning as mentioned above using well-validated psychometric assessments, questionnaires, and direct observation. Assessments administered include diagnostic evaluations, intelligence and developmental assessments, assessments of adaptive behavior, motor and visual-motor skills, psychoeducational tests, assessments of speech and language, social skills, play, executive functioning or neuropsychology, and other assessments. Measures are selected based on each child's unique needs. Refer to Table. 7.1 for a complete list of assessments administered at CARD. After determining a child's individual skills and needs, supervisors can begin the process of curriculum design, choosing what to teach based on the child's assessment results and creating customized lessons to teach each target skill.

CARD has developed eight curricula to address all eight of the developmental areas of functioning (social, motor, language, adaptive, play, executive functions, cognition, and academic skills). The Social curriculum emphasizes teaching the child skills that will maximize successful social functioning. The child learns social rules, social interaction and relationship-building skills, and how to use social language successfully. The Motor curriculum focuses on teaching fine motor (e.g., hand skills, such as twisting, and finger skills, such as the pincer grasp), gross motor (e.g., jumping, catching), and visual motor skills (e.g., tracking, scanning). The Language curriculum focuses on teaching the child to understand language by teaching concepts such as matching and receptive identification and to use language functionally by teaching concepts such as using language to request, label, and converse. The Adaptive curriculum teaches personal (e.g., teeth brushing, toileting), domestic (e.g., making the bed), safety (e.g., stranger safety, using safety equipment), and community skills (e.g., restaurant skills). The Play curriculum starts by teaching the child appropriate toy play skills (e.g., sensorimotor and manipulative play, constructive play, pretend play) and then progresses to teaching the child to use his or her play skills socially in play with peers. The Executive Functions curriculum teaches the child skills that are necessary for goal-directed behavior. This includes teaching skills related to inhibition, attention, flexibility, memory, problem solving, planning, and self-management. The Cognition curriculum focuses on teaching the child to understand and respond to the mental states of others, thereby allowing the child to predict others' behavior and modify his or her interactions with others in order to make the interactions more effective (perspective taking or Theory of Mind). Some example topics covered in the Cognition curriculum include desires, emotions, senses, physical states, thinking, preferences, knowing, beliefs, deception, sarcasm, and intention. Finally, the Academic curriculum emphasizes skills related to math and language arts. In total, the CARD curricula are made up of almost 4,000 individual activities that teach skills comprised of over 40,000 individual instructional targets.

Treatment Procedures are Rooted in ABA

EIBI programs utilize scientifically validated intervention techniques based on the principles of behavior analysis (Love et al. 2009). CARD programs incorporate a

Table 7.1 Assessment instruments

Type of measure	Instrument	Reference
Diagnostic	Autism Diagnostic Interview Revised (ADI-R)	Rutter et al. 2003
	Autism Diagnostic Observation Schedule (ADOS)	Lord et al. 1999
	C.A.R.D Autism Symptoms Questionnaire (CARD ASQ)	
	Childhood Autism Rating Scale (CARS)	Schopler et al. 1988
	Checklist for Autism in Toddlers (CHAT)	Baron-Cohen et al. 2000
	Gilliam Asperger's Disorder Scale (GADS)	Gilliam 2001
	Gilliam Autism Rating Scale—Second Edition (GARS-II)	Gilliam 2006
	Pervasive Developmental Disorders Behavior Inventory (PDDBI)	Cohen and Sudhalter 1999
Intelligence	Differential Abilities Scales (DAS)	Elliott 1990
	Leiter International Performance Scale—Revised (Leiter-R)	Roid and Miller 1997
	Merrill-Palmer-Revised Scales of Development (M-P-R)	Roid and Sampers 2004
	Wechsler Intelligence Scale for Children—Fourth Edition (WISC-IV)	Wechsler et al. 2004
	Wechsler Preschool and Primary Scale of Intelligence—Third Edition (WPPSI-III)	Wechsler 2002
Developmental	Bayley Scales of Infant and Toddler Development—Third Edition (Bayley-III)	Bayley 2006
	Brigance Diagnostic Inventory of Early Development—Second Edition (IED-II)	Brigance 2004
	The Developmental Profile II (DP-II)	Alpern et al. 1980
Adaptive behavior	Vineland Adaptive Behavior Scales—Second Edition (Vineland-II)	Sparrow et al. 2005
Motor	Test of Gross Motor Development—Second Edition (TGMD−2)	Ulrich 2000
Visual-motor	Beery-Buktenica Developmental Test of Visual-Motor Integration—Fifth Edition (Beery VMI−5)	Beery and Beery 2004
Psycho-educational	Psychoeducational Profile—Third Edition (PEP—3)	Schopler et al. 2005
Speech and language	Clinical Evaluation of Language Fundamentals—Third Edition (CELF—4)	Semel et al. 2003
	Clinical Evaluation of Language Fundamentals—Preschool (CELF—P)	Wiig et al. 1992
Speech and language	Goldman—Fristoe—Woodcock—Test of Auditory Discrimination	Goldman et al. 1970
	Peabody Picture Vocabulary Test—Third Edition (PPVT-III)	Dunn and Dunn 1997
	Preschool Language Scale—Fourth Edition (PLS—4)	Zimmerman et al. 2002
	Rossetti Infant—Toddler Language Scale	Rossetti 1990
	Test of Language Development: Intermediate—Third Edition (TOLD-I:3)	Hammill and Newcomer 1997
	Test of Language Development—Fourth Edition (TOLD-P:4)	Newcomer and Hammill 2008
	Test of Problem Solving—Third Edition (TOPS-3)	Bowers et al. 2005

Table 7.1 Continued

Type of measure	Instrument	Reference
Pragmatic language	Test of Pragmatic Language—Second Edition (TOPL-2)	Phelps-Terasaki and Phelps-Gunn 2007
Social skills and play	Social Behavior Assessment Inventory (SBAI)	Stephens and Arnold 1992
	Social Skills Improvement System Rating Scales (SSIS)	Gresham and Elliott 2008
	Social Responsiveness Scale (SRS)	Constantino and Gruber 2005
	Symbolic Play Scale	Westby 1991
Executive functioning/ neuropsychology	Behavior Rating Inventory of Executive Function—Preschool Version (BRIEF-P)	Gioia et al. 2003
	Behavior Rating Inventory of Executive Function (BRIEF)	Gioia et al. 2000
	Children's Color Trails Test (CCTT)	Llorente et al. 2003
	The Auditory Sequential Memory Test	Wepman and Morency 1973
	Test of Auditory Discrimination (ADT)	Wepman and Reynolds 1987
	The Stroop Color and Word Test	Golden 1978
	Wisconsin Card Sorting Test	Grant et al. 1993
Treatment evaluation	Autism Treatment Evaluation Checklist (ATEC)	Rimland and Edelson 1999
Achievement	Johnson III Tests of Achievement	Woodcock et al. 2001
Other	Aberrant Behavior Checklist (ABC)	Aman and Singh 1986
	Behavior Assessment System for Children (BASC-2)	Reynolds and Kamphaus 2004
	Clinical Global Impression (CGI)	Guy and Bonato 1970
	Parenting Stress Index (PSI)	Abidin 1995

variety of behavior analytic procedures shown to be effective with children with autism and common to all good ABA programs (Tarbox and Granpeesheh 2011). Procedures include prompting and fading, discrimination training, preference assessment, shaping, chaining, and explicit programming for maintenance and generalization. Procedures are always selected and tailored according to each child's individual needs. A full review of the different behavioral procedures used at CARD is beyond the scope of this chapter, but we provide an outline describing the most commonly used procedures for those new to ABA techniques. The most common teaching techniques used at CARD are discrete trial teaching (DTT), natural environment training (NET), and fluency-based instruction (FBI). DTT, a scientifically supported teaching procedure for children with autism (Tarbox and Granpeesheh 2011), is a therapist-led procedure delivered in a 1:1 setting and is frequently used to teach discrimination skills (e.g., how to vocally label objects and how to receptively identify objects). DTT involves breaking down complex skills into basic units of behavior that are taught through a series of discrete teaching trials. In this way, multiple learning opportunities are presented to the child within a short period of time. Blocks of discrete trials are continuously presented until the child reaches a predetermined mastery criterion (e.g., 80–100 % correct over a predetermined number of trial blocks).

The beginning of each discrete trial is signaled by an instruction. The child then has the opportunity to respond (usually within 3–5 s). The therapist uses prompts to guide the child to the correct response, fading the prompts as the child begins to acquire the target skill. Immediately following the child's response, a consequence is delivered, signaling the end of the trial and providing feedback to the child regarding his or her response (i.e., whether he or she was correct). A desired response typically results in deliverance of a favored item, activity, and/or praise. Inappropriate responses, on the other hand, are followed by vocal feedback (e.g., "no" or "try again") and are usually followed by an error correction procedure.

Unlike DTT, NET procedures are considered child led and involve therapists capturing and contriving teaching opportunities within the child's natural environment (e.g., during play activities, mealtimes, or routines such as getting dressed). Further, the natural consequence of the behavior acts as the reinforcer where possible (Cowan and Allen 2007; Delprato 2001). Therapists use prompting and fading as necessary to guide the child to demonstrate the target skill successfully. An advantage of NET is that skill generalization is encouraged, thus decreasing the need for additional generalization programming (e.g., Cowan and Allen 2007; Delprato 2001). NET is often used to teach language skills (e.g., Charlop-Christy and Carpenter 2000; Charlop-Christy and LeBlanc 1999; Koegel et al. 1998), play skills (Stahmer 1995; Stahmer et al. 2003; Thorpe et al. 1995), and social skills (e.g., Harper et al. 2008; Kaiser et al. 2000; Kohler et al. 2001; Krantz and McClannahan 1998).

FBI involves the use of a free operant procedure which essentially means that the child is given the opportunity to respond freely and as quickly as possible, undertaking a task for a period of time (usually anywhere from 10 s to 1 min). This procedure is employed to increase both the child's accuracy and speed in an attempt to allow the child to become fluent at a skill. Fluent performance is defined as the rate of responding necessary for competent performance (Binder 1996). FBI is commonly used to teach math and reading skills but can also be relevant to other skills (e.g., tying shoes, buttoning, speaking). FBI is often implemented once the child is performing accurately during DTT or NET sessions with the goal of now getting the child to perform the skill automatically and without hesitation (fluently).

Younger CARD clients aged between 1 and 3 years typically have programs containing more social and play-based targets, taught mostly through NET and an errorless learning approach, which involves providing the child with guidance to ensure that he or she is successful during every teaching opportunity, fading the level of guidance provided as the child becomes proficient at the target skill. CARD programs for children aged 3 and 5 years typically involve a broader range of skill targets taught via a combination of DTT and NET. FBI techniques are generally used once the child has demonstrated accuracy with a DTT or NET procedure in an effort to promote accuracy combined with speed (fluency).

In addition to teaching new skills, a goal of all CARD programs is the reduction of challenging behaviors, such as stereotypy, self-injury, aggression, and noncompliance, and the replacement of these with adaptive behaviors. This process begins with an assessment to identify the function of the behavior (i.e., the conditions under which the behavior occurs). Supervisors are then able to design an individualized behavior intervention plan based on the results of the functional assessment (for a discussion of function-based interventions, readers should refer to Filter and Horner 2009 and Ingram et al. 2005). CARD behavior intervention plans involve not only strategies for reducing challenging behavior when they occur but, also, strategies for *preventing* the behavior from occurring, as well as strategies for teaching appropriate replacement behaviors. CARD supervisors train both therapists and family members to implement behavior management protocols consistently and closely monitor the behavior to ensure the plan is effective.

Once the skills have been taught and challenging behavior has been reduced, the final step of the CARD treatment process is to ensure that maintenance and generalization are achieved (i.e., taught skills continue to be used over time and occur in the natural environment across people and in different settings, etc.). Generalization and maintenance rarely happen on their own; thus CARD supervisors design an individualized maintenance and generalization plan for each child and continuously monitor the plan to ensure that the strategies employed are successful (see Brown and Odom 1994; Ghezzi and Bishop 2008; Stokes and Baer 1977; and Stokes and Osnes 1989 for in-depth reviews of strategies for generalization and maintenance).

Ultimate Goal is Integration into a Classroom Setting

The ultimate goal of EIBI programs is most often the successful integration of the child into the classroom (Howard et al. 2005; Sallows and Graupner 2005). At CARD, treatment is typically conducted in the child's home initially and then generalized into classroom and community settings as appropriate for the child's age. The first year of CARD treatment typically consists of intensive work on language and behavior management. The second year involves a progression into social skills, developing into a focus on more abstract cognitive and executive functioning skills in the third year. The fourth and final year emphasizes a gradual fade out of services. However, children with less severe diagnoses of PDD-NOS or Asperger's Syndrome may require a focus on social, cognitive, and executive functioning skills, delivered through a more cognitive behavioral format. Ultimately, the progression of a child's treatment program will depend on his or her initial profile.

Other Features of CARD Treatment Programs

In addition to the above core EIBI features, all CARD programs incorporate a holistic philosophy emphasizing a need to treat the whole child, including acknowledging health and sensory needs. We believe that optimal learning occurs with stable health, adequate sleep, and functional regulation of sensory input. Therefore, the assessment process includes assessing sensory dysregulation in the visual, auditory, tactile, and proprioceptive modalities and conducting full medical and health evaluations wherever possible in order to identify any underlying or comorbid medical, sensory, or dietary issues that might destabilize the child's health, sleep, and ability to attend. CARD supervisors are then able to make adjustments to treatment procedures and materials wherever appropriate, so as to maximize treatment outcome.

Finally, at CARD we believe that every child has personal dignity, individuality, and self-determination; thus CARD treatment programs aim to continuously encourage the expression of personal beliefs, feelings, interests, and preferences.

Format of Service Delivery

Home-Based

For those children who reside within 30 miles of a CARD office, CARD offers home-based services. This format of service delivery involves CARD therapists conducting 1:1 therapy sessions in the child's home at regularly scheduled times. The majority of therapy is conducted in a designated "therapy room" with skills being targeted throughout the child's home where more appropriate. Home-based sessions provide excellent teaching opportunities by allowing increased access to the child's home environment, including his or her toys, daily living materials, and family routines.

Workshop-Based

For those families who are located outside the 30-mile radius or reside in a state or country without a CARD office, CARD offers remote clinical services. Remote clinical services begin with an initial 2–3-day workshop conducted in the child's home. The aim of this workshop is to assist the family in setting up a home-based CARD ABA treatment program with periodic consultation with a CARD clinical supervisor. The supervisor spends the first day of the initial workshop training family members and therapists in behavior principles, skill acquisition, and maintenance, behavior management techniques, and data collection. The next 1–2 days are spent teaching parents and therapists how to implement the child's CARD ABA treatment program successfully. Following the initial workshop, the supervisor continues to provide periodic consultation through face-to-face visits; phone or video conferences; and correspondence via fax, e-mail, or mail.

Outcome of the CARD Treatment Model

CARD's research and development department has published over 60 research articles in peer-reviewed scientific journals and has contributed over 25 chapters to edited scientific texts. CARD's scientific work spans several programs of research, including (a) assessment and treatment of challenging behavior, (b) procedures for teaching basic language and verbal behavior, (c) social skills interventions, (d) teaching independent living skills, (e) treatment of feeding disorders, (f) factors affecting outcome of EIBI, (g) teaching higher-order cognition and executive function skills,

(h) procedural and methodological innovations, (i) the role of technology in autism treatment, and (j) recovery from autism. Next, we briefly describe publications from each of these programs of research.

CARD research on challenging behavior has innovated nonintrusive treatment procedures for a variety of behaviors, such as rumination (Rhine and Tarbox 2009), bruxism (Barnoy et al. 2009), and domestic pet mistreatment (Bergstrom et al. 2011). CARD's research on basic language and verbal operants addresses a variety of topics including procedures for increasing the complexity of verbal imitation (Tarbox et al. 2009). CARD's research on social skills addresses areas of complex social cognition and understanding, including teaching foundational perspective-taking skills (Gould et al. 2011). CARD's research on independent living skills endeavors to produce new information on how children with autism can be taught to implement useful life skills independently, such as home safety skills (Summers et al. 2011) and pill-swallowing skills (Yoo et al. 2008). CARD's research on feeding disorders focuses on the application of nonintrusive treatments in real-life environments, such as parent-implemented home-based interventions for food refusal (Tarbox et al. 2010a). Research on the outcome of EIBI at CARD is oriented toward identifying how a multitude of variables impinges on the general outcome of EIBI, such as age and treatment intensity (Granpeesheh et al. 2009a). CARD's research on higher-order skills is focused on developing and evaluating behavioral teaching procedures for helping children with autism improve in areas such as executive functioning, including working memory (Baltruschat et al. 2011). CARD's research on procedural and methodological innovations investigates topics that hold promise for streamlining the treatment process and/or enhancing its efficiency, such as evaluating expedited data collection procedures (Najdowski et al. 2009). CARD researchers also maintain an active interest in the role of technology in autism treatment, including its potential for helping to aid in dissemination. CARD's research on technology includes studies on eLearning methods for staff training (Granpeesheh et al. 2010), electronic data collection during discrete trial training (Tarbox et al. 2010b), and validation of web-based curriculum assessments (Dixon et al. 2011).

We believe recovery from autism (as defined earlier in the chapter) is possible and have observed it with a substantial minority of CARD clients. Granpeesheh et al. (2009c) reported the results of a retrospective evaluation of 38 CARD children who had reached an optimal outcome by achieving a lack of clinically significant impairment and loss of ability to qualify for any ASD diagnosis. In line with previous findings in the published literature, we found that an intensity of 25 or more hours per week of behavioral intervention for 2 or more years, beginning at a young age (mean under 3.5), optimizes positive outcome, resulting in complete remediation of clinical symptoms for some children. Prospective research on the topic of recovery from autism is still very much needed, and such research is currently underway.

Maximizing Global Access to the CARD Model

Given the breadth of CARD's services to children with autism, robust staff training, and comprehensive scope of treatment as outlined up to this point, the demand for CARD services has reached an insatiable altitude creating the inability of CARD to service everyone through a CARD office or workshop model. In an effort to meet the level of demand through dissemination of the CARD model and to reach its mission of helping as many families affected by autism as possible, CARD has developed web-based versions of its training (called CARD eLearning™) and its skills assessment and curricula (called Skills™). Both CARD eLearning™ and Skills™ can be accessed on the Internet at www.skillsforautism.com.

CARD eLearning™

CARD eLearning™, a web-based version of the didactic portion of the therapist-level training conducted at CARD over the last 20 years, began development in 2002 and was completed in 2010. Therapists are the individuals delivering the one-to-one ABA-based intervention to children with autism. CARD eLearning is designed to train anyone (including parents, teachers, and other professionals) how to implement ABA-based techniques with children with autism in order to teach the children the skills they need and to decrease their challenging behavior. It is not necessary to have a college education to take the course. CARD eLearning™ assumes that the user has no previous knowledge about autism, ABA, or how to teach skills using ABA-based techniques.

CARD eLearning™ is a web-based interactive program that provides the equivalent of a 40-h training course. It is broken into nine modules with training in topics such as "What is Autism?," "What is ABA?," "Skill Repertoire Building," and "Behavior Management." Training is provided using narrated storyboards, which include videotaped demonstrations and examples of what is being taught so that trainees can view the techniques actually occurring with live therapists and children. Users can watch videos as many times as they want and pause to take notes which can be reviewed at anytime. Each module has an accompanying quiz which is taken to ensure that the user understands the material before moving to the next module. After the completion of the last module, the user is presented with a final exam. Upon passing the final exam at 85 % or better, the user is presented with a certificate of completion.

After completion of CARD eLearning, one can expect to have foundational knowledge in the principles and application of behavior analysis to the treatment of autism. In fact, research has demonstrated this outcome. In 2010, a study was published which demonstrated that CARD eLearning™ effectively increased the academic knowledge of newly hired staff in principles and procedures of ABA for autism (Granpeesheh et al. 2010).

In addition to the training that a direct user can get from CARD eLearning™, other ABA providers, schools, or other autism intervention providers can benefit from the ability to give the training to their staff. This makes CARD eLearning™ a useful time-saving tool for many organizations with the desire or need to train staff on the use of ABA to treat children with autism. Organizations that choose to utilize CARD eLearning™ in this manner are provided with reports that allow them to determine the performance of their staff in terms of their quiz and final exam scores, as well as how many times users take each quiz and the final exam before they pass. Likewise, the CARD eLearning™ final exam can be taken as a pretest to determine baseline levels of staff knowledge and as a posttest, after training, to measure the level of staff improvement. The final exam could also be used as a tool to weed out potential candidates applying for clinical positions within organizations.

One limitation of CARD eLearning™ is that it does not provide training in the hands-on practical application of what is taught during the course. Thus, it is recommended that CARD eLearning™ graduates obtain additional hands-on training from a qualified professional with a track record in delivering ABA-based intervention to children with autism. However, that said, current research underway at CARD is showing that therapists trained using CARD eLearning™ are able to perform sufficiently under hands-on, real-world conditions. The field performance of these therapists is being compared to a group of therapists who received a traditional in-person version of CARD eLearning on the same topics. So far, no significant difference between the groups has been found, suggesting that therapists trained through an eLearning format are performing equally as well during their hands-on training experience as individuals who are trained using an in-person version of CARD eLearning™.

Skills™

Skills™ is an online tool delivering CARD's comprehensive assessment and curriculum and providing a globally accessible repository for data storage and analysis allowing the progress to be tracked by all members of the child's treatment team (including parents, speech language pathologist, occupational therapists, and physicians). Based on CARD's comprehensive set of curricula, which have been in continuous development and use internally for the past 20 years (with new phases released regularly), the development of Skills™ was initiated in 2003 and was completed in 2010. The creation of Skills™ has now allowed for assessment to be directly linked to lesson activities within CARD's curricula and, thus, for progress within curricular areas and lessons to be tracked both at the level of lesson activities (e.g., labeling emotions), as well as at the level of each new target behavior learned (e.g., happy, sad, angry).

Skills™ was created as a tool for any individual involved in the assessment and treatment planning of a child with autism. This could include professionals (ABA providers, speech language pathologists, occupational therapists, physicians, etc.), school teachers, and parents. Skills™ was created with the aim of promoting a multidisciplinary approach in which everyone on a child's treatment team is able to input data on the interventions they are implementing with the child and view their effects on learning all at once.

It is highly recommended that at least one person on a child's treatment team using Skills™ is a BCBA or an equally qualified professional with a track record of designing ABA-based interventions for children with autism. The role of this individual is to design and direct the child's curriculum program within Skills™.

Five Steps to Skills™

There are five steps involved in using Skills™: (1) Create a profile, (2) start assessment, (3) choose activities, (4) start treatment, and (5) evaluate effects of different treatments on progress.

In step 1, the user creates the child's profile. This involves inputting basic demographic information about the child. The single most important piece of information that is inputted is the child's birth date. This is because Skills™ uses the child's birth date to generate a pool of age-appropriate assessment questions for the child.

When creating the child's profile, the user has the ability to give access to the account to other members of the child's team and to give them either viewing rights only or rights to enter data into various sections of the child's account. The nice thing about this is that various team members can be assigned to work on different assessments or parts of the treatment plan. For example, the speech language pathologist might be assigned to the assessment and treatment of the language domain, the occupational therapist to the assessment and treatment of the motor domain, and the behavior analyst to the remaining areas. In addition, the account manager might choose to share the account with the child's physician who enters data into the account indicating when changes have been made to the child's biomedical treatments.

In the second step, the user starts the process of assessment. The Skills™ assessment is the most comprehensive assessment of skills ever created for children between the age of 0 and 8 years. In developing the Skills™ assessment, its creators researched every possible skill that develops between that timeframe across all areas of human functioning. In addition to its breadth and scope, in 2010, research demonstrated that the Language subscale of Skills™ has high test-retest and inter-rater reliability (Dixon et al. 2011).

Filling out this assessment is essential to identify the child's level of skills compared to his or her typical peers across all areas of development. This involves an individual who is very familiar with the child answering a series of "yes" or "no" questions regarding the child's skills across the eight developmental areas: Social, Motor, Adaptive, Play, Executive Functions, Cognition, and Academic skills.

The user first chooses which developmental area he or she would like to assess (e.g., the user might choose to assess Cognition). Then, the user chooses a concept area to assess within the developmental area (e.g., within the developmental area of cognition, the user might choose between "intention," "deception," or "emotions"). This flexibility of breaking the assessment into subsections allows users either to complete the entire assessment before beginning to design a treatment plan or to search for concepts they want to assess and immediately begin to treat only those.

Once a concept area is chosen for assessment, the user begins to answer questions for that area. Every question has an assigned age and questions are presented in the order of typical development starting with infant level skills and building up to the child's current chronological age. The assessment is built on an intelligent system in that when early questions are answered "no," later questions that build on that skill are also automatically answered "no," saving the user's time spent answering assessment questions.

Completing the assessment results in the generation of a set of bar graphs depicting where the child is functioning within each curriculum and concept area in comparison to where he or she should be functioning for his or her age, as well as a list of age-appropriate activities that the child needs to learn.

In step 3, the user begins the process of choosing activities to place into the child's treatment plan. As highlighted in the previous step, the activities from which the user can choose are linked directly to the results of the assessment. This means that the user is automatically presented with a pool of available activities to teach the child which are relevant to the child's age.

In addition to this, the user is provided with five tools to help him or her make good choices when deciding which activities to teach. The five tools include the following:

1. Teaching levels: Each lesson is assigned to a teaching level between 1 and 12 with 1 being the most basic lesson and 12 being the most advanced. Users might want to start with lessons in lower teaching levels before working on lessons in higher teaching levels.
2. Assigned activity numbers: Each lesson is composed of multiple activities which are numbered in a suggested order for teaching.
3. Assigned skill ages: Posted with each activity is the age at which the skill is observed to occur in typically developing children. Users will likely start with younger skills before moving to older skills.
4. Prerequisites: Each activity lists whether it has any prerequisite lessons. Users should consult those prerequisite lessons and introduce any activities from those lessons that are needed in order for the child to begin working on the current activity.
5. Building block, fundamental skill, or expansion skill designations: Each activity is labeled as being a building block, fundamental skill, or expansion skill. Fundamental skills are considered the milestones. Building blocks are activities that may or may not be needed (depending on how quickly the child learns) as a step to help the child learn the fundamental skill. Expansion skills are also not essential for every child because they are not necessarily required for daily living but are considered skills that might enrich the child's functioning within the associated skill area.

The user employs all of these tools to design an individualized treatment plan for the child and adds activities on which he or she would like to focus to the child's treatment plan.

In step 4, the user begins the process of teaching. CARD eLearning™ becomes very helpful at this point. The user implements the strategies and teaching procedures that he or she learned during CARD eLearning™ to teach the skills related to the activities that are placed into the child's treatment plan.

In addition to applying the knowledge learned from CARD eLearning™ to begin teaching, the user is also given an assortment of materials for teaching each of the activities that are placed in the child's treatment plan. For example, the user is provided with an activity guide which provides step-by-step instructions, such as teaching tips, goals, and benchmarks that can be used in the child's individual education plan and ideas to ensure that what the child learns during the teaching session is maintained and generalized to the child's real-life settings. The teaching guide is editable in order to be customized for the individual child. Specifically, the user can change the teaching tips to pertain to the child at hand and can make some custom settings with respect to which ABA-based teaching paradigm to use (i.e., DTT, NET, or FBI) and which prompting hierarchy he or she wants therapists to follow.

In addition to the activity guide, the user is given a video demonstration of a therapist and child performing the target activity, as well as access to a variety of handouts, including worksheets, visual aids, data tracking forms, and target checklists. The target checklists are also customizable. The idea is that the user will be able to print everything needed and then begin teaching and/or present the materials to a therapist who will do the teaching.

As the teaching is initiated and the child starts to acquire skills, the fifth step of "progress tracking" begins. Each time the child learns a new target or learns and masters an entire activity, the user marks off that the item was mastered. In doing so, several different graphs are automatically fed data and updated to show the child's progress.

Users can view bar graphs depicting where the child was functioning during assessment and compare it to how much the child has learned since starting Skills™. The comparisons are made both at the level of each developmental or curriculum area (e.g., social skills, motor skills, and so on) and at the level of the lesson or concept (e.g., within the social skills curriculum area, one can see performance within lessons such as "Apologizing," "Initiating Conversation," and so on). The child's mastery of skills is also depicted within a multidisciplinary timeline which depicts the child's acquisition of skills over time on a line graph.

Multidisciplinary Timeline

In addition to depicting the child's learning curve over time, the multidisciplinary timeline allows for all members of a child's treatment team to track the initiation of treatment components and detect effects they might have on the child's acquisition over time. For example, users can input when the child starts an alternative intervention, such as a biomedical intervention, onto the timeline. Then, the user can evaluate whether this change in the child's treatment program has had an effect on the child's learning by either increasing or decreasing skills acquired. Other events can also be plotted onto the timeline, such as life events (e.g., decrease in treatment hours, child is ill) and challenging behaviors (e.g., aggression, stereotypy, tantrums, self-injury). This allows correlation between life events and changes in skill acquisition or challenging behavior to be made, and, in addition to tracking changes in skill acquisition, the user can track whether challenging behaviors are decreasing or increasing concomitantly with the introduction of an alternative treatment.

Analytics

Individuals or organizations that continuously use this system by entering data into the Skills™ website will have access to a series of quantitative analyses derived from the database that supports Skills™. These analytics will allow projections such as predicting probable outcomes for children, evaluation of team performance, and cost analysis. In terms of predicting probable outcomes for children entered into Skills™, given certain child parameters, Skills™ will be able to predict the child's best expected outcome as a result of receiving ABA-based intervention. Additionally, Skills™ will be able to predict how many activities within the Skills™ curriculum the child should be able to learn given a hypothetical number of treatment hours per week and how many years of ABA-based intervention will be needed at that number of hours in order to reach the predicted optimal outcome.

Furthermore, given the child's progress (rate of learning, skills acquired, etc.) under the care of various treatment supervisors and agencies, Skills™ will be able to score and rank treatment supervisors and agencies in terms of what kinds of outcomes they achieve with their children. Comparisons of performance across children will be able to be made among treatment supervisors. Likewise, comparisons of effectiveness between treatment supervisors and agencies can be made. Given this, interested parties will be able to choose to place children under the care of treatment providers with the highest impact values, as well as conduct a cost analysis to determine the number of treatment hours they will fund and for what length of time for a given child.

Support

Skills™ offers support through a multitude of modalities. Navigational support is provided on each page of the website via a video-based tutorial, and tips that are clinical in nature are provided both in written and video library formats. If users still have questions, they can enter into the Skills™ support community. Here, the user can search frequently asked questions and answers, post a new question, report bugs, share ideas with others, and give praise. Answers to users' questions are posted and then added into the question and answer library for other users to utilize. Skills™ also offers live assistance through "on camera" support via web chat with a "Skills™ Live" host. The "Skills™ Live" host answers live questions each day and provides presentations on important topics and areas that will help users to be successful with their treatment programs.

Conclusion

CARD's global mission is the provision of the highest quality ABA-based intervention to as many families affected by autism spectrum disorders as possible. We are continuously developing our curriculum, services, internal staff training, and parent training, while keeping abreast of the latest published research and conducting our own treatment evaluation research. With the creation of CARD eLearning™ and Skills™, CARD is now in a position to accomplish its mission of disseminating over 20 years of knowledge and experience in treating and recovering children with autism by sharing its treatment model with the world. When moving forward with the execution of the CARD mission, quality and quantity cannot be compromised. We continue to improve and refine CARD eLearning™, Skills™, and our high-quality behavioral treatment model. In doing so, CARD remains at the forefront of effective treatment for autism spectrum disorders.

References

Abidin, R. R. (1995). *Parenting stress index: Professional manual*. Odessa: Psychological Assessment Resources.

Alpern G. D., Boll T. J., & Shearer M. S. (1980). *Developmental profile II*. Aspen: Psychological Development Publications.

Aman, M. G., & Singh, N. N. (1986). *Aberrant behavior checklist: ABC*. New York: Slosson Educational Publications.

Baltruschat, L., Hasselhorn, M., Tarbox, J., Dixon, D. R., Najdowski, A. C., Mullins, R. D., Gould, E. R. (2011). Addressing working memory in children with autism through behavioral intervention. *Research in Autism Spectrum Disorders, 5,* 267–276.

Barnoy, E. L., Najdowski, A. C., Tarbox, J., Wilke, A. E., & Nollet, M. D. (2009). Evaluation of a multicomponent intervention for diurnal bruxism in a young child with autism. *Journal of Applied Behavior Analysis, 42,* 845–848.

Baron-Cohen, S., Wheelwright, S., Cox, A., Baird, G., Charman, T., Swettenham, J., Drew A., & Doehring, P. (2000). The early identification of autism: The Checklist for Autism in Toddlers (CHAT). *Journal of the Royal Society of Medicine, 93,* 521–525.

Bayley, N. (2006). *Bayley scales of infant and toddler development* (3rd ed.). San Antonio: PsychCorp.

Beery, K. E., & Beery, N. A. (2004). *The Beery-Buktenica developmental test of visual-motor integration* (5th ed.). Bloomington: Pearson.

Bergstrom, R., Tarbox, J., & Gutshall, K. A. (2011). Behavioral intervention for domestic pet mistreatment in a young child with autism. *Research in Autism Spectrum Disorders, 5,* 218–221.

Binder, C. (1996). Behavioral fluency: Evolution of a new paradigm. *The Behavior Analyst, 19,* 163–197.

Bolton, J., & Mayer, M. D. (2008). Promoting the generalization of paraprofessional discrete trial teaching skills. *Focus on Autism and Other Developmental Disabilities, 23,* 103–111.

Bowers, L., Huisingh, R., & LoGiudice, C. (2005). *Test of problem solving 3 (TOPS 3: Elementary): A test of reasoning in context*. East Moline: LinguiSystems.

Brigance, A. H. (2004). *Brigance diagnostic inventory of early development-II*. North Billerica: Curriculum Associates.

Brown, W. H., & Odom, S. L. (1994). Strategies and tactics for promoting generalization and maintenance of young children's social behavior. *Research in Developmental Disabilities, 15,* 99–118.

Charlop-Christy, M. H., & Carpenter, M. H. (2000). *Modified incidental teaching sessions: A procedure for parents to increase spontaneous speech in their children with autism. Journal of Positive Behavior Interventions, 2,* 98–112.

Charlop-Christy, M. H., & LeBlanc, L. A. (1999). Naturalistic teaching strategies for acquisition, generalization, and maintenance of speech in children with autism. In P. M. Ghezzi, W. L. Williams, & J. E. Carr (Eds.), *Autism: Behavior analytic perspectives* (pp. 167–184). Reno: Context.

Cohen, I. L., & Sudhalter, V. (1999). *Pervasive Developmental Disorder Behavior Inventory (PDDBI-C).* New York: NYS Institute for Basic Research in Developmental Disabilities.

Cohen, H., Amerine-Dickens, M., & Smith, T. (2006). Early intensive behavioral treatment: Replication of the UCLA model in a community setting. *Developmental and Behavioral Pediatrics, 27,* S145–S155.

Constantino, J. N., & Gruber, C. P. (2005). *Social Responsiveness Scale (SRS).* Los Angeles: Western Psychological Services.

Cowan, R. J., & Allen, K. D. (2007). Using naturalistic procedures to enhance learning in individuals with autism: A focus on generalized teaching within the school setting. *Psychology in the Schools, 44,* 701–715.

Delprato, D. J. (2001). Comparisons of discrete-trial and normalized behavioral language intervention for young children with autism. *Journal of Autism and Developmental Disorders, 31,* 315–325.

Dixon, D. R., Tarbox, J., Najdowski, A. C., Wilke, A. E., & Granpeesheh, D. (2011). A comprehensive evaluation of language for early behavioral intervention programs: The reliability of the SKILLS™ language index. *Research in Autism Spectrum Disorders, 5,* 506–511.

Dunn, L. M., & Dunn, L. M. (1997). *Peabody picture vocabulary test* (3rd ed.). Circle Pines: American Guidance Service.

Elliott, C. (1990). *Differential abilities scales.* Pensacola: Psychological.

Fenske, E. C., Zalenski, S., Krantz, P. J., & McClannahan, L. E. (1985). Age at intervention and treatment outcome for autistic children in a comprehensive intervention program. *Analysis and Intervention in Developmental Disabilities, 5,* 49–58.

Filter, K. J., & Horner, R. H. (2009). Function-based academic interventions for problem behavior. *Education and Treatment of Children, 32,* 1–19.

Ghezzi, P. M., & Bishop, M. R. (2008). Generalized behavior change in young children with autism. In J. K. Luiselli, D. C. Russo, W. P. Christian, & S. M. Wilczynski (Eds.), *Effective practices for children with autism: Educational and behavioral support interventions that work* (pp. 137–158). New York: Oxford University Press.

Gilliam, J. (2006). *Gilliam autism rating scale* (2nd ed.). Minneapolis: Pearson.

Gilliam, J. E. (2001). *Gilliam Asperger's disorder scale.* Austin: Pro-Ed.

Gioia, G., Isquith, P., Guy, & Kenworthy (2000). *The behavior rating of executive function (BRIEF).* Odessa: Psychological Assessment Resources.

Gioia, G. A., Espy, K. A., & Isquith, P. K. (2003). *The behavior rating inventory of executive function: Preschool version (BRIEF-P).* Odessa: Psychological Assessment Resources.

Golden, C. J. (1978). *The stroop color and word test: A manual for clinical and experimental uses.* Chicago: Stoelting.

Goldman, R., Fristoe, M. S., & Woodcock, R. W. (1970). *Test of auditory discrimination.* Circle Pines: American Guidance Service.

Gould, E., Tarbox, J., O'Hora, D., Noone, S., & Bergstrom, R. (2011). Teaching children with autism a basic component skill of perspective-taking. *Behavioral Interventions, 26,* 50–66.

Granpeesheh, D. (2008). Recovery from autism: Learning why and how to make it happen more. *Autism Advocate, 50,* 54–58.

Granpeesheh, D., Dixon, D. R., Tarbox, J., Kaplan, A. M., & Wilke, A. E. (2009a). The effects of age and treatment intensity on behavioral intervention outcomes for children with autism spectrum disorders. *Research in Autism Spectrum Disorders, 3,* 1014–1022.

Granpeesheh, D., Tarbox, J., & Dixon, D. R. (2009b). Applied behavior analytic interventions for children with autism: A description and review of treatment research. *Annals of Clinical Psychiatry, 21,* 162–173.

Granpeesheh, D., Tarbox, J., Dixon, D. R., Carr, E., & Herbert, M. (2009c). Retrospective analysis of clinical records in 38 cases of recovery from autism. *Annals of Clinical Psychiatry, 21,* 195–204.

Granpeesheh, D., Tarbox, J., Dixon, D. R., Peters, C. A., Thompson, K., & Kenzer, A. (2010). Evaluation of an eLearning tool for training behavioral therapists in academic knowledge of applied behavior analysis. *Research in Autism Spectrum Disorders, 4,* 11–17.

Grant, D. A., Berg, E. A., & Heaton, R. K. (1993). *Wisconsin card sorting test.* Odessa: Psychological Assessment Resources.

Green, G. (1996). Early behavioral intervention for autism: What does research tell us? In C. Maurice, G. Green, & S. C. Luce (Eds.), *Behavioral intervention for young children with autism: A manual for parents and professionals* (pp. 29–44). Austin: Pro-Ed.

Gresham, F. M., & Elliott, S. N. (2008). *Social skills improvement system rating scales manual.* Minneapolis: Pearson.

Guy, W., & Bonato, R. (1970). CGI: Clinical Global Impressions. In W. Guy & R. Bonato (Eds.), *Manual for the ECDEU Assessment Battery.* Chevy Chase: National Institute of Mental Health pp. 12-1–12-6.

Hammill, D. D., & Newcomer, P. L. (1997). *Test of Language Development: Intermediate (TOLD-I: 3)* (3rd ed.). Austin: Pro-Ed.

Harper, C. B., Symon, J. B. G., & Frea, W. D. (2008). Recess is time-in: Using peers to improve social skills of children with autism. *Journal of Autism and Developmental Disorders, 38,* 815–826.

Howard, J. S., Sparkman, C. R., Cohen, H. G., Green, G., & Stanislaw, H. (2005). A comparison of intensive behavior analytic and eclectic treatments for young children with autism. *Research in Developmental Disabilities, 26,* 359–383.

Ingram, K., Lewis-Palmer, T., & Sugai, G. (2005). Function-based intervention planning: Comparing the effectiveness of FBA function-based and non-function-based intervention plans. *Journal of Positive Behavior Interventions, 7,* 224–236.

Kaiser, A. P., Hancock, T. B., & Nietfeld, J. P. (2000). The effects of parent-implemented enhanced milieu teaching on the social communication of children who have autism. *Early Education and Development, 11,* 423–446.

Koegel, R. L., Camarata, S., Koegel, L. K., Ben-Tall, A., & Smith, A. E. (1998). Increasing speech intelligibility in children with autism. *Journal of Autism and Developmental Disorders, 28,* 241–251.

Kohler, F. W., Anthony, L. J., Steighner, S. A., & Hoyson, M. (2001). Teaching social interaction skills in the integrated preschool: An examination of naturalistic tactics. *Topics in Early Childhood Special Education, 21,* 93–103.

Krantz, P. J., & McClannahan, L. E. (1998). Social interaction skills for children with autism: A script-fading procedure for beginning readers. *Journal of Applied Behavior Analysis, 31,* 191–202.

Leblanc, M. P., Ricciardi, J. N., & Luiselli, J. K. (2005). Improving discrete trial instruction by paraprofessional staff through an abbreviated performance feedback intervention. *Education and Treatment of Children, 28,* 76–82.

Llorente, A. M., Williams, J., Satz, P., & D'Elia, L. F. (2003). *Children's color trails test professional manual.* Odessa: Psychological Assessment Resources.

Lord, C., Rutter, M., DiLavore, P., Risi, S. (1999). *Autism diagnostic observation schedule manual.* Los Angeles: Western Psychological Services.

Lovaas, O. I. (1987). Behavioral treatment and normal educational and intellectual functioning in young autistic children. *Journal of Consulting and Clinical Psychology, 55,* 3–9.

Love, J. R., Carr, J. E., Almason, S. M., & Petursdottir, A. I. (2009). Early and intensive behavioral intervention for autism: A survey of clinical practices. *Research in Autism Spectrum Disorders, 3,* 421–428.

Moes, D. R., & Frea, W. D. (2000). Using family context to inform intervention planning for the treatment of a child with autism. *Journal of Positive Behavior Interventions, 2,* 40–46.

Moes, D. R., & Frea, W. D. (2002). Contextualized behavioral support in early intervention for children with autism and their families. *Journal of Autism and Developmental Disorders, 32,* 519–533.

Myers, S. M., & Plauché Johnson, C. (2007). Management of children with autism spectrum disorders. *Pediatrics, 120,* 1162–1182.

Najdowski, A. C., Chilingaryan, V., Bergstrom, R., Granpeesheh, D., Balasanyan, S., Aguilar, B., & Tarbox, J. (2009). Comparison of data collection methods in a behavioral intervention program for children with pervasive developmental disorders: A replication. *Journal of Applied Behavior Analysis, 42,* 827–832.

National Research Council. (2001). *Educating children with autism. Committee on Educational Interventions for Children with Autism. Division of Behavioral and Social Sciences and Education.* Washington: National Academy.

Newcomer, P. L., & Hammill, D. D. (2008). *Test of language development primary* (4th ed.). Austin: Pro-Ed.

New York State Department of Health, Early Intervention Program. (1999). *Clinical practice guideline: Report of the recommendations: Autism/pervasive developmental disorders: Assessment and intervention for young children (age 0–3 years).* Albany: New York State Department of Health.

Phelps-Terasaki, D., & Phelps-Gunn, T. (2007). *Test of pragmatic language* (2nd ed.). Austin: Pro-Ed.

Reed, P., Osborne, L. A., & Corness, M. (2007). Brief report: Relative effectiveness of different home-based behavioral approaches to early teaching intervention. *Journal of Autism and Developmental Disorders, 37,* 1815–1821.

Reynolds, C. R., & Kamphaus, R. W. (2004). *BASC 2, Behavior assessment system for children.* Circle Pines: American Guidance Service.

Rhine, D., & Tarbox, J. (2009). Chewing gum as a treatment for rumination in a child with autism. *Journal of Applied Behavior Analysis, 42,* 381–385.

Rimland, B., & Edelson, S. M. (1999). *Autism Treatment Evaluation Checklist (ATEC).* San Diego: Autism Research Institute.

Roid, G. M., & Miller, L. J. (1997). *Leiter international performance scale–revised: Examiners manual.* Wood Dale: Stoelting.

Roid, G., & Sampers, J. (2004). *Merrill-Palmer-revised scales of development.* Wood Dale: Stoelting.

Rossetti, L. (1990). *The Rossetti infant-toddler language scale.* East Moline: LinguiSystems.

Rutter, M., Lord, C., & LeCouteur, A. (2003). *Autism Diagnostic Interview—Revised* (3rd ed.). Chicago: Department of Psychiatry, University of Chicago.

Sallows, G. O., & Graupner, T. D. (2005). Intensive behavioral treatment for children with autism: Four-year outcome and predictors. *American Journal on Mental Retardation, 6,* 417–438.

Sarokoff, R. A., & Sturmey, P. (2004). The effects of behavioral skills training on staff implementation of discrete-trial teaching. *Journal of Applied Behavior Analysis, 37,* 535–538.

Schepis, M. M., Reid, D. H., Ownbey, J., & Parsons, M. B. (2001). Training support staff to embed teaching within natural routines of young children with disabilities in an inclusive preschool. *Journal of Applied Behavior Analysis, 34,* 313–327.

Schopler, E., Reichler, R. J., & Rochen Renner, B. (1988). *Childhood Autism Rating Scale (CARS).* Los Angeles: Western Psychological Services.

Schopler, E., Lansing, M. D., Reichler, R. J., & Marcus, L. M. (2005). *Psychoeducational profile examiner's manual* (3rd ed.). Austin: Pro-Ed.

Semel, E., Wiig, E. H., & Secord, W. A. (2003). *Clinical evaluation of language fundamentals* (4th ed.). San Antonio: PsychCorp.

Sparrow, S. S., Cicchetti, D. V., & Balla, D. A. (2005). *Vineland Adaptive Behavior Scales survey forms manual* (2nd ed.). Circle Pines: American Guidance Service.

Stahmer, A. C. (1995). Teaching symbolic play skills to children with autism using pivotal response training. *Journal of Autism and Developmental Disorders, 25,* 123–141.

Stahmer, A. C., Ingersoll, B., & Carter, C. (2003). *Behavioral approaches to promoting play. Autism, 7,* 401–413.

Stephens, T. M., & Arnold, K. D. (1992). *Social behavior assessment inventory: Professional manual.* Odessa: Psychological Assessment Resources.

Steven's Law (2008), Ariz. Rev. Stat. Ann. § 20–826.04, § 20–1057.11, § 20–1402.03, and § 20–1404.03.

Stokes, T. F., & Baer, D. M. (1977). An implicit technology of generalization. *Journal of Applied Behavior Analysis, 10,* 349–367.

Stokes, T. F., & Osnes, P. G. (1989). An operant pursuit of generalization. *Behavior Therapy, 20,* 337–355.

Sturmey, P. (2008). Best practice methods in staff training. In J. K. Luiselli, D. C. Russo, W. P. Christian, & S. M. Wilczynski (Eds.), *Effective practices for children with autism: Educational and behavioral support interventions that work* (pp. 159–178). New York: Oxford University Press.

Summers, J., Tarbox, J., Findel-Pyles, R. S., Wilke, A. E., Bergstrom, R. & Williams, W. L. (2011). Teaching two household safety skills to children with autism. *Research in Autism Spectrum Disorders, 5,* 629–632.

Tarbox, J., & Granpeesheh, D. (2011). What makes a great ABA program? Sorting through the science, the brands, and the acronyms. In K. Siri & T. Lyons (Eds.), *Cutting-edge therapies for autism: 2011–2012.* New York: Skyhorse Publishing.

Tarbox, J., Madrid, W., Aguilar, B., Jacobo, W., & Schiff, A. (2009). Use of chaining to increase complexity of echoics in children with autism. *Journal of Applied Behavior Analysis, 42,* 901–906.

Tarbox, J., Schiff, A., & Najdowski, A. C. (2010a). Parent-implemented procedural modification of escape extinction in the treatment of food selectivity in a young child with autism. *Education and Treatment of Children, 33,* 223–234.

Tarbox, J., Wilke, A. E., Findel-Pyles, R. S., Bergstrom, R. M., & Granpeesheh, D. (2010b). A comparison of electronic to traditional pen-and-paper data collection in discrete trial training for children with autism. *Research in Autism Spectrum Disorders, 4,* 65–75.

Thomson, K., Martin, G. L., Arnal, L., Fazzio, D., & Yu, C. T. (2009). Instructing individuals to deliver discrete-trials teaching to children with autism spectrum disorders: A review. *Research in Autism Spectrum Disorders, 3,* 590–606.

Thorpe, D. M., Stahmer, A. C., & Schreibman, L. (1995). Effects of sociodramatic play training on children with autism. *Journal of Autism and Developmental Disorders, 25,* 265–282.

Ulrich D. A. (2000). *Test of gross motor development* (2nd ed.). Austin: Pro-ed.

U.S. Department of Health and Human Services. (1999). *Mental health: A report of the Surgeon General.* Rockville: U.S. Department of Health and Human Services, Substance Abuse and Mental Health Services Administration, Center for Mental Health Services, National Institutes of Health, National Institute of Mental Health.

Vismara, L. A., & Rogers, S. J. (2010). Behavioral treatments in autism spectrum disorder: What do we know? *Annual Review of Clinical Psychology, 6,* 447–468.

Wechsler, D. (2002). *WPPSI-III administration and scoring manual.* San Antonio: PsychCorp.

Wechsler, D., Kaplan, E., Fein, D., Kramer, J., Morris, R., Delis, D., et al. (2004). *Wechsler Intelligence Scale for Children integrated administration and scoring manual* (4th ed.). San Antonio: PsychCorp.

Wepman, J. M., & Reynolds, W. M. (1987). *Auditory discrimination test* (2nd ed.). Los Angeles: Western Psychological Services.

Wepman, J., & Morency, A. (1973). *Manual of the auditory sequential memory test*. Los Angeles: Western Psychological Services.

Westby, C. E. (1991). A scale for assessing children's pretend play. In C. E. Schaefer, K. Gitlin, & A. Sandgrund (Eds.), *Play diagnosis and assessment* (pp. 131–161). New York: Wiley.

Wiig, E. H., Secord, W., & Semel, E. (1992). *CELF-Preschool: Clinical evaluation of language fundamentals-preschool*. New York: Psychological Corp.

Woodcock, R. W., McGrew, K. S., & Mather, N. (2001). *Woodcock-Johnson III*. Rolling Meadows: Riverside Publishing.

Yoo, J. H., Tarbox, J., & Granpeesheh, D. (2008). Using stimulus fading to teach a young child with autism to ingest wireless capsule endoscopy. *Gastrointestinal Endoscopy, 67*, 1203–1204.

Zimmerman, I. L., Steiner, V. G., & Pond, R. E. (2002). *Preschool Language Scale* (4th ed.). San Antonio: PsychCorp.

Part III
Strategic Interventions

Chapter 8
Social Competence Intervention Program

Margaret Semrud-Clikeman, Laura Guli and Elizabeth Portman Minne

> The [socially] competent individual is one who is able to make use of environmental and personal resources to achieve good developmental outcome. (Waters and Sroufe 1983, p. 81)

The Social Competence Intervention Program (SCIP) is an innovative, manualized, group intervention for children on the autism spectrum (Guli et al. 2008). It uses fun and cooperative creative drama techniques to address skills that make social interactions difficult for this population. These include the giving and taking of nonverbal cues, perspective taking, and cognitive flexibility. The group format allows social difficulties to be addressed in the moment they occur, and so children in the program begin to experience the feelings of social success. SCIP is founded on several models of social competence and social perception described in following sections.

Models of Social Competence

Social competence develops over time and experience of the infant and child. Basic building blocks include joint attention, eye contact, shared enjoyment of experiences, flexibility, the ability to apply learning from previous experiences, perspective taking, and emotional adaptability (Semrud-Clikeman and Schaefer 2000). Generally, attachment to significant others underlies social competence and sets the stage for the development of trust, skill in social interaction, and understanding of emotions, which later develop into appropriate interpersonal relationships. The link between social competence, social skills, and social communication involves the use of verbal and nonverbal language as well as accurate perception of the other and motivation knowledge to perform the requisite skill in their relationships (Spitzberg 2003).

M. Semrud-Clikeman (✉)
Division of Pediatric Clinical Neuroscience, University of Minnesota, 420 Delaware Street, Minneapolis, MN 55455, USA
e-mail: semru002@umn.edu

L. Guli · E. P. Minne
University of Texas at Austin, SZB 5800 Austin, TX 78712, USA

S. Goldstein, J. A. Naglieri (eds.), *Interventions for Autism Spectrum Disorders*,
DOI 10.1007/978-1-4614-5301-7_8,

The ability to recognize the appropriate context and what behaviors are to be represented in that context is also important. For children with social competence problems, social communication is difficult to understand, and it is also likely that due to this misunderstanding, the appropriate behaviors are not selected on the basis of the context. Behaviors that are appropriate in one setting are likely not appropriate in another (Guli et al. 2008). When there is a mismatch between the behavior and the context, the child often has difficulties with social behaviors and may be referred for assistance in developing these skills. Difficulty with social competence may arise from problems with perception as discussed above as well as with behavioral difficulties with attention and behavioral control. One theory of how social competence deficits are present across various diagnoses has been suggested by Voeller.

Voeller's Clusters Voeller (1994) suggests three types of deficits that can lead to social competence difficulties: (1) a group with aggressive and hostile behavior, (2) a perceptual deficits subgroup, and (3) a group with difficulty with self-regulation. Children in the first group tend to act out their aggression and hostility and are often rejected by their peers. Problems are present in which they frequently interrupt others' games, have difficulty waiting for their turn, and become extremely unpleasant when thwarted. These children are often diagnosed with oppositional defiant disorder or conduct disorder. At the heart of this type of social competence problems are deficits in social information processing and poor social problem-solving strategies. The strategy that is most often chosen is either aggressive behavior or verbal abuse. A particularly intriguing finding from the research is that negative interactions appear to be more salient to them and are sought out more often compared with the perceptions of typically developing children (Crick and Dodge 1994).

The second diagnostic cluster includes children with significant perceptual difficulties that lead to significant misinterpretations of interpersonal interactions. Difficulties are frequently present in their ability to understand social information, to read facial and voice cues, and to misunderstand body language. The most common diagnosis is pervasive developmental disorder, Asperger's disorder, and/or nonverbal learning disabilities.

The final diagnostic cluster includes those children who have classic difficulties in executive functioning. A key difficulty for these children is disorganization and significant executive function deficits. Some children in this group may be diagnosed with attention deficit hyperactivity disorder, whereas others may not show the full clinical syndrome. Children with social perceptual difficulties may also show problems with executive functioning and attention (Hala et al. 2003). The co-occurrence of two disorders (attention and perceptual difficulties) has been found to be significantly related to a more severe disorder than a sole diagnosis (Semrud-Clikeman et al. 2010). Not only do they experience difficulty with their perception but also problems with attention often lead them to quickly scan their environment and miss important cues (Semrud-Clikeman et al. 2010). These children may be able to decipher facial expressions in isolation, but when asked to understand dynamic social interactions, they have significant difficulties (Fine et al. 2008).

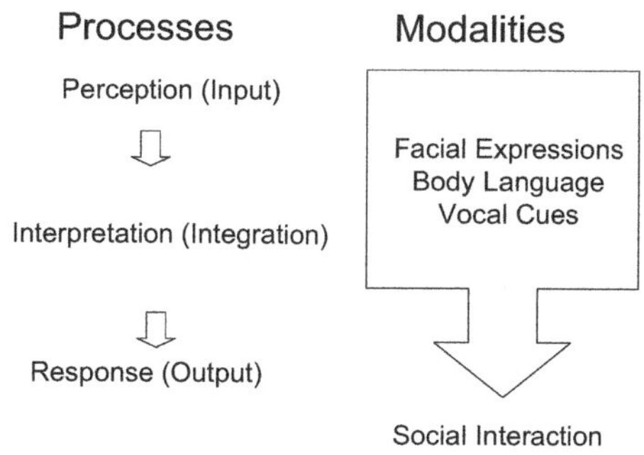

Fig. 8.1 A model for social perception

Crick and Dodge's Model Crick and Dodge (1994) proposed a six-step social information-processing model for understanding social competence. Difficulty at any level results in problems with social interaction and thus social competence. Included in these steps are the following aspects:

1. *Encoding of relevant stimuli*—Important skills are attention to nonverbal and verbal social cues both obvious and covert.
2. *Interpretation of the cues*—An understanding of what has happened as well as the cause and intent underlying the interaction.
3. *Establishing a goal*—The ability to determine what the child wants from the interaction and how to put forth an understanding of what is required.
4. *Being able to represent and remember the situation*—This ability allows the child to compare his or her past experience to the situation at hand. In addition, he or she must recall the reaction in the past to his or her actions. This step requires working memory.
5. *Selecting the most appropriate behavior*—In this step, the child selects from all possible responses on the basis of his or her perception of the event and what skills he or she possess.
6. *Acting and evaluating*—The child acts and then determines how successful he or she is.

Figure 8.1 shows the relationship between perception, interpretation, and response (Guli 2005). As one can see from Fig. 8.1, facial expressions, body language, and voice intonation provide information about the success of these skills; with inaccurate perception, these modalities do not provide the feedback needed to perform appropriately socially.

To evaluate a social situation, a great deal of information needs to be processed simultaneously in a dynamic and ever-changing context. One way to simplify the perceptual field is to select the most important aspect of the situation and respond accordingly. This selection is an important aspect, as keying in on a less important aspect or perceiving it incorrectly often leads to difficulties in relating to others (Guli et al. in press). Moreover, a child's past memory of his or her previous experiences and what worked or didn't work is a crucial information for the selection of what behavior to employ in the present situation. There are emotional and physiological aspects to this memory with children who have experienced significant difficulties related to others having biological and emotional reactions to situations that are similar (Damasio 1994). These emotional and physiological components, in turn, influence how the child or adolescent responds to the current scenario. Thus, the child's past social learning experiences come into play in his or her interpretation of the current event and color his or her resulting reactions (Semrud-Clikeman 2007).

Another aspect important to consider is whether the developmental level of the child matches the expectations of parents, peers, and teachers. Generally, this level is commensurate with the child's age; however, when not commensurate, the child is frequently socially rejected, seen as "odd," and isolated from peers. This isolation further restricts the child's ability to relate to others and to develop appropriate skills. Without the development of appropriate skills, the child will often flounder socially and have much fewer opportunities to practice social interactions.

Perspective taking and theory of mind are important contributions to social competence. The ability to understand another person's perspective has been implicated in autism as well as related disorders (Ozonoff and Rogers 2003). When there is limited self-awareness and other-awareness, difficulties with social interactions are likely and limit the child's ability to share thoughts and feelings with others (Happe and Frith 2006). This difficulty in establishing the understanding of differing perspectives for different people has been found related to problems with conversational ability and poor social functioning in children with autism. It is highly likely that difficulty with language skills impairs social communication (Barrett et al. 2004). This is a dynamic skill that children develop. When a child is taught directly to look at another's motives and feelings, the child is able to complete this task within a defined setting. However, the ability to translate this knowledge into less structured and dynamic settings does not occur readily and likely relates back to the difficulty experienced with flexibility and social information processing present in many children with social competence disorders (Corbett 2003).

Recently, various social competence programs have been developed for higher functioning children with autistic spectrum disorders that have an emphasis on assisting the child in developing an understanding of emotions and body language through the use of creative drama. Creative drama is an effective medium to use for this type of program, as drama activities originated as a means for actors to become skilled in reading each others' nonverbal cues for the stage. Thus, this process directly addresses the difficulties experienced by individuals on the autism spectrum (Lerner et al. 2010). Drama is grounded in a belief in discovery-in-this-moment and has a great potential for helping children with autism spectrum disorder (ASD) by teaching them to better understand interactions with others (Sherratt and Peter 2002) and solve social disagreements in context (Guli et al. 2008).

Program Description

The SCIP was developed by Laura Guli as part of a dissertation emphasizing creative drama as a basis for teaching social perspective as well as developing social skills.

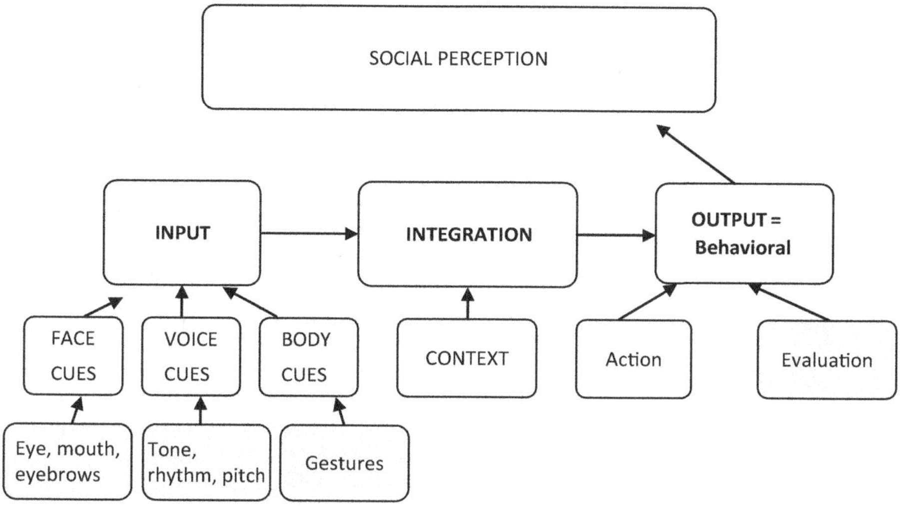

Fig. 8.2 SCIP model of social competence

SCIP is a 16-session intervention based on creative drama and process drama activities. The activities have been modified for children with autistic spectrum disorders as well as those with nonverbal learning disabilities. Some of the content consisting of cooperative drama activities was modified and derived from existing sources (Cresi 1989; Neelands and Goode 2001; O'Neill and Lambert 1994; Spolin 1986), whereas the original process dramas were created specifically for the program. A major goal of the SCIP program is to teach children the fundamental skills of social perception in such a way as to provide practice in foundational skills using a framework that includes cooperative play and allows many opportunities for practice.

The program consists of three stages that were developed to parallel the steps theorized to be involved in social competence: input, integration, and output. See Fig. 8.2 (Guli et al. 2008).

Modules

There are 16 manualized modules incorporated in SCIP. Sessions 1–7 target input and focus on the following:

1. Establishing the group and learning about the leaders and the children participating.
2. Teaching knowledge about emotions; what makes up the emotions, how they are expressed, and how to understand the emotions.
3. Learning how to focus attention appropriately.
4. Learning how to understand and interpret facial expressions and body language.
5. Learning how to understand and interpret vocal cues.

Table 8.1 Outline of the SCIP

Session no.	Social perception stage	Topic
1	Input	Establishing group identity
2	Input	Focusing attention
3	Input	Emotional knowledge
4	Input	Facial expressions and body language
5	Input	Facial expressions and body language
6	Input	Vocal cues
7	Input	Putting cues together
8	Integration	When cues do not match
9	Integration	When cues do not match (part 2)
10	Integration	Point of view
11	Integration	Understanding interactions
12	Integration	Understanding interactions (part 2)
13	Output	Becoming fluent in conversation
14	Output	Dealing with teasing
15	Output	Content review
16	Output	Goodbye and closure

6. Learning how to put together facial expressions, body language, and vocal cues in a social interaction.
7. Learning how to handle situations where nonverbal cues do not match the words being said.

Sessions 8–13 target the integration and interpretation processes. These sessions include the following modules:

1. Perspective taking
2. Interpretation of nonverbal body language, facial expressions, and gestures.
3. Introduction and use of process dramas involving role playing. During this time, participants are assisted in breaking down complex social interactions into sequential parts and to discuss the emotions present.
4. Exploring various outcomes that can occur during a social interaction as well as how to determine the most appropriate behaviors.

Finally, sessions 14–16 address output and focus on techniques that can be used to resolve conflict as well as how to respond to teasing. The organization of the activities moves from an initial emphasis on the child's experience and emotions surrounding social interaction to an understanding of how others may interpret the same situation in an alternative manner. Target emotions progress from general emotions (happy, sad, and angry) to subtler emotions (shame, embarrassment, and annoyance).

Each session includes a warm-up activity, followed by a review of home assignment, discussion of the topic of the day and activities along that line, and then a wrap-up discussion of the day's experience. Peer feedback is the key throughout the sessions as well as leader guidance. If conflicts arise, each participant's needs are addressed and resolved. This intervention has a manual, which is necessary when working with children; the format is flexible and may need to be changed as required by individual children (Table 8.1).

Behavior Management and Manual Flexibility

Working with children with autism and social competence problems is rewarding as well as challenging. As discussed in other chapters in this volume, behavioral management is an important part of working with any child in a group. As the program is fun, it is not unusual for children to become too active or loud during activities. Some of the "rowdiness" is to be welcomed, as it reflects the fact that children are making friends with each other. Also, while flexibility may not be one of the strengths of the children in these groups, it is essential for the leaders of the group to be able to put the individual child's needs on a particular day ahead of the manual. This program is not meant to be a cookbook intervention that is to be followed rigidly. Rather, it is meant to work with the creativity of the leaders and the children to provide the best of all worlds; structure and flexibility. With this in mind, peer conflicts and individual difficulties should be used as therapeutic opportunities to teach participants about problem solving and help them recognize their role in a social interaction. For example, in the initial groups of SCIP, one child accidentally mispronounced "fork" and it sounded like a bad word. When the other children laughed in response, he was mortified, and began to cry. A group leader took him out of the room briefly to give him some privacy, to help him process his feelings, and to reassure him that he could successfully return to the group. At the same time, other group leaders worked with the remaining children regarding sensitivity to others' feelings and how to respond to the child who was upset.

Examples of Drama Activities

Gift Giving In the "gift giving" game, children pantomimed giving and receiving gifts to each other. The "giver" is allowed to give anything, regardless of size or sense, and the "receiver" has to accept the gift with great gratitude and enthusiasm. The game often results in laughter and giggles from participants, who enjoy thinking of all the funny things they could give, such as an elephant or an old piece of chewing gum. Although children with ASDs are often characterized as being unable to engage in or enjoy pretend play, group leaders observed that the children loved this activity, which stresses cognitive flexibility, cooperation, and increasing intensity of nonverbal cues. Although some children have a difficult time accepting absurd and imaginary gifts with enthusiasm, they usually respond positively with leader encouragement.

Gibberish In the "gibberish" game, children are asked to have a conversation with a partner in a made-up language called "gibberish." Group leaders give participants topics that have emotionally laden content to talk about; for example, "describe the scariest dream you ever had" or "tell about your favorite vacation." Although participants cannot understand the actual words that their conversation partner is saying, they have to try to understand and respond, in gibberish, with appropriate facial expression and vocal tone. By taking away actual verbal content, participants are forced to focus on the nonverbal cues to determine how to respond, and practice the natural reciprocal give and take of conversation in a fun context.

Process Dramas

Process dramas refer to largely unscripted group improvisations that allow group participants to solve problems within a given context. Process dramas written for and enacted in this intervention included "Miss Gibber and the Stolen Dog" and "Spaceship Mission" for younger children (8–10 years) and "Scotland Yard and the Case of the Stolen Cake," "Theft at the Computer Store," and "Ad Agency" for older children (11–14 years). In the initial dramas, group leaders present participants with a context in which they have to take dramatic roles and solve a problem by decoding nonverbal cues. For example, in "Miss Gibber and the Stolen Dog," "Theft at the Computer Store," and "Scotland Yard" dramas, children take the roles of detectives in an agency, while group leaders take the roles of head detectives needing help from his or her team. Participants are asked to interview suspects played by group leaders, one of whom speaks with incongruent nonverbal and context cues, and determine who is guilty. For example, the guilty party in each drama can smile while saying that he or she is innocent, but speak very nervously and angrily. In "Miss Gibber and the Stolen Dog," children have to determine what happened to a dog on the basis of the facial and vocal tone cues of a witness who can only speak in Gibberish. In "Space Station" and "Ad Agency," participants pretend to be members of a team presented with a mission. In "Space Station," children develop roles of members of a space station traveling around the universe to learn about other beings. After being introduced to the drama, the children receive an urgent message from aliens threatening to destroy earth because it cannot decipher the confusing emotional meanings in human communication. With group leader assistance, the participants decide to develop a videotape that will help the aliens understand how to read and express nonverbal cues better. In "Ad Agency," older children take the roles of members of an ad agency faced with a new contract. The task asks them to produce a video to help parents understand how preteenagers interact with each other. By filming improvised interactions between peers and then watching them on tape, participants practice integrating the skills they have learned in earlier sessions.

Qualitative and Quantitative Support for SCIP Intervention research is not difficult to complete for several reasons. One major reason is the nature of this type of research, which requires commitment on the part of the participants as well as the leaders of the group to come to the sessions. In most cases, children came to the sessions twice a week for approximately 2.5 h. In addition, the type of data is very important. Relying solely on quantitative data for this type of research robs the richness of the experience as well as deprives a full picture of the results. Relying solely on qualitative data similarly gives an incomplete picture. For that reason, we have utilized both a qualitative and quantitative methodology. In the following section, we include both types of data as support for SCIP. The following section provides some portions of interviews with parents and children who participated in this program to assist the reader in fully understanding the program. In addition, it also provides an inside look as to what occurred in some of the sessions. Names and ages have been changed throughout to protect identities. These excerpts are adapted from Dr. Guli's dissertation (Guli 2005) and Dr. Minne's dissertation (Portman 2006).

Feedback from Parents

David's mother noticed that her son used his body and face more to communicate with others. She explained:

> The other day my husband was saying that... [David's] making a lot of different faces that he's never seen before.... [David] came into the kitchen and shrugged his shoulders and blew out this big breath like (heavy sigh sound), 'just waiting for me to,' [my husband] was saying, 'waiting for me to notice him.' And [my husband] didn't know what to do. He just didn't do anything, and [David] did it again (heavy sigh sound). 'Dad?' And so [my husband] turned around and said 'What [David]?,' and he goes 'Don't you see that something's wrong?' And he would have never done that before.

One parent reported that her and her child's involvement in this program had allowed her to have conversations with her son, which was a "big deal," and that it helped her and her husband feel hopeful that they can "increase him [the child] socially more than we thought." A parent also noted that her child's teacher reported that her son's "social skills have improved greatly in the last two months."

By the program's mid-point, group leaders reported: "She pays attention and always participates," and "Her facial expressions are becoming even more expressive." Lee's mother speculated that her daughter's increasing comfort in the group may have been related to her daughter's sense of belonging, as she explained, "I think she knows that people are speaking her language..."

Her mother explained:

> Um, well I know at dinner we do something called Sunshine and Clouds, and we talk about different things that happened in our day. And a lot of times I'll talk about something, that, that when she came out of group... that she was smiling and she was happy. And I try and connect the fact that she's like anxious sometimes when she first walks in and then it goes okay and she's okay. My hope... is just that she'll remember that. You know, maybe a little less anxiety each time. She can just self talk 'Okay, I've been through this, I'll be okay.'

The above excerpt and data demonstrate that Lee's participation in the intervention group was an exercise of overcoming social anxiety. Seven months after the end of the intervention program, Jake's mother and I corresponded. She reported:

> I am happy to report that [Jake] is having the best year ever at school.... Here we are half way through the school year and he has not had a problem one single day. He has had... no incidents with other kids, no refusing to do what they are doing, no getting upset and not recovering. He is like a new kid this year and we are loving it! He talks to us more now about his day and tells us he is happy. But better than that, he tells us when he is upset too, with words, appropriately... I think that counting and breathing is the most valuable tool he learned (for us too!) from the class because it works for all different situations. Just

> last week he was reading a book with his dad and he got stuck on some words and became frustrated . . . he counted and took some breaths and then he was fine and could read the words.

All parents reported that, to some degree, the home assignments allowed them to be more involved in their children's social development. David's mother explained that "I think it helped me help him," as she added that her increased involvement with her son's positive social development would continue even after the intervention ended. Lee's and Kyle's mothers reported that their involvement with this program raised their awareness of the weak areas of their children's social development that were in need of focused attention from their parents. One parent expressed gratitude that the program gave her the tools to take "the first step in teaching empathy."

Jake's mother felt that her involvement helped her to ask her son the right questions, which helped him to relate better to his mother and to communicate with her. The new, "opened up" line of conversation between her and her son was a big deal for Jake's mother because Jake now shared new enjoyable experiences that he had gained through the intervention. For instance, his mother reported that he was finally having the experience of friendships with other children in the group, which impacted both her and her son positively because now: "We can talk about his friends; something we've never been able to do. So that's been nice."

Lee's mother explained that this group provided her opportunity to bond with her daughter. She reported that their participation in the intervention allowed them to have more one-on-one time together and opportunities to talk together about ideas. She explained:

> Um, it's sort of become a bonding experience for [Lee] and I because we'll go have ice cream . . . right before we come here. And sometimes we'll either have time to talk about what's, you know, what's coming up in the session, what she might be doing. And so just having the time with her is really good, and then being able to bring it home and talk at the dinner table about what the subject matter was . . .

Lee's mother was impressed by her daughter's developing ability to properly greet others, a skill specifically taught during intervention sessions. Her mother felt that this was one of the three most important things that her daughter learned during the social skills program. Lee demonstrated to her mother the steps that she had learned in introducing herself, such as "how you should say hello, and look in their eyes and shake their hands." Furthermore, Lee's mother observed her doing the greeting with her grandfather, as she reached out for his hand when saying goodbye.

Mary's mother noted that: "Before the intervention she would sit in the car with me, but since the intervention she goes 'I'm not afraid anymore' and she runs out and that was a big deal for her, real big . . . I know she wouldn't be where she is without the intervention. I'm very proud of the changes." Jacob's mother reported that: "My sister . . . said it was like night and day. She said his face seemed a lot more animated and he seemed to make a big effort to communicate and actually do a give and take in communication . . . he carried on a conversation with her and asked her questions about herself and prompted her to continue the conversation . . . . she was surprised." Additional parent comments included: "I've noticed that he seems to be reaching out more to kids in the neighborhood to try to befriend them . . . I think the thing that I see is that he is more interested in people, in relating to them, and that's a positive thing. I would say a year ago he could care less," and "He has seemed more interested in seeking out friends more. He has talked about that . . . having friends over more." "He seems to have improved in being able to perhaps think about what the other person may be feeling, something that never entered his mind before. He even showed compassion yesterday for a friend with severe learning disabilities."

A couple of parents noticed changes in the expression of nonverbal cues as well as perception: "He was looking at her, making faces to her, making her laugh, he was laughing. I noticed his face shows more expression." The same parent noted that "Well one day he got mad at me so he frowned and made a mad face and I said, 'Oh, you're mad.' And he said, 'Yes.' Another parent noticed that her son Michael appeared to be showing more congruent affect and not laughing at sad topics anymore. Anne's mother stated, "I have seen her showing more empathy toward (her sister) . . . if she falls down or hurts herself and is crying I have noticed that she is showing more attention to her." Two parents reported that their children were greeting them and making conversation more spontaneously. "It seems like after this class he has made a very big effort to ask 'how was your day.' Now, he may do it three or four times in a row because he doesn't know how to lead a conversation any further along, but he knows that 'this is one of the things I'm supposed to do now when I meet someone.' "

Feedback from Child Participants

Child participants were also very positive about their group experience. When an 11-year-old boy with Asperger's syndrome first came to the group, he expected a very negative experience: ". . . kind of like a psycho hospital 'cause I've been inside a therapy office . . . where there are a bunch of quote-unquote 'problem kids.' " Instead of being similar to his past therapeutic experiences, the group normalized his difficulties: "It made me feel that I wasn't alone in the world . . . made me feel that there were other people going through the same things that I was, and understood what was going on." Another child learned that, "I just remember if I want to talk to someone I got to look at them." The same child realized that he had to get permission before hugging someone, because otherwise it might scare them.

The majority of children interviewed (68 %) believed that they learned how to perceive nonverbal cues better, especially facial expressions and body language, as the following quotes indicate: "I can focus on other people's body language a little bit clearer; I can understand what they're saying with their body language a little bit clearer." "I learned a lot like about feelings and stuff. I know mostly all those dolls (points to dolls on shelf) look sad . . . like their lips are kind of drooping." "If somebody were happy and they were showing that they were sad I could figure out how they were doing that . . . . they said they were happy and they weren't 'cause they looked sad and I could tell they were sad." "Besides learning about how people feel we learned about how people act."

Many of the children (43 %) reported making friends in the group. Several children also explained that being in the group was helping them in school with peers. One 9-year-old child learned to "ignore people that tease you a lot and stuff, and try to find out how feelings are by seeing faces and just hearing them." Another child reported, "Now, I know a lot about feelings and I can talk to my friends more easily". An 8-year-old girl explained, "It helped me to feel more that I had more confidence, so that I could say hi to people without being scared." A 12-year-old boy said, "I'm a little bit calmer. I can understand people now. I have a social life now."

Quantitative Empirical Support

The SCIP program has been completed well by more than 100 children aged 6–14 in a variety of contexts, including school districts and speech and language programs. Two studies have been completed on the manualized version of SCIP and a developmentally adapted version that show excellent promise in reliability and validity. In the first study, led by the main developer of SCIP (Guli 2005), children with diagnoses of Asperger's syndrome, High Functioning Autism, nonverbal learning disabilities, and/or ADHD completed a 16-week intervention (Guli et al. in press). These children were aged 8–14 and divided into two groups: 18 in the treatment group and 16 in the clinical control group. The children in the clinical comparison group were children who were unable to attend the sessions. Pre- and posttesting on measures of social perception, social competence, and direct observations in the school setting found that the treatment group showed both significant increases in positive interactions as well as significant decreases in solitary behaviors in comparison with the clinical control group. Additionally, postintervention interviews with parents and children indicated that the majority of parents and participants saw marked changes in one or more areas of social competence.

A further study utilizing younger children (aged 6–8) used a qualitative methodology (Minne and Semrud-Clikeman 2011), which was based on Dr. Minne's dissertation. Findings were of the key changes in social interactions, particularly in emotional understanding and behavioral improvement. Although the pattern of rigid interests and behavior patterns continued following the intervention, the ability of these children to participate in social interaction improved drastically as reported by parents and teachers. These two studies are just the beginning of studies with SCIP. Additional study has now been completed in Barcelona, Spain, with favorable results (Querol and Piera 2011, personal communication).

Conclusion

The purpose of this chapter was to describe the SCIP and to provide preliminary evidence for its ecological validity and effectiveness. The SCIP is a group program that uses drama activities to help children accurately perceive and respond to social cues. Intervention programs that are based in creative drama have just begun to be developed and show promise for working with children with ASDs as well as those with similar social difficulties (Guli et al. in press; Lerner et al. 2010; Minne and Semrud-Clikeman 2011). By allowing children to develop social competence in a real-time and playful context, the program provides a unique opportunity for children to experience the feelings of social success. The emerging empirical support for programs, and particularly SCIP, which utilize creative drama, is very promising. Additional research is currently being conducted to continue to empirically validate this program.

References

Barrett, S., Prior, M., & Manjiviona, J. (2004). Children on the borderlands of autism. *Autism, 8*(1), 61–87.

Corbett, B. A. (2003). Video Modeling: A window into the world of autism. *The Behavior Analyst Today, 4*, 1–10.

Cresi, M. M. (1989). *Creative dramatics for children*. New York: Scott Foresman.

Crick, N. R., & Dodge, K. A. (1994). A review and reformation of social-information processing mechanisms in children's social adjustment. *Psychological Bulletin, 115*(1), 74–101.

Damasio, A. R. (1994). *Descartes' Error: Emotion, reason, and the human brain*. New York: Grosset/Putnam.

Fine, J. G., Semrud-Clikeman, M., Butcher, B., & Walkowiak, J. (2008). Brief report: Attention effect on a measure of social perception *Journal of Autism and Developmental Disorders, 38*, 1797–1802.

Guli, L. A. (2005). The effects of creative drama-based intervention for children with deficits in social perception. *Dissertations Abstracts International, 65*, 3690 (UMI No. 3151245).

Guli, L. A., Semrud-Clikeman, M., Lerner, M., & Borich, M. (in press). Use of creative drama as intervention for children with social competence deficits. *Arts in Psychotherapy*.

Guli, L. A., Wilkinson, A., & Semrud-Clikeman, M. (2008). *Social Competence Intervention Program*. Champaign: Research Press.

Hala, S., Hug, S., & Henderson, A. (2003). Executive function and false-belief understanding in preschool children: Two tasks are harder than one. *Journal of Cognition and Development, 4*, 275–298.

Happe, F., & Frith, U. (2006). The weak coherence account: Detail-focused cognitive style in autism spectrum disorders. *Journal of Autism and Developmental Disorders, 36*(1), 5–25.

Lerner, M. D., Mikami, A. Y., & Levine, K. (2010). Socio-dramatic affective-relational intervention for adolescents with Asperger syndrome and high functioning autism: Pilot study. *Autism, 15*(1), 21–42. doi:10.1177/1362361309353613.

Minne, E., & Semrud-Clikeman, M. (2011). A social competence intervention for young children with High Functioning Autism and Asperger Syndrome. *Autism*. doi:10.1177/1362361311423384.

Neelands, J., & Goode, T. (2001). *Structuring drama work: A handbook of available forms in theatre and drama*. Cambridge: Cambridge University Press.

O'Neill, C., & Lambert, A. (1994). *Drama structures: A practical handbook for teachers*. Portsmouth: Stanley Thornes.

Ozonoff, S., & Rogers, S. J. (2003). Autism spectrum disorders: A research review for practitioners. In S. Ozonoff, S. J. Rogers, & R. L. Hendren (Eds.), *Review of psychiatry* (pp. 3–33). Washington, D.C.: American Psychiatric Publishing.

Portman, E. (2006). A social competence intervention program for children with high functioning autism and Asperger's Syndrome: A qualitative study. *Dissertations Abstracts International, 68,* 212 (UMI No. 3294420).
Querol, M. G. & Piera, E. (personal communication) from Centre Salut Mental Infantil I Juvenil.
Semrud-Clikeman, M. (2007). *Social competence in children.* New York: Springer.
Semrud-Clikeman, M., & Schaefer, V. (2000). Social competence in developmental disorders. *Journal of Psychotherapy in Independent Practice, 4,* 3–20.
Semrud-Clikeman, M., Walkowiak, J., Wilkinson, A., & Christopher, G. (2010). Neuropsychological findings in nonverbal learning disabilities. *Developmental Neuropsychology, 35,* 582–600.
Semrud-Clikeman, M., Walkowiak, J., Wilkinson, A., & Minne, E. (2010). Behavior and social perception in children with Asperger's Disorder, Nonverbal Learning Disability, or ADHD. *Journal of Abnormal Child Psychology, 38,* 509–519.
Sherratt, D., & Peter, M. (2002). *Developing play and drama in children with autistic spectrum disorders.* London: David Fulton.
Spitzberg, B. H. (2003). Methods of interpersonal skill assessment. In J. O. Greene & B. R. Burleson (Eds.), *Handbook of communication and social interaction skills* (pp. 93–134). Mahwah: Erlbaum.
Spolin, V. (1986). *Theater games for the classroom.* Evanston: Northwestern University Press.
Voeller, K. K. S. (1994). Techniques for measuring social competence in children. In G. R. Lyon (Ed.), *Frames of reference for the assessment of learning disabilities* (pp. 523–554). Baltimore: Brookes Publishing.
Waters, E., & Sroufe, L. A. (1983). Social competence as a developmental construct. *Developmental Review, 3,* 79–97.

Chapter 9
Progress for Remediating and Expanding Social Skills (PROGress)

Lori Krasny

The better part of one's life consists of his friendships . . . —Abraham Lincoln

Social interactions form the building blocks for much of human development. Children learn from other people and through play with peers. Their ideas, skills, and interests are shaped by these exchanges. For persons with autism spectrum disorders (ASD), interactions and friendships may be no less valuable, but they are far more difficult to establish. The ability to connect with others, participate in exchanges, learn from interactions, and enjoy relationships with others is impaired (American Psychiatric Association 2000; Bauminger and Kasari 2000; Bauminger and Shulman 2003; Daniel and Billingsley 2010; Locke et al. 2010).

Social difficulties are a core deficit of autism. Research has consistently documented social deficits common to autism spectrum disorders, including: difficulty understanding or deciphering subtle social cues such as facial expressions, tone of voice, and body language; deficits in joint attention; difficulty joining peer conversations or interactions; struggles with fully processing verbal and nonverbal communication; and/or uncertainty regarding expectations in different social environments (American Psychiatric Association 2000; Siegal and Blades 2003; Tager-Flusberg 1999; Wetherby et al. 1998; Wetherby and Prutting 1984). For most people with ASD, these difficulties define their most challenging experiences. Because of them, attempts at navigating peer and social settings often result in confusion, anxiety, and depression (Barnhill 2001; Bellini 2006; Myles et al. 2001; Wing 1981). Repeated failed attempts at social interaction may lead to decreased social interest, and/or an aversion or avoidance of social situations. In general, persons with ASD are often uncertain as to how to read their social environment, inappropriate in engaging in it, or excluded by peers from participating in it.

Difficulty and failure in peer social interactions are frequently experienced from a very early age. Their impact is far reaching, often negatively affecting the interpersonal relationships of persons with ASD, across their entire lifetimes (Howlin

L. Krasny (✉)
The Children's Center, 350 South 400 East, Salt Lake City, Utah 84111, USA
e-mail: lkrasny@tccslc.org

S. Goldstein, J. A. Naglieri (eds.), *Interventions for Autism Spectrum Disorders*,
DOI 10.1007/978-1-4614-5301-7_9, © Springer Science+Business Media New York 2013

2000; Levy and Perry 2011; McGovern and Sigman 2005; Seltzer et al. 2003). Furthermore, these negative experiences become highly difficult to impact or change (Bellini 2006; Farrugia and Hudson 2006).

Traditional behavioral interventions for children with ASD, including social skill development, are typically provided in individual therapy sessions, one-on-one with an adult. Individual skills or behaviors are often taught in isolation and outside of a social context. In these programs, intervention in peer settings does not begin until late in a child's therapeutic program, when generalization of the isolated skills becomes the goal. More recent behavioral interventions offered within natural environments typically focus on acquisition and use of specific behaviors important in interactions. Similarly, group social skills interventions typically teach and practice specific skills using adult instruction or peer mentoring strategies. While these models are highly valuable, there are few published group curricula for young children with ASD and those reported do not commonly utilize the genuine social peer environments in which these children typically participate or wish to join. Furthermore, they tend to lack critical emphasis on the affective and/or social emotional experiences of the child. Also, lacking is a therapeutic opportunity to regularly experience natural peer groups as fun, positive, enjoyable, and successful.

This chapter will discuss a group social skills intervention model that aims to change the cycle of social failure often experienced by children with ASD by creating an environment that fosters successful peer engagement. In this model, a positive peer environment is created within which children with ASD experience a sense of belonging, joy, and excitement at attending, as well as satisfaction and success in engaging with peers. This environment sets into motion a completely different and far more facilitating experience than is usually experienced by children with ASD in group peer settings. By creating an environment that fosters natural and successful peer engagement and interactions early on, young children with autism spectrum disorders can experience, learn, and succeed in peer play much as their typical peers do. As a result of these early positive experiences, children with ASD can develop positive social foundations with which to learn needed skills, seek continued friendships, and experience social successes. Furthermore, by providing environmental supports such as structure, predictability, language scaffolding, and visual instruction, described later in this chapter, the participants are supported in and freed from the typically confusing and anxiety-producing elements that usually challenge them. They are then "freed up" to recognize, practice, and experience success with social interactions and needed skills. In such an environment, the children can experience the natural and often unpredictable social elements of peer group interactions. They can learn what to do, how to do it, and with whom. They can develop motivation to engage with peers, learn to seek interactions, perceive peer social experiences positively, and establish genuine friendships. Support and structure can help them understand and manage the situations as they arise. Ultimately, they can experience success in authentic and intrinsically motivating peer interactions, and can experience the joys of friendship and interaction often achieved by their typical peers.

The PROGress Model and Curricula

The PROGress Model (*PROG*ram for *R*emediating and *E*xpanding *S*ocial *S*kills) described in this chapter is designed for early school-age children, ages 4–9, with autism spectrum disorders. The concepts presented incorporate intervention strategies demonstrated as effective in clinical and research literature. This model can be easily adapted for children and young adults of varying ages and abilities. Furthermore, while this model has been implemented with hundreds of children in an after-school clinical setting, it can also be easily adapted for school settings as well. Adaptations to the model described are discussed later in the chapter.

The PROGress Model is designed as a 25-week curriculum, consisting of up to five units that each last for 5 weeks. The first 4 weeks of each unit introduce and build skills, while the fifth week is designed as a generalization session, typically involving a community outing. This format is designed to parallel a typical school year, giving children an opportunity to settle into their classroom settings prior to beginning the group. Similarly, the sessions run weekly and thus end just before the school year also ends. The 25-week curriculum is successful in providing needed time for genuine friendships and relationships to develop, as well as ample time for the basic skills to be repeatedly practiced and honed, while additional skills can be added and developed.

Each session typically lasts for 75–90 minutes. This provides adequate time to include organized opening and closing routines, skill development and practice, and snack time to further enhance social skills and generalization. The PROGress Model also utilizes a 1:3 or 1:4 adult to child ratio within the groups, with a maximum of 12 children enrolled. Both the group size and the adult child ratio are dependent upon the needs of the participants. Groups with children needing more individualized support are often grouped in smaller configurations of six to eight children, with a 1:3 adult to child ratio. Groups of children with more independence and self-regulation typically benefit from a larger peer group and a 1:4 adult to child ratio is provided to support their success.

Group and Curricular Planning

In this section, features, factors, and elements critical to forming groups and determining curriculum will be addressed.

Forming Groups

Many aspects of group social skills intervention require careful attention and planning. First and foremost in the planning process is the careful determination of the group and the peers with whom a child is placed. Social skills group placement in the PROGress Model requires different consideration than is often applied to classroom placements.

In most school settings, academic placements typically group children with same-age, same-grade peers, based upon their emerging skills. This allows children to perpetually work on skill *acquisition*. In the PROGress Model, skill *use,* rather than acquisition, is the primary emphasis and focus. A child's social ability and use is highly dependent upon his personal willingness, desire, and comfort in interacting. Regardless of what social skills a child possesses, he can only truly be successful with them when he is willing to utilize them. Thus, placement in a group where a child can experience comfort, ease, and enjoyment in social interactions is a critical first step to both the planning of the group and to the child's social success. Social interest, motivation, and skills are all primary placement concerns. An unstructured social play observation by a skilled clinician is generally adequate for assessing this. First, the child's social use and comfort with peers is carefully determined. Only after that should consideration be given to the developmental, cognitive and language abilities, and age of the group participants. This careful matching and placement results in the greatest social fit for participants, and the greatest ability to adapt the group format, expectations, and instruction. This careful matching of social comfort and individual skills maximizes engagement and success. Once social comfort and skill use is achieved, further skill development can then be addressed.

> Anthony is $5^1/_2$ years old and has a diagnosis of autism. He uses one- and two-word utterances to communicate. He typically plays and works in isolation but often watches his peers when he is in a group activity. Anthony will initiate to a peer only when given a physical prompt and a verbal model.
>
> Eric is 4 years old with a diagnosis of High Functioning Autism. He can spontaneously engage with adults using complete sentences in one-on-one interactions. He enjoys many toys and activities with adults or at home and can follow simple directions and sequenced play activities. When Eric is in a peer group setting, he covers his ears, runs around the room, and will not join in group activities.

- In the PROGress Model, both these boys would be placed in the same group. While they are in different grades at school, and their verbal and cognitive skills differ, both are working on maintaining regulation and simple engagement with peers in a group setting.

> Evan is 6 years old and has a diagnosis of PDD-NOS. He is highly verbal at home but is very reserved and quiet outside of his home and rarely engages verbally in any other settings. He is in a half-day regular education kindergarten and has age-appropriate cognitive and receptive language skills. In class, he follows all classroom instructions and engages in all activities, albeit nonverbally.
>
> Jacob is 7 years old and has a diagnosis of autism. He is in a special education classroom at his neighborhood school. His academic skills range in ability from first grade (language) through third grade (math). Jacob is friendly with peers and adults and is willing to join in teacher-led classroom activities but he has no friends in the class. He often plays alone at recess and sits alone at lunch.

- In the PROGress Model, both these boys would be placed in the same group. They are a year apart in school, are in different academic settings, and have very different abilities. Both boys can follow simple directions and participate in structured, concrete activities. They both need significant assistance and support in engaging successfully with peers.

Group Levels

Once children are matched based upon their social comfort and use, the appropriate curriculum level and focus must be determined. The PROGress Model is designed with four different levels of curricular focus. Each level is intended to meet the general social and developmental needs of the group. That noted, however, each grouping of children brings with it its own issues, balance, and flow. Thus, each group of children must be carefully observed and assessed, and adaptations to each group's schedule, activities, and curriculum must be made. These adaptations will be discussed in the next section.

The four curricular levels of PROGress Model include:

- Play-based
- High structure
- Low structure
- Thematic activities

Each level addresses different social and developmental needs that are described below.

Play-Based This curriculum is designed for children with ASD who exhibit an interest in engaging with peers but who are primarily challenged to remain calm and regulated when in a group of peers. The activities within this curriculum are play-based in nature, allowing the participants to engage in motivating activities and materials at the level of engagement with which they are most comfortable. Once engaged in play, the goals within the curriculum should include playing in close proximity of peers, participating in activities with others, using a common set of materials, attending to peers, imitating peers, initiating and responding to simple requests, and playing together with peers.

High Structure This curriculum is designed to meet the needs of children with ASD who demonstrate interest in interacting, who have at least some spontaneous language abilities, and who can participate in and follow structured, concrete activities. This curriculum is intended to provide needed scaffolding to children who require structure and support to process language, to participate in activities, and/or to interact with peers.

Low Structure This curriculum is intended to support the social interactions of children who have both the interest and ability to interact spontaneously with peers, but who may need some guidance and support in understanding the most appropriate ways to do so. This curriculum provides opportunity for independent interactions and supports the practice and use of skills in semistructured or natural social opportunities.

Thematic Activities This curriculum is designed for children who have already benefited from and mastered participation in the Low Structure Groups and/or for children who function fairly well in typical peer activities but need some support to understand appropriate interaction skills or with negotiating social problems. This curriculum offers multisession thematic activities that involve social peer skills such as negotiation, cooperation, compromise, acceptance, and joint planning and participation. Support, coaching, and teaching is provided and practiced within the context of the activities, as needed.

It is vital to the success of the children in the group that they are following the curriculum level at which they are most able and comfortable engaging, rather than at a level that requires abilities they have not yet mastered or are not at ease using in peer groups.

Ryan is a 6-year-old boy with autism who has spontaneous, independent language that he uses at home with his siblings and family. Ryan is considered very shy and demonstrates significant anxiety when in social peer groups. Upon enrolling in the social skills group, Ryan was willing to participate in activities, but required his mother to remain in the room, and refused to verbally engage with peers. Although he had language skills consistent with the children in the Low Structure group, that group required him to use his language abilities in order to participate. This social demand was not consistent with his social comfort and typical engagement. Thus, Ryan was placed in a High Structure group. His mother remained in the room for the first 5 weeks, until a planned exit at the predictable snack time was implemented. Three weeks later, he told his mother she could leave after the opening Hello Song. Ryan participated in this group for the 25-week session, becoming increasingly more comfortable with his peers as the weeks progressed. By the end of group, he was both at ease with his peers and was independently using his spontaneous language skills in all activities. The following session, Ryan participated in the Low Structure Group and was able to independently engage with peers while practicing and learning new skills throughout the session. By the end of this second group, Ryan considered the Thematic Activity Group (called "The Kids' Club") but felt he no longer needed to attend the social skills groups and began inviting peers over to his house for play dates. He was highly successful in these small, planned social opportunities and his classroom teacher also reported that he was engaging in small groups of peers spontaneously at school.

Determining the Curriculum

Relevance to ASD

Children with ASD are often unable to recognize or understand the subtle social cues that their peers intuitively use and depend upon when engaging with each other. For example, cues from peers that signal such subtleties as interest, disinterest, openness, and engagement are frequently missed by the child with ASD. Failure to recognize these cues often results in the child with ASD being unaware of whether peers are engaged or interested. As a result, the child with ASD may experience difficulty joining in, may be unaware of when to stop a behavior or conversational topic, or may lack understanding of what the social expectations are. Ultimately, this can lead to personal confusion, peer rejection, social isolation, and/or group exclusion commonly experienced by children with ASD.

Although autism-specific curricula such as the PROGress Model are being developed and offered, most commercially available social skills curricula designed to meet the needs of children with social difficulties often do not adequately address these underlying social difficulties that make social interactions so challenging for children with ASD. In a social skills intervention specifically aimed at meeting the social needs of this population, it is imperative that the goals addressed are salient, relevant, and central to the underlying deficits common in autism. For children without ASD such goals may seem foolish and obvious, but for children with ASD the goals addressed and skills developed must help these children to recognize and understand the present and at times subtle social information that often eludes them.

Research has demonstrated that skill awareness and daily use is facilitated when children understand the importance and relevance of the skill and its use (Gray 1995). Thus, it is also important that information about not only the behaviors but the variables critical to appropriately using those behaviors is embedded in the teaching and rehearsal opportunities provided within the groups. Children with ASD must learn more than just how to perform the targeted skills. If simply teaching a behavior or skill was sufficient to change the social deficits commonly seen in autism, this chapter would be unnecessary and the social skill deficits of children with ASD would be easily remediated. Rather, it is commonly understood that these deficits are complex and difficult to eliminate. Perhaps that is because learning a skill is only the first part of what needs to be taught. Children with ASD must learn not only what they need to do and how to do it, but also why they need to do it, with whom they should and should not use a skill, when and when not to use the skill, and why. Taught in the context of the interactions, the relevance of the instruction is authentic and motivating. The likelihood of the skill becoming a part of the child's social repertoire is enhanced.

> Carly is a 7-year-old girl with ASD who enjoys being with peers and is easily engaged in social activities. She easily enters the group each week and will willingly interact with adults and peers. Carly is very soft-spoken, however, and is barely audible when she interacts. In group, activities are designed to require initiating, requesting, and responding to peers in highly motivating activities. When Carly first began spontaneously engaging her peers, she was reminded "Justin can't hear you. You need to change your voice to a 'medium voice' so he knows what you want." (Note: this was only offered after voice volumes were concretely defined and taught). Following repeated practice, Carly is now only reminded "this room is pretty noisy!" or "Do you think he heard you?" to which she is able to independently problem solve and change her volume to one that is more audible and successful.

Group Goals and Skills

The goals identified for a group must be dependent upon many factors: the abilities of the children within the group, the rate and pace at which they can understand and acquire skills, and the amount of time available in the group to learn, practice, and gain skills. In the PROGress Model, the goals for each of the groups are included below.

Play-Based

Interaction basics Learning peers' names, greeting, observing others.

Communication basics Greeting, initiating, showing, asking, listening.

Play and friendship skills Playing alongside and with, using materials together, sharing space, taking turns.

High Structure
Interaction basics Learning peers' names, using an appropriate volume, maintaining an appropriate distance, and observing and listening to others.

Communication basics Commenting or "telling," questioning or "asking"; commenting and questioning with peers, "checking in" with peers in a conversation; initiating a conversation, participating in a peer's conversation topic, maintaining a conversation, ending a conversation, staying on a conversation topic, switching a conversation topic.

Play and friendship skills Defining a "Friend" versus "Not a friend," joining in play, sharing materials and equipment, taking turns, compromising, negotiating, following group rules, fairness, winning and losing.

Emotions and feelings Developing an emotional vocabulary, recognizing varying emotions in others, recognizing varying emotions in self, understanding what causes emotions and feelings, dealing with emotions, taking others' perspective, and developing and showing empathy.

Self and others awareness Identifying unique and important characteristics of self and of others, recognizing similarities and differences in people, playing and working cooperatively, sharing different interests, cooperating and compromising.

Low Structure The first four units described above are also addressed with the Low Structure groups, although it is done so in ways that facilitate and utilize greater independence and spontaneous engagement. In addition, because these children experience and are able to understand and negotiate greater abstract social issues, the following unit is also included:

Social problem solving Being told "no"; dealing with things you don't like, feeling left out, being teased, saying or being told "I don't know," and self-advocating in social situations.

Thematic Activities The children in this group work on skills needed as they work together on thematic units such as science experiments, building projects, cooking, games, etc. Although the goals may vary, dependent on each particular group of children, they commonly work on maintaining a conversation topic, checking in with and engaging peers, negotiating, decision making, consensus building, cooperating, compromising, self-advocating, winning and losing, and dealing with disappointment.

Sequential and Progressive Instruction

It is commonly known that repetition and practice are critical to skill mastery. However, it is perhaps all too common that children are taught social skills as a series of isolated behaviors with little ongoing reinforcement or skill coordination. In planning social skills interventions, it is important to consider the order in which activities and skills are introduced and rehearsed to maximize the opportunities for coordinated skill development and use. A fluid and connected learning continuum should be provided in which the most relevant skills needed are continually addressed and practiced. As described below, this sequential and progressive programming should occur for each session, for each set or unit of lessons, and across the entire skill content provided. It is important to teach basic skills first, then continue to practice them as later skills are introduced and practiced. Activities and skills should build upon each other and be interrelated. Intervention should intentionally utilize a natural context within which the authentic social motivation and learning can occur. By doing so, one can carefully ensure that not only are the appropriate skills addressed, but also that they are taught in a coordinated manner that supports, reinforces, and builds upon earlier skills. Such programming promotes social awareness and skill development, ensures necessary practice and repetition needed to develop mastery, and increases the likelihood of maintenance and use of the skills. Below, a description of how the PROGress Curricula planfully accomplishes this is provided.

Curricular Sequence

Within each set of skills or skill unit, the way in which the skills are presented and taught must also be considered and carefully planned so that the earliest and most fundamental skills are practiced with greatest frequency and repetition, while new skills are added. The Introductory, Skill Development, Integration and Generalization Phases detailed below can also be built in to the design of skill units within a curriculum. In the PROGress curricula for the High and Low Structure Groups, the first 2 weeks of a 5-week unit comprises the Introductory Phase. In these sessions, the basic concepts and skills of the unit are introduced and practiced. The next two sessions make up the Skill Development portion of the unit. During these weeks, the skills from the first 2 weeks continue to be practiced while additional skills are added. In the fourth week of the unit, all the skills are combined and integrated into typical, semistructured, age-appropriate activities and games that require the coordinated use of those skills previously taught. The fifth and last week of the unit is dedicated to generalization of the skills. A community outing is scheduled at a location or event that requires the use of the skills addressed in the unit just completed.

- In the High Structure Group of the PROGress curriculum, the Conversation Skills Unit begins with activities that teach and reinforce greetings, using peers names to engage them, and initiating a topic or interaction. Next, "telling" and "asking" are practiced individually. This is followed by coordinating the acts of telling a designated number of comments and then engaging or asking a peer to join in. Next, strategies and tools to blend these together into a conversation are taught and rehearsed. For the final week, we meet at a pizza restaurant to eat and talk with each other.

Finally, the coordination of all sessions and units should be considered in a sequential manner when determining the flow of instruction for the entire curricula. The sequence of skills taught across the entire group curriculum should also be carefully determined so that those concepts and skills taught first are prerequisite to the subsequent skills addressed. With such planning, the earlier skills addressed at the beginning of the curriculum continue to be practiced and used as the next skills are introduced and learned.

- In the Low Structure PROGress Curriculum, the children focus on learning peers' names in the first and second weeks in the group curriculum so that when in the sixth week of the curriculum they address Conversation Skills they learn to say the person's name and then initiate a topic.

If skills are carefully planned, then those taught first are practiced as needed throughout the course of the group. Skill development and mastery can thus be planfully designed.

- Learning the concept of "friend" versus "not a friend" is addressed in the 13th week of the Low Structure PROGress Curriculum. Awareness of whether someone's social attention is intended as friendly or not and mastery of recognizing and evaluating these advances must be learned before the participants can be expected to use self-advocacy strategies, to apply, for example, when someone is not being a friend. This is addressed in the 21st week of the curriculum in the Social Problem-Solving Unit.
- Children learn to identify other people's emotions and their own emotions in weeks 17 and 18 of the Low Structure PROGress Curriculum. A child must be able to identify that he is becoming frustrated, before he can be expected to implement a skill or strategy to deal with frustration. In the Social Problem-Solving Unit, taught in weeks 21 through 24, the children then learn strategies for what to do when they feel frustrated.

Session Sequence

Within a group session, it is important to consider and plan the sequence and progression of the many activities and experiences to be provided. The order of activities and events should carefully assist the participants in both learning and practicing skills. Thus, each session should be designed to include the greatest structure and adult input at the beginning of the session, when the skill is first being introduced and taught. This would be an Introductory Phase. Activities are designed to provide clear and concrete instruction and examples of the skills being introduced. Practice is incorporated in natural and age-appropriate activities to enhance understanding, awareness, and skill development. As the session progresses, the activities are designed with decreased instruction and structure as well as increased practice so that the participants can learn to use the skill more independently with each other. This is the Skill Building Phase. Group leaders provide assistance as needed or identify the importance of the skill within the activity or interaction. As the session progresses, the children use the skills within a familiar game, event, or routine, such as snack. This is the Integration Phase. Natural opportunities to practice must be designed, incorporated, and encouraged. Last, the children practice the skill in a semistructured game or event that closely resembles typical peer activities but is adapted to include, emphasize, or highlight the skill for the day. This is the Generalization Phase. Throughout this session, the use of skills previously taught and relevant to the interaction are reinforced, highlighted, and encouraged as well.

Group Structure and Flow

The design of a group's schedule and activities can be as individual as the group itself. Each purposefully chosen set of children create their own group character, pacing, flow and group energy. The personality of the group as a whole is important to identify, as the planning of a session must be responsive to it.

- When Opening circle for a Play-Based Group began, the children were seated on carpet squares on the rug in a semicircle. Unlike most groups, it was noted that this particular group of children had a very difficult time focusing and remaining regulated during this highly structured task. Visual and spatial cues such as carpet squares and an identified corner of the carpeted area were utilized to better structure the activity; however, the children demonstrated continued difficulty focusing and engaging when seated on the floor. Recognizing that the large open space on the carpet may have been the dysregulating factor, the opening circle and hello time was moved to the table, where the children sat in chairs around the table. This arrangement was far more facilitating and they easily participated in the opening activity when this change was made.
- The children enrolled in a particular High Structure class were more easily distracted and required significantly more support and adult assistance than typical to fully participate in small group activities. Thus, rather than enrolling 12 children in the group, only 9 were enrolled. These 9 children were regularly divided into three groups of 3 children to participate in most learning activities and games. These smaller more focused groups increased the amount of individual structure that could be provided, increased the child's time on task, decreased the amount of waiting time they had to navigate, and provided more opportunities for hands-on practice of the skill. Once the children began developing skills and becoming more comfortable within the group routine and with peers, we were able to divide the group into two slightly larger groups to include the addition of interactive games in the second half of the group sessions.
- Following the opening circle, a group of 12 children in the Low Structure group were divided into three small groups comprising of 4 children each to work on skill development. As was typical for the Low Structure groups, the small groups of children rotated together through three activities in order to practice the day's target skill in three different ways. One particular group, however,

found the small groups very distracting. Regardless of the activity presented, the attention and focus of most of the children was on what was occurring in the other small groups, rather than their own. As a result, the group flow was changed and the 12 children were divided into two groups of 6 children each. These two groups did identical tasks to decrease distraction and increase participation.

Techniques and Strategies for Group Intervention

In the next section, specific techniques and strategies that facilitate the success and appropriateness of group interventions and activities will be discussed. Many of the techniques discussed throughout this chapter have been consistently reported in the research literature and are commonly used in individual and classroom interventions. When utilized within the group social skills setting, they help guide the children in knowing what is expected of them and how and when they are being successful. While not an exhaustive list of best practices, they are techniques that can be universally helpful in group intervention. Implementation of these techniques in newly developed curricula or in conjunction with already published social skills curricula may prove useful in implementing group intervention for children with ASDs.

Predictability and Routine

Research and practice has demonstrated the importance of predictability and routine in easing anxiety and in promoting understanding and participation for children with ASD. For these reasons, the use of predictable routines is equally important to include in the group social skills planning. Providing a consistent routine followed each time, the group meetings allows the participating children to understand in advance what will occur and what they will be expected to do. By doing so, anxiety caused by uncertainty, anticipation, fear, and/or a feeling of helplessness is addressed. A group routine that incorporates a consistent opening routine, instructional events, routines and rituals, and a closing routine help the children anticipate, know, and join in with the flow of the session. By consistently following such a routine or series of consistent events, the specific activities within each event can vary to meet the curricular needs. For example, small group instructional activities always occur following the opening circle and greeting routine. Once the children are in these small groups, the activity they engage in may be an art project, a story, a game, or a construction task, depending upon the skill being taught. Each week the activity may change but it will consistently occur within the regular routine of dividing into small learning groups.

- Each week of the High Structure group, the session schedule includes: an opening hello song on the floor, then they divide into small work groups on the floor. Next, they move to a large group activity at the table, and then have snack or a snack activity at the table. Last, they move to a large group activity on the floor, and then end with a closing goodbye song sung on the floor.

- The Play-Based Group enters the room and engages with free play toys on the rug. After 10 minutes, the children put their toys in the bucket and are given 10 stickers to put on a sticker sheet set out at the table. After stickers, an opening hello song or routine is planned. The children then remain at the table for a sensory activity, followed by a group construction or art project. Once finished, the children are given a transition object to bring to the interactive book circle on the carpet. While on the carpet, a large motor or group interaction activity occurs next, then the children move to the table to have snack or a snack activity. Next is a group table activity and then a closing goodbye song or routine.

Make Abstract Concepts Concrete

Children with ASD typically interpret information literally and concretely. Unfortunately for them, most social information and concepts are not only abstract but they may also be person-specific, context-dependent, and/or situation-related. Many of the social skills with which children with ASD struggle are skills that are subtle, implied, and/or abstract. Concepts such as kindness, conversation, frustration, and friendship are highly abstract and difficult to fully grasp. Such skills are both difficult for children with ASD to recognize and difficult for educators and parents to explain. In order for children with ASD to understand exactly what is expected of them socially, these abstract tasks must be taught and practiced in the most concrete ways possible. Children with ASD must be able to define the skill or situation in order to recognize whether it is present or absent. The child must have concrete rules or strategies to use. This often takes thoughtful consideration on the part of those teaching the abstract skills, to take into account what is understood, or misunderstood, by the child with ASD. Some skills that are naturally intued by many are often unknown or unrecognized by a child with ASD.

To help children with ASD understand these abstract concepts, it is critical that the concept is first defined in clear, concrete terms that allow children to understand if the behavior is present or absent, yes or no, true or untrue. An operational definition must be developed that allows the child to clearly identify the behavior. In the PROGress Curriculum groups, we make sure the children can concretely identify the behavior, for example, a soft versus a medium voice. With consideration for the abilities of the children in the group, tools can be developed to address complex social situations. This may include developing a definition, creating a concrete list, using a visual model, or defining behaviors. The children can then practice identifying positive and negative examples based on the tool developed. In the context of a peer social group, these behaviors can then not only be learned but more importantly, children can be shown or taught why it is important to apply the skills as they practice using them with each other.

- A “Hug List” can be developed for children who indiscriminately hug people with whom they come in contact. If a name is on the list, that person can be hugged; but, if the person is not on the list, hugging is not permitted.
- Social concepts such as standing too close may be operationally defined as “you need to stand an arm away.” Children can then determine whether they are at the desired distance or not by outstretching his or her arm and measuring his/her own distance from a peer, and make any corrections needed.
- Eye contact is commonly targeted skill. To make such a skill concrete, we use the concrete concept of pointing, as in “point your eyes,” rather than “look at me” to help children understand what is expected. This is taught by offering arrows and asking the children to point to various named objects or people with their arrows. Then, the children are asked to place the arrows beside their eyes and point both arrow and eyes at the named object and peers. This then uses the concrete task of pointing to help understand directing or pointing your eyes to the person talking to you or to whom you are talking.
- The same strategy can be used for more abstract and complicated social situations. Teasing, for example, must be defined in terms the child can understand, and that will provide as clear a distinction as possible between teasing and not teasing. In this example, children might learn that teasing is: not nice, using mean words, doing something mean, trying to make you mad or get you in trouble, trying to make you sad or mad, etc. This concrete definition helps a child differentiate between teasing and a neutral comment, or even teasing versus being told something you are not happy about. Once the child can detect that teasing is occurring, he or she can be taught strategies to respond appropriately to the social problem.

Visual Instruction and Support

Providing visual support is another tool in making abstract or difficult concepts more concrete and comprehensible. Children with ASD often find it much easier to follow visual rather than verbal information and prefer or learn best with visually cued instruction. Visual supports can be used to augment verbal instruction and information provided. Unlike language, visual supports are concrete and remain present and available over time and thus can be frequently referred to. This helps to make verbal instruction more tangible and more easily understood. In the PROGress groups, this is referred to as “see it first, say it second.”

Visual supports then, are an important tool in helping the children in a group to know what is expected and what will occur. Visual supports can be offered in a number of ways and to support or explain a variety of events. A picture schedule corresponding with the consistent group routine can be displayed to remind and support the children in knowing what is expected and joining the routine. Visual supports can also be used to provide an explanation of what is expected within each of the group events or activities. For example, a template can be provided to show a child where he is expected to glue on his selected pictures; carpet squares placed in a semicircle on the floor show the children in the group where they are expected to sit; giving two children the same colored circle shows them who their partner is; and, showing a finished art product may show the children how to do the art project. These visual supports can be offered and the verbal instruction or explanation can be offered secondary to the visual information provided.

Promoting "Other Focused" Engagement

Healthy peer interaction typically involves cooperation and shared participation. For some young children in general, and for children with ASD in particular, it is often easier, more comfortable, and more desirable to focus on one's own self-interests and desires than to attend to the interests and desires of others. For children with ASD, deficits or challenges with theory of mind, or understanding and attending to the perspectives and interests of others, makes engaging fruitfully with them all the more challenging. However, participating in a social skills group is an opportunity for social rather than independence skill building. Yet, group camaraderie and belonging will likely not occur without actively planning and repeatedly practicing opportunities to attend to, engage with, and positively experience interactions with others. In the PROGress Model, all planning follows the rule that the children neither do things for or by themselves that they can instead do for or with someone else. By adopting this practice, all activities are altered to ensure that the children participating in them are focused or engaged with or on their peers. This can be accomplished in a number of ways depending upon the activity. As previously detailed, children may be paired with peers to complete a task together, rather than alone. When doing projects, children may share a common set of materials rather than be given their own materials. For example, if building a city with blocks, children may be required to use a common base to add their structure to so that the city created is built by all four children in the instructional group. Similarly, if painting a picture, children in pairs may share a large piece of paper rather than have their own. At snack, peers can ask each other to get their desired items for them. All activities can be designed to have the children work together, either on the same task or by sharing materials. The children are regularly and consistently encouraged to watch or interact with their partners or their friends and if a child is working alone, she typically is doing so to make something for another peer, rather than for herself. These strategies foster group camaraderie, shared interests, and reciprocal friendships that would not necessarily occur naturally amongst this population.

Another feature of healthy friendship and community is that participants are generally familiar with and cooperatively engage in each others' individual interests and preferences. In other words, friends know what their friends like or what their interests are. However, theory of mind deficits commonly found in children with ASD impact their ability to take on the perspectives of others. Furthermore, their heightened and restrictive interests often impact their ability to share in the interests of others. Another way to develop friendships and promote a positive group culture within a social skills group is by creating opportunities for regular and repeated practice engaging in and becoming familiar with each other's interests. This may be done in a number of ways. In the PROGress Model groups, regularly scheduled opportunities are provided for the children in the group to be "In the Spotlight" as well as being paired with a peer who is a "Spotlight Partner." Both roles are planned a week in advance. One child is chosen to be "In the Spotlight." This child picks a topic of interest to share with peers in the subsequent week. The "Spotlight" is welcomed to bring in props and materials to show to peers, teach about the interest, or encourage others to also be interested in the topic. The challenge for this child is to share his heightened interest or chosen topic for only a designated and somewhat brief amount of time. A peer is then chosen as a "Spotlight Partner." In this role, the child must also share information about his peer's chosen topic of interest. He may choose to do so in any way that is appealing to him. For example, children find books on the topic, search the web for pictures or information, draw pictures, or find toys or props. The challenge for the "Spotlight Partner" is to engage in a topic of interest that is not his or her own. This task aims to build an early foundation for engaging in others' interests, learning friendship skills, and developing empathy and understanding of others.

Attending to the interests of peers might also be practiced with activities that require the children to select an activity, object, or gift that the child thinks his peer may like. This might be facilitated by sharing a list of the child's favorites such as color, foods, and activities. This list can be used to guide in the selection of the object or gift.

In social skills groups where children are regularly and frequently supported to engage together, a culture of positive peer interaction is created. Peers in the group regularly experience positive and successful peer engagement and can learn that such group camaraderie can be both enjoyable and rewarding.

Scaffolded Language and Support

As described above, social skills groups are most successful when the social needs, cognitive abilities, and language skills of the participants are most closely matched. The more similar the needs of the group, the better able a group leader is to appropriately gear the level of instruction and the expectations of the activity. In addition, the language support or scaffolding used to meet the developmental and social abilities of the children in each group can be more uniformly provided. In other words, the way a skill is taught and practiced for one group of children may be very different than how the same skill is taught and practiced with another group of children.

- In a Conversation Unit for a High Structure group, children are working on developing the skill of commenting or telling. These children have limited independent verbal skills. Thus, they are given a tray of small objects and a simple verbal script: "I have a _______." The first child is required to choose an object and comment on or tell what they have. The next child uses the same phrase to share what she has and the task and language are repeated for each child.

- In a Conversation Unit for a Low Structure group, the children have independent language skills and thus are required to pick an object and comment on or tell two things about it before passing it to the next child.

Within and across groups, regardless of how similar the children are in their social skills, the participation required and the amount of support can and should be carefully varied for each child. By doing so, the same skill can be practiced by each child regardless of their individual language or cognitive skills. Children with minimal verbal skills can participate in an activity gesturally, by pointing to or giving a picture or object. Some children can be asked to provide very specific and circumscribed responses, while others can respond to open-ended questions, based upon their abilities. By individualizing the level of support and the expectations required, all children within a group can participate in activities that practice and use important skills, at a level that best meets their abilities, in a setting with peers who share a similar level of understanding and engagement.

- During snack in Play-Based group, Dylan requested to Lucy "I want a marshmallow." Lucy, who has limited expressive language, gave Dylan the marshmallow then handed him a picture of popcorn to request her snack.
- At an art activity in a High Structure group, Alex had the markers and turned to Justin. The group leader modeled for him "What color?" Alex repeated "What color?" and Justin responded with "I want yellow." Alex handed Justin the yellow marker then passed the marker box to Sam. Sam turned to Eliza and spontaneously asked, "Do you want blue or orange?"
- A Low Structure group was practicing questions, or asking, in group one day. Each child had an interview sheet with picture icons to help them think of topics to ask about with their peers. Derrick approached a peer and asked, "How many pets do you have?" while Austin asked his partner, "Can you tell me all about who is in your family? But only the ones that live within 20 miles!"

Multiple and Varied Learning Opportunities

Not all children are interested in the same activities or learn in the same ways. Some children need to be moving in order to learn, while others must be still to take it all in. Some children love to hear stories read and others are motivated by building and construction projects. The work done by Howard Gardner, Mel Levine, and others (Gardner 2006; Levine 1998) demonstrates that children have different ways of engaging in learning and different strengths and preferences in doing so. We incorporate this knowledge into our planning and implementation of social skills interventions for children with ASD. In the PROGress Model, we try to reach all the children participating by varying the ways in which we engage the children in learning. Within and across the sessions, we can better ensure that motivation and learning is occurring for all the children if we are using a variety of activities and events to engage them and facilitate their social interactions. We utilize movement, stories, construction projects, imaginative play, object play, role playing, writing and drawing, art projects, and many other activities. We also vary the learning environment to include floor activities, table activities, sitting events, standing and moving activities, as well as large group, small group, and dyadic pairings. These variations are carefully included in hopes that all the children in the group will be engaged in at least some if not most of the learning and social opportunities available.

- In a single Play-Based group session practicing "Playing Together," activities included toy play with cars and trucks, making a single large Styrofoam structure with assorted items poked into the Styrofoam, coloring on a large tin foil with markers, listening to a book interactively using coins in a container to match the story, going down slides and crawling through tunnels together, making popcorn together for snack, and looking at pictures taped inside boxes with flashlights.
- The High Structure Group regularly begins with an opening routine that involves rhythm and memory. They then rotate through three stations, one that is an art or construction project, one that is a game, and one that involves a book or song. The eat snack or participate in a snack making activity, participate in a game or project in two small groups, then play a social game as a large group, ending with a goodbye song and movement routine.
- The Thematic Group, over the course of the entire session, typically engages in units that involve building and construction, story telling, dramatic play, cooking, game playing (cards, board games, and interactive games), hands on exploration, and outdoor play events.

Engaged Transitions

Children with ASD are often challenged by changes in schedule and activity. With any schedule, transitions are plentiful and thus should be planned for and addressed as carefully as the planning of the activities themselves. For children with ASD, the difficulty of ending a known activity and moving to an unknown event can cause notable anxiety, fear, resistance, and consequently, behavioral repercussions that can derail the child and thus, also derail the flow of a group. Thus, planned support of these transitions is critical for many children.

Transitions occur as children leave their classroom or home to come to group, as they enter the group room, between each activity and schedule change, and as they leave the group. Each should be considered and programmed for as needed. Specific transition activities can be planned that focus the children on a task, action, or item that then naturally guides them from the current activity to the next. With this technique, which in the PROGRess Model is called "engaged transitions," the goal is to focus the child's attention on the concrete task rather than on the change of activity.

> Garrett struggled to come to group each session. He often cried and tantrumed once arriving in the parking lot and it was very difficult to get him from the car to the group room. Once in the room, however, he readily calmed and fully participated for the entire group. Recognizing

that the transition to group, rather than the group itself, was anxiety producing, a transition plan was designed. At the end of each session, Garrett and all the other children in the group were given a picture to take home. The picture identified an object that each child had to find and bring in the following week that would be incorporated into an activity. These included items such as a big rock, a stuffed animal, a red leaf, a picture of an ocean animal. With this in place, Garrett eagerly entered the group each week, excited to show his peers and group leaders the wonderful item he brought.

Eric often entered the group room so excited to arrive that he often ran around the perimeter of the room for about 15 minutes, highly dysregulated and unable to focus. Knowing that he loved Star Wars, he was instead met in the lobby and given an assortment of Star Wars pictures from which to choose one. His peers were also given favorite pictures to select. Upon entering the room, identical pictures were placed on the carpet squares set in the opening circle. Eric eagerly entered the room, searched for his match, sat on the corresponding carpet square, and was ready to begin the opening routine.

Abby was the only girl in the Low Structure group. Upon entering, toys were offered on the rug for the group to play with until all the participants arrived. The high level of activity, energy, and noise that the boys in the group shared were very aversive for Abby. Recognizing this, and knowing that she loved to write, a journal was provided to her at a table on the opposite side of the room. While the boys played on the rug, Abby was able to sit quietly with a group leader and write in her journal. Once the toys were cleaned up, and the boys were sitting in the opening circle singing the hello song, Abby independently stopped writing and came over to join the group.

Transitions can be similarly addressed within the group routine. For example, children transitioning from the large group "hello song" to smaller instructional groups may be asked to select an object. The group leader can generate interest and intrigue regarding what will happen next with the item selected. Examples may include sets of identical objects used to group children into their instructional groups. For example, some children may select a bear while others select a fish. The group leader then instructs "find two friends who have an animal just like yours." Children may also be given items or objects that will be used in the next activity, and then be engaged with "I wonder what we will be doing with that bag of eyeballs!"

In PROGress Model groups, the transition from opening circle to work groups is accomplished with an activity called "Pick and Pass" which is included in the regular daily routine and on the schedule. For this transition, items are placed in a large "Pick and Pass" can. When Pick and Pass is next on the schedule, the children chant "Pick and Pass," clapping their hands or patting their legs to the chant. This is usually met with great joy and anticipation as each child selects an item from the can and then passes the can to the child beside him. Once all children have an object, they typically are eager to know what to do with it. Doing something with the selected object, such as grouping with the peers who have the same object, taking the objects to a designated area, etc. serves to complete the transition and begin the next activity.

Another strategy often used in PROGress groups for children able to follow simple directions is to provide the children with tasks that must be completed in a particular order before the next activity can occur. In some of the PROGress groups, this is accomplished by a planned transition activity called "job teams" which is included on the regular group schedule each week. For this transition, four to six tasks, depending upon the size of the group, are listed on the wall with pairs of children assigned to each task. The first pair of children may pick up all the carpet squares, the next may move the table to the center of the room, the next may set up chairs, etc. Once all tasks are completed in order, the room is set up for the next activity.

Transitions between activities for children who cannot follow complex or sequential directions or activities must also be carefully planned but with more concrete and developmentally appropriate activities. Simple rituals or routines can be regularly embedded at each transition to help the children understand or recognize what is expected of them. Concrete visual cues can be provided as needed. The key to such transitions is to plan, schedule, and include them consistently and regularly, just as you do the instructional activities.

- A simple song is sung every time the children are asked to move from the floor to the table. The song is: "find a chair and sit at the table, find a chair and sit at the table, find a chair and sit at the table, let's all have some fun!" This song, when regularly included, makes the act of moving from floor to table an activity in and of itself and once quickly completed, the next activity can begin.
- When asking children to move to new or different areas of the room, masking tape was placed on the floor to show the children where they needed to go. The activity "Walk on the tape" was included at a regular time in the schedule and was cued by repeatedly chanting and clapping "Walk on the tape. Walk on the tape. Walk on the tape." This fun activity was familiar and simple to follow and the children eagerly walked on the tape to the desired destination and the next activity then began.
- When the hello routine ended, the Pick and Pass can was passed and each child chose a small object, that was either red or yellow. All the children with yellow objects went to the yellow paper and all the children with red objects went to the red paper. On each paper was a board game, and the small objects were used as each child's marker as they played the game.

Incorporating Individual Goals

Research has demonstrated that skill awareness and daily use is facilitated when children understand the importance and relevance of the skill and its use. Thus, it is important that information regarding the skills being taught is embedded in the teaching and rehearsal opportunities provided within the groups. Group social interactions and activities offer supportive and highly motivating, natural peer interactions within which to learn and practice new skills. Thus, the activities within the social skills groups are the ideal context within which to help children recognize the skill being practiced, understand in a genuine interaction why it is important, and experience the benefit or natural reinforce that results from using the skill.

In addition to the group goals addressed within the curriculum, it is also important to help each child recognize and understand his own deficits within a social context. Thus, in addition to the group goal, each child should be assisted in working on specific individual goals as well, that will improve his/her social participation. Each child should be clear and aware of the goal they need to improve, and should be reminded of and reinforced for it throughout the session. This can be done by using a token reinforcement system highlighted throughout the session. As a child demonstrates awareness and attention to their individual goal, the group leaders can provide immediate feedback to the child that they are doing exactly as expected by immediately giving them a sticker or mark on their individual goal chart. Similarly, a child can wait to be reinforced until she/he demonstrates the skill, with or without support as required. Group leaders can then help the child to understand why it is important to use the targeted skill, within the natural social context. Thus, the immediate reinforcement allows the child to recognize what is being expected, along with how and why the skill is important. Individual goals may remain constant throughout the course of the group or may change as needed to learn and use skills.

Fostering Self-Awareness, Self-Esteem, and Self-Advocacy

Children with autism, as mentioned at the beginning of this chapter, often struggle to participate in peer groups and to feel confident and competent when in them. Peer groups are often avoided and even if attempts to participate are made, failure and rejection is commonly the result. In social skills groups where safe and positive peer relations are developed, the curriculum can provide regular and frequent opportunities to highlight and reinforce the positive aspects of interaction as well as the strengths and abilities of the children in the group. Positive individual and group attributes and successes should be frequently identified and reinforced. These opportunities lay a positive foundation of self-esteem. For example, children within the group can learn the concept of complimenting, and why it is an important skill. Group leaders can reinforce for each child the skill of attending to the achievements and abilities of others. Opportunities for regular and frequent peer-to-peer compliments can be facilitated. Thus, children can build positive self-perceptions from both the adult and peer input regularly encouraged

Safe and positive peer group environments also provide the opportunity for participants to take social risks. Children can safely practice and understand how and why to use new skills, and experience success in doing so. Children in positive peer social skills groups can practice both positive and negative social examples. The children can be given an opportunity to try out strategies within the safe confines of the group. Participants can begin to understand what the strategies are, why they might use them, how to use them, and what the positive or negative outcomes might be. This "safe" peer practice can help the child to better understand and acquire skills that they may otherwise not be able to practice. As the children with ASD learn that they can use social skills and strategies successfully, they may be more willing and able to implement these strategies more often with peers.

Once children with ASD can recognize a social situation, they can then utilize a learned skill or strategy to address the situation. The strategies the children learn must be those that she or he is able to understand and use independently and successfully. For example, if a child with ASD is being maliciously targeted by peers, that child would no doubt be unsuccessful if his or her only strategies were to reason or talk their way out of the negative peer situation. Clearly, trying to use these skills for which s/he is less capable would most likely not stop or not improve the situation for that child. Instead, the child with ASD might be taught proactive strategies, for example, to positively remove himself or herself from a situation in which he or she is being targeted. To make this abstract concept more concrete and accessible, the child can be taught that if X happens, you do Y. The child learns that if a negative situation occurs (e.g., teasing, being left out, responding to something she/he does not like), he can remove himself from the situation by, for example, taking a break alone, or finding another person (a peer to play with, an adult to ask for help). Such self-advocacy can teach the child that he can independently improve his negative situations.

Designing and Adapting Group Intervention

Designing and/or revising curricula to meet the needs of a group of children is an ongoing task and must be considered specifically for each and every group. The adaptations needed for any given group are dependent on the collective abilities and social engagement of that group. However, there are some general areas that any curricula must consider. These include adaptations based on the developmental level of the group, the skills and abilities the participants have, the skills needed in order for the participants to engage and participate, the amount of structure and support required, and the session parameters of time and frequency. Adaptations based upon each of these factors are addressed below.

- **Developmental Level of Group**
  As described earlier in this chapter, skills can be addressed in a number of different ways, depending upon how much scaffolding is provided, how independent the children can be in practicing and using skills, and what their interests and other abilities are. In this regard, the following questions must be considered in adapting both the goals and activities to meet the needs of the children in the group: What is appropriate play for the age and development of the children in the group? What are appropriate materials for the ages and interests of the children in the group? What are appropriate expectations for these children? These considerations are critical in ensuring that the environment in which the children are learning with each other is appropriate to their needs and appropriately similar to those found with their typical peers.
- **Goals and Skills Addresses**
  For each group, it is important to identify the skills that are most important for that group to learn, and how many can be addressed in the amount of time the group runs. For young children learning the most basic interaction skills, fewer skills practiced over a longer period of time might be most appropriate, whereas for

older, more skilled students, they may target a much wider range of skills over time that build upon and enhance each other. Thus, a group of young children working on maintaining regulation while engaging with each other may focus on only a few goals repeated over time in a variety of learning activities. However, children with adequate receptive and expressive language who are socially motivated to interact may address a new skill each week while continuing to practice those already addressed in previous weeks. Thus, a greater number of different goals will be targeted or addressed for this group of children over the course of the group intervention.

- **Supports Required**
  The level, type, and amount of supports provided to the children are critical in engendering their understanding, interest, motivation, participation, and success. In both activities and transitions, the children must be engaged at an appropriate level, be given needed support and be provided the guidance and reinforcement necessary to understand what is expected, why and whether or not they are doing what is expected of them. Thus, for each group, it is important to evaluate, prior to presenting the activity, how the children will know what is expected of them. Instruction presented verbally will make it more difficult for some children to understand the task, whereas visual supports may greatly impact participation.
  Group leaders must develop skill and timing to know when to intervene and when to wait; when to reinforce and when to allow for natural peer reinforcers to occur; when to scaffold and support; and when to let the child process independently. This is difficult but critical for the successful learning experiences of the children in the groups.
- **Level of Participation**
  It is also critical to identify what are reasonable expectations for participation in planned activities. Can the children verbally engage independently or will they require verbal models? Depending upon their abilities, activities must be planned that allow them to participate in ways that are reasonable, motivating, and developmentally appropriate. Even with the most well-formed group, the children within it will have varied skills. Thus, for each activity, one must consider how each of the children might be able to socially participate in the most appropriate and naturally motivating way possible. For example, three children may be interested in making a caterpillar while one may be responsible for handing out the materials requested by each child.
- **Time on Tasks**
  Taking into consideration the age and abilities of the children in the group, how long are they collectively able to remain on a task? Based upon this, how many tasks will you need to plan for the amount of time you have for the children in group? This may be dependent upon the types of activities presented. For example, the children may be able to remain in sensory activities for 20 minutes but in motor activities for only 10 minutes. Knowing the interests and abilities of the children in the group is important to consider when planning sessions and activities.

- **Environmental Space**
  The environmental space in which the social skills groups are conducted plays an important role in the successful facilitation of the group activities. Some children, who are highly regulated and independent, can work and move freely and competently in a variety of settings. Other children, however, may be far more affected by the space in which they are playing. For example, some children demonstrate great difficulty in open, unstructured environments, such as on the floor of an open space. For these children, organizing themselves and participating in activities in such an unstructured space may be very challenging. For them, moving to a more enclosed corner, or sitting at a small table may best help to regulate and facilitate participation. For each group of children, attending to the subtle contributions made by the environment are important and should be carefully considered when designing the group schedule and activities.
- **Group Size**
  The number of participants in a group is another important consideration for adaptation. The size of the group presents opportunities and challenges for social interaction, negotiation, and variety that are vital to each group's needs. Group size affects the amount of support and attention available to each child. A group of children needing a high level of support and assistance may require a smaller group size or smaller teacher-to-child ratio than a group more able to function independently and with less support. Group size may also vary based upon the individual preferences and needs of the children in group. For example, some children, such as those who are particularly anxious or shy may feel a greater sense of comfort and belonging in a group that has fewer peers with whom to interact and navigate. Others, who may be very outgoing and social, may benefit more from a larger group with different peer preferences and styles to negotiate and integrate. Finally, group size may also vary based upon the goals or requirements of an activity. Lessons that require practice and repetition may best be conducted in smaller subgroups of children. Likewise, group games or social activities may be better rehearsed in larger subgroups of children. Finally, children with age-appropriate abilities may be best served practicing specific social skills with a wider variety of children and groups of children to more closely mirror interactions he will encounter in his typical peer environments.
- **Length of Each Group and Overall Session**
  The time available to conduct a social skills group session may be determined by the children in the group or by the setting in which groups are offered. Typically, children who are younger in age or who are more challenged by sensory and self-regulation issues may be able to participate and engage in group events for a shorter period of time than their peers who are perhaps older, more regulated, and capable of longer periods of interaction. Such factors should be carefully considered and the group length and activities should be planned according to the abilities of the participants. The length of some groups, however, might be determined by the times children are available, such as when their school or after-school schedules allow. The amount of time each session will run and the frequency and regularity of the group sessions is critical to the planning of activities and opportunities

provided within the groups. The number of sessions that make up the group curriculum is also dependent on both child and scheduling issues. In general, the longer the children are able to participate in groups together, the more comfortable and familiar they become with each other and the more progress they can make in learning, practicing, and incorporating skills into their social interactions and exchanges together. That said, the planning of the length of each social skills curricula should be considered in light of the availability of the children in the group, external scheduling considerations such as the length of the school year or summer break, the affordability of running a group for an adequate amount of time, and the interest and commitment of those participating.

Generalization of Social Skills

Much can be accomplished in a social skills group. The children in it can experience social success and pleasure. They can participate in motivating and fun activities with others, and they can acquire and practice new skills within this context. Generalization can be practiced as part of the social skills groups by scheduling opportunities for practice outside of the group setting or with new people. Community outings can be regularly scheduled into the curriculum. Opportunities to invite peers to group events can also be intentionally planned. However, the ability to generalize these experiences is difficult and often reported as the shortcoming of social skills group intervention (Barnhill et al. 2002; Marriage et al. 1995; Ozonoff and Miller 1995). However, with continued learning and practice beyond the group setting, the ability to acquire and use new social skills may be significantly impacted.

In order to achieve this in a clinical setting, parents and caregivers must be knowledgeable of the skills being taught and must be engaged in continuing to identify, shape, practice, and use the skills developed in group in other settings outside of group. An important component of the PROGress Model is the parent involvement and participation. Parents bringing their children to group observe the group through a one way window, see their child's successful experiences within the group, receive information and instruction clarifying skills and how to facilitate them, and receive information and support on how to continue to practice those skills most relevant to their child's social success. This is facilitated by providing written and verbal information regarding the processes and strategies implemented in group, techniques and ideas for practicing the skills within the natural context of home, and if appropriate for the group, providing assignments or activities that the child can practice between group sessions.

By having parents present and observing in a clinical setting, a wonderfully supportive phenomenon also occurs. Parents meet other parents who understand their situation and child, and who may have had similar experiences. These parents support each other, share stories, successes and challenges, share resources and information, and support each other as no professional can. Positive social relationships are then developed not only amongst the children, but amongst the parents too. This support is vital and powerful for many parents. In fact, PROGress Groups, at the end of 25 weeks together, regularly and typically leave with close friendships and connections forged between both children and families. The families are highly encouraged to continue to meet, on their own, at a regularly scheduled time and place, to continue to facilitate the learning, generalization and support they have developed. Many groups continue to meet for months and even years following the end of group.

Social skills interventions offered in a school setting enable children to learn needed skills within the environment where they are most likely to use them. The peers with whom the children are regularly grouped will, in the best of situations, be peers with whom they will have regular opportunities to engage throughout the day. Skills taught within the group setting can be practiced and supported in naturally occurring events throughout the school day. This might be accomplished by providing opportunities for kids from group to play and socialize together at school but outside of the group. This can also be accomplished by providing information to the teacher, aide, playground attendant, or peer buddies regarding the goals a child is working on and the strategies and ways in which a child can be reminded to use them. Information can be shared across teachers and with parents through written correspondence and chatting. Overall, the school setting offers an ideal social skills intervention venue within which children are most familiar, where peer interactions occur naturally and regularly, where trained staff and social peers can be monitored and educated regarding goals and techniques, and ultimately, where a daily positive impact on a child's social life can be made.

Beyond Social Skills Groups

Generalization of skills learned and more importantly perhaps, of continued positive experiences in peer group settings are ongoing and sometimes lifelong focuses for persons with ASD. Once positive peer experiences have been created, many children will recognize and seek such interactions with others. Maintaining success, however, will most likely require structure and support.

Young children may seek to have play dates with new and varying friends. These play dates may require careful planning, at least, initially. The concepts and techniques described in this chapter can be applied as appropriate to a home play setting. Predictability can be provided by planning in advance a schedule of activities with which the child with ASD can be familiar. Within those plans, variations and variety can occur, just as they do in the groups. For example, the child may be prepared in advance that first, the children will play outside. Activities that may occur during that time can be listed, using visual supports, and rehearsed if necessary. Next, the children may have a snack together. The choices of snack options can also be reviewed by the child with ASD, and offered to his peer. Last, the children may come inside the house to play. The child with ASD may be prepared in advance that he will pick one game or activity and then the friend will pick the next game or activity, but both children will participate in all activities. As needed, a picture schedule of the play date can be provided. When carefully planned and with reasonable time limits set, children can begin to experience positive peer interactions at home.

Community settings often impose a greater challenge. Less predictability and control are often involved. However, children with ASD may find groups, clubs, or classes within the community that focus or organize around special interests that are shared by the person with ASD and others. These community groups may provide motivation and purpose to join. Furthermore, engagement around a highly preferred topic or activity may reduce the pressure often felt to know what or how to participate. Community groups or courses may offer a stimulating, motivating, and purposeful setting to more easily join and participate.

References

American Psychiatric Association (APA). (2000). *Diagnostic and statistical manual of mental disorders: DSM-IV-TR.* Washington: American Psychiatric Association.

Attwood, T. (1998). *Asperger's syndrome: A guide for parents and professionals.* Philadelphia: Kingsley.

Ballaban-Gil, K., Rapin, I., Tuchman, R., Shinnar, S. (1996). Longitudinal examination of the behavioral, language, and social changes in a population of adolescents and young adults with autistic disorder. *Pediatric Neurology, 15*(3), 217–223.

Barnhill, G. P. (2001). Social attributions and depression in adolescents with Asperger syndrome. *Focus on Autism and Other Developmental Disabilities, 16*(1), 46.

Bauminger, N., & Kasari, C. (2000). Loneliness and friendship in high-functioning children with autism. *Child Development, 71*(2), 447–456.

Bauminger, N., & Shulman, C. (2003). The development and maintenance of friendship in high-functioning children with autism: Maternal perceptions. *Autism, 7,* 81–97.

Bellini, S. (2006). The development of social anxiety in adolescents with autism spectrum disorders. *Focus on Autism and Other Developmental Disabilities, 21,* 138–145.

Daniel, L. S., & Billingsley, B. S. (2010). What boys with an autism spectrum disorder say about establishing and maintaining friendships. *Focus on Autism and Other Developmental Disabilities, 25*(4), 220–229.

DeRosier, M. E., Swick, D.C., Davis, N., McMillen, J., Matthews, R. (2011). The efficacy of a social skills group intervention for improving social behaviors in children with high functioning autism spectrum disorders. *Journal of Autism and Developmental Disorders, 41*(8), 1033–1043.

Farrugia, S., & Hudson, J. (2006). Anxiety in adolescents with Asperger syndrome: Negative thoughts, behavioral problems, and life interference. *Focus on Autism and Other Developmental Disabilities, 21*(1), 25–35.

Gardner, H. (2006). *Multiple intelligences: New horizons.* New York: Basic Books.

Gray, C. (1995). Teaching children with autism to "read" social situations. In K. A. Quill (Ed.), *Teaching children with autism: Strategies to enhance communication and socialization* (pp. 219–241). Albany: Delmar.

Gutstein, S. E., & Whitney, T. (2002). Asperger syndrome and the development of social competence. *Focus on Autism and Other Developmental Disabilities, 17*(3), 161–171.

Howlin, P. (2000). Outcome in adult life for more able individuals with Asperger syndrome. *Autism, 4,* 63–83.

Krasny, L., Williams, B. J., Provencal, S., Ozonoff, S. (2003). Social skills interventions for the autism spectrum: Essential ingredients and a model curriculum. *Child and Adolescent Psychiatric Clinic of North America, 12,* 107–122.

Landa, R. J., Holman, K. C., Garrett-Mayer, E. (2007). Social and communication development in toddlers with early and later diagnosis of autism spectrum disorders. *Archives of General Psychiatry, 64,* 853–864.
Levine, M. D. (1998). *Developmental Variation and Learning Disorders* (2nd ed.). Cambridge: Educators Publishing Service.
Levy, A., & Perry, A. (2011). Outcomes in adolescents and adults with autism: A review of the literature. *Research in Autism Spectrum Disorders, 5,* 1271–1282.
Lincoln, A. (1849). Letter to Joseph Gillespie. In R. Basler (Ed.), *The collected works of Abraham Lincoln* (p. 57). New Brunswick: Rutgers University Press.
Locke, J., Ishijima, E. H., Kasari, C., London, N. (2010). Loneliness, friendship quality and the social networks of adolescents with high-functioning autism in an inclusive school setting. *Journal of Research in Special Educational Needs, 10*(2), 74–81.
Marriage, K. J., Gordon, V., Brand, L. (1995). A social skills group for boys with Asperger's syndrome. *Australian and New Zealand Journal of Psychiatry, 29,* 58–62.
McGovern, C. W., & Sigman, M. (2005). Continuity and change from early childhood to adolescence in autism. *Journal of Child Psychology and Psychiatry, 46*(4), 401–408.
Mundy, P., Sigman, M., Kasari, C. (1990). A longitudinal study of joint attention and language development in autistic children. *Journal of Autism and Developmental Disorders, 20*(1), 115–128.
Myles, B., Barnhill, G., Hagiwara, T., Griswold, D., Simpson, R. (2001). A synthesis of studies on the intellectual, academic, social/emotional and sensory characteristics of children with Asperger syndrome. *Education and Training in Mental Retardation and Developmental Disabilities, 36,* 304–311.
Ozonoff, S., & Miller, J. N. (1995). Teaching theory of mind: A new approach to social skills training for individuals with autism. *Journal of Autism and Developmental Disorders, 25,* 415–433.
Parker, J. G., & Gottman, J. M. (1989). Social and emotional development in a relational context: Friendship interaction from early childhood to adolescence. In T. Brendt, & G. Ladd (Eds.), *Peer Relationships in Child Development* (pp. 95–131). New York: Wiley.
Seltzer, M., Krauss, M., Shattuck, P. T., Orsmond, G., Swe, A., Lord, C. (2003). The symptoms of autism spectrum disorders in adolescence and adulthood. *Journal of Autism And Developmental Disorders, 33*(6), 565–581.
Siegal, M., & Blades, M. (2003). Language and auditory processing in autism. *Trends in Cognitive Sciences, 7*(9), 378–384.
Tager-Flusberg, H. (1999). A psychological approach to understanding the social and language impairments in autism. *International Review of Psychiatry, 11*(4), 325–334.
Tager-Flusberg, H., & Joseph, R. M. (2003). Identifying neurocognitive phenotypes in autism. *Philosophical Transactions of the Royal Society of London Series B: Biological Sciences, 358,* 303–314.
Wetherby, A. M., Prizant, B. M., Hutchinson, T. (1998). Communicative, social-affective, and symbolic profiles of young children with autism and pervasive developmental disorder. *American Journal of Speech-Language Pathology, 7,* 79–91.
Wetherby, A., & Prutting, C. (1984). Profiles of communicative and cognitive-social abilities in autistic children. *Journal of Speech and Hearing Research, 27,* 364–377.
Wetherby, A. M., Woods, J., Allen, L., Cleary, J., Dickinson, H., Lord, C. (2004). Early indicators of autism spectrum disorder in the second year of life. *Journal of Autism and Developmental Disorders, 34*(5), 473–493.
White, S. W., & Roberson-Nay, R. (2009). Anxiety, social deficits, and loneliness in youth with autism spectrum disorders. *Journal of Autism and Developmental Disorders, 39*(7), 1006–1013.
Wing, L. (1981). Asperger's syndrome: A clinical account. *Psychological Medicine, 11,* 115–129.

Chapter 10
Peer and Adult Socialization

Katherine Walton, Allison Wainer, Natalie Berger and Brooke Ingersoll

Impairments in social interaction are a hallmark feature of autism spectrum disorders (ASD). Deficits in social behaviors are often present by the end of the first year of life (Ingersoll 2011), and are one of the first recognizable signs of the disorder (e.g. Zwaigenbaum et al. 2005). In addition, studies examining the course of ASD symptoms over the lifespan suggest that most individuals with ASD continue to show significant social difficulties in adolescence and adulthood, and these symptoms are closely related to community inclusion (Orsmond et al. 2004) and other quality of life indicators (Howlin et al. 2004). Social symptoms appear to show less improvement over time (see Seltzer et al. 2004 for review) and may be less responsive to traditional treatments than symptoms in the other core ASD domains, such as language skills (Strain and Schwartz 2001). For these reasons, a variety of interventions have been developed that are specifically focused on increasing socialization in children with ASD.

Social skills interventions may be generally classified into three broad approaches, parent-mediated interventions, peer- and sibling-mediated interventions, and direct instruction in social skills. Although each of these approaches can be used with children with ASD at any stage of development, the different approaches are often targeted toward different developmental stages. For example, increasing early social-communication skills—such as social engagement, imitation, language, and play—with significant others is a primary goal for young children with ASD (Rogers 1999). Thus, many social skills interventions developed for toddlers and preschoolers with ASD utilize a parent-mediated approach, which teaches parents to use techniques to increase their child's social-communication skills during parent–child

K. Walton (✉)
Michigan State University, 316 Physics Rd., East Lansing, MI 48824, USA
e-mail: Ktmeyer15@gmail.com

A. Wainer · N. Berger · B. Ingersoll
Department of Psychology, Michigan State University, 316 Physics Rd., East Lansing, MI 48824, USA
e-mail: ingers19@msu.edu

S. Goldstein, J. A. Naglieri (eds.), *Interventions for Autism Spectrum Disorders,* 197
DOI 10.1007/978-1-4614-5301-7_10, © Springer Science+Business Media New York 2013

interactions. As children with ASD enter school, social skills with peers become more important. Thus, peer- and sibling-mediated interventions are often used with school-aged children with ASD in order to promote social interaction and friendships with other children. Direct instruction in social skills, in which the child with ASD is taught to engage in specific social behaviors with adults or other children, has been used with children with ASD across development; however, the specific strategies used often differ depending on the age of the child. This chapter will provide an overview of these different approaches to improve socialization in children with ASD. The reader is referred to several, recently published comprehensive reviews of social skills interventions for children with ASD (Bellini and Peters 2008; McConnell 2002; Reichow and Volkmar 2010; Rogers 2000; Scattone 2007) for a more detailed discussion of these approaches and their research base.

Parent-Mediated Interventions

Young children with ASD typically present with significant delays in early nonverbal social-communication skills—such as social engagement, joint attention, and imitation—as well as language and play skills (Wetherby et al. 2004). These behaviors are fundamental for establishing early social interactions with others (Tomasello 1995), and thus deficits in these skills often lead to interaction difficulties with caregivers and other adults (Sigman et al. 1986). Parent-mediated interventions provide caregivers with direct instruction in intervention strategies to manage their child's behavior and support their child's social-emotional development (Mahoney et al. 1999). A number of studies, including several recent randomized control trials, have demonstrated that parent-mediated intervention is an effective approach to improve social-communication skills in young children with ASD (McConachie and Diggle 2007) and can improve the quality of parent–child interactions (Green et al. 2010).

There are numerous benefits associated with parent-mediated interventions for children with ASD. Teaching parents to use specific intervention techniques provides children with more hours of intervention in daily settings with natural interaction partners. Learning in such natural contexts has been shown to be associated with increases in generalization and maintenance of child skill (e.g., Koegel et al. 1982). Participation in parent-mediated intervention programs has also been associated with improvements in parental and family functioning. For example, research suggests that training parents in intervention techniques can lead to reductions in parental stress and depression (Tonge et al. 2006), which is particularly important given the high levels of stress and depression experienced by parents of children with ASD (e.g. Estes et al. 2009; Quintero and McIntyre 2010). Furthermore, participation in parent-mediated intervention programs has been found to be associated with increases in family leisure and recreation time, and increases in parents' optimism about their child's future (Koegel et al. 1982). Additionally, when parents are trained in intervention techniques, they can teach other important individuals in the child's life (e.g. siblings, grandparents) how to use these strategies, thereby producing more opportunities for the entire family's involvement in the child's education and intervention (Symon 2005).

Although there is considerable agreement that early, intensive intervention, including parent-mediated approaches leads to improvements in children's functioning (NRC 2001), there is debate in the field as to which intervention approach is best for the promotion of child's skill and long-term outcomes (Ingersoll 2010a). Traditionally, behavioral interventions based on the principles of applied behavior analysis have had the largest evidence-base for promoting social-communication skills in young children with ASD (NRC 2001). The literature examining parent implementation of these behavioral techniques in more naturalistic settings—such as Pivotal Response Training (PRT; Schreibman et al. 1991), Naturalistic Language Paradigm (NLP; Koegel et al. 1987), and Milieu Teaching (e.g. Kaiser et al. 2000)—suggests that such programs are effective to increase social-communication skills in children with ASD. Another body of research has indicated that parent-mediated intervention programs which take a developmental or social-pragmatic approach to intervention, such as Relationship Development Intervention (RDI; Gutstein 2001), Responsive Teaching (Mahoney and Perales 2003), and Hanen's More Than Words (Sussman 1999) can also produce significant improvements in a variety of child social-communication skills. With the recognition that parent training in both behavioral and developmental strategies can be effective intervention approach, investigators have begun to examine ways to integrate techniques from both approaches into parent training curricula. Initial evaluations of such programs, like Project ImPACT (Ingersoll and Dvortcsak 2010) and the Early Start Denver Model (ESDM: Rogers and Dawson 2009), suggest that the use of these "blended" parent-mediated intervention programs can be effective for increasing child social-communication skills.

Parent Training in Naturalistic Behavioral Intervention

Naturalistic behavioral parent training programs have traditionally focused on teaching parents prompting and reinforcement strategies to increase their child's use of core social-communication skills such as language and imitation. In one of the earliest studies of parent training for children with autism, Laski et al. (1988) examined the efficacy of training parents of children with ASD to use the Natural Language Paradigm to promote their children's spontaneous speech. Results from this study indicated that all parents increased their use of the intervention techniques, and all children increased their rate of vocalizations. Parents and children generalized their newly learned skills to additional non-training environments (Laski et al. 1988). In a different study, Kaiser and colleagues (2000) taught six mothers of children with autism to implement Enhanced Milieu Teaching (EMT) strategies to promote their children's spontaneous verbal language. All parents increased their correct use of the EMT techniques from baseline to intervention sessions, with five out of the six mothers achieving criterion level fidelity of implementation during the 24-session training program. Moreover, all six children showed increases in their total use of communication targets; however, increases in spontaneous use of communication targets were variable across individual children. Most parents and children in this study were able to generalize use of skills across the majority of situations and over a period of time (Kaiser et al. 2000). Nefdt and colleagues (2009) created a computerized self-directed learning program for parents of children with ASD that taught motivational techniques from pivotal response training (PRT) to increase their children's social-communication, primarily verbal language. After the use of the computerized training program, parents were able to implement PRT strategies with fidelity, provided more language opportunities for their children, and displayed greater confidence when interacting with their children. Moreover, children of these parents demonstrated increases in their use of verbal language (Nefdt et al. 2009). Finally, Ingersoll and Gergans (2007) evaluated the efficacy of training parents to use a naturalistic behavioral intervention, reciprocal imitation training (RIT), in order to improve imitation skills in children with ASD. Parents were able to increase their use of intervention techniques in a lab setting as well as during play interactions with their children at home. Additionally, children in the study increased their spontaneous imitation with objects during lab sessions and were able to generalize these skills to their home environments. Taken together, these studies suggest that parents can be taught to implement naturalistic behavioral techniques with a high degree of fidelity to promote gains in their child's use of core social-communication skills.

Parent Training in Developmental/Social Pragmatic Intervention

A different, and growing, body of research suggests that parent-mediated developmental or social-pragmatic interventions can also lead to important gains in social-communication skills in children with ASD. These developmental parent training programs typically focus on enhancing the parent-child relationship and promoting child skills such as social engagement, shared affect, and social reciprocity (Brookman-Frazee et al. 2009). Many of the early evaluations of developmental parent-mediated intervention programs did not use experimental designs; although changes in important outcome measures were observed, it was difficult to attribute these changes to the parent training directly (Ingersoll 2010a). For example, Mahoney and Perales (2003) examined the effect of Responsive Teaching, a parent-mediated intervention, for 20 children with ASD using a pre-post study. Results from this study indicated that a majority of parents became more responsive with their children during participation in the program and a majority of children demonstrated significant gains in social-emotional skills, including social competence. Improvements in parents' responsiveness was associated with child gains in social-emotional skills. However, there were no controls in this particular study making it impossible to parse out maturational and other effects from the impact of the parent training program (Mahoney and Perales 2003). Recently, a handful of controlled trials of parent-mediated developmental interventions have been conducted to address limitations of the early work in this area. For example, McConachie and colleagues (2005) evaluated the effect of Hanen's More than Words curriculum (Sussman 1999), a developmental parent-mediated intervention, on parents' ability to facilitate social-communication in their children with ASD. Parents who participated in the program used significantly more facilitative strategies during parent-child interactions than did parents in the control condition. Moreover, parents who received training indicated larger gains in child vocabulary than did parents in the control group. Green and colleagues (2010) evaluated the effect of a parent-mediated communication-focused intervention, Preschool Autism Communication Trial (PACT), on parent and child outcomes. Results from this study suggest that parents in the PACT group improved their parental synchrony with their child and rated their children as having greater improvements in language and social-communication skills than did the parents of children in the treatment as usual group. The results of investigations of developmental parent training programs suggest that parents can learn to increase their responsiveness in order to facilitate the development of social-communication skills in their children with ASD.

Parent Training in Blended Approach to Intervention

Although the underlying theoretical tenets of naturalistic behavioral and developmental approaches differ, they are actually quite similar in terms of the intervention techniques utilized to help parents promote their child's social-communication skills (Ingersoll 2010a). Appreciating these similarities, researchers have begun to examine parent-mediated interventions that integrate intervention techniques from both approaches in order to further enhance the social-communication skills of children with ASD (Ingersoll and Dvortsack 2006). In a pilot study of the Early Start Denver Model (Vismara et al. 2009), investigators examined the impact of participation in a blended program on parental skill acquisition and child social-communication skills. Seven out of eight parents were able to achieve mastery of implementation of the intervention techniques after participating in the program for 6 weeks. Moreover, these parents retained high levels of implementation fidelity over the next several months. Additionally, children whose parents completed the program demonstrated increases in social-communication skills including expressive language. A pilot study of another blended parent training program, Project ImPACT (Ingersoll and Dvortscak 2010), found similarly encouraging results for the use of such an approach (Ingersoll and Dvortsak 2006). The format of this particular parent training program was developed to be compatible with classroom-based intervention models, and thus the parent training can be conducted by clinicians as well as classroom teachers. Results from the pilot study revealed that parents increased their understanding of the intervention techniques, were highly satisfied with training format, and attributed gains in their child's social-communication skills to the program. A follow up study of Project ImPACT (Ingersoll and Wainer in press) found that the parent training program could be effectively implemented by educators in early childhood classroom settings to produce improvements in parent's fidelity of intervention implementation, decreases in parental stress, and improvements in child social-communication skills.

Summary

The majority of empirical research on parent-mediated interventions for children with ASD has examined the efficacy and effectiveness of teaching various intervention techniques to parents to promote social-communication, and thus early socialization skills. Across studies, there is emerging evidence to suggest that these approaches can increase early social-communication skills in young children with ASD and that gains are maintained over time. As such, teaching parents how to promote their child's social-communication during daily routines and activities is recommended practice for ASD intervention (NRC 2001). Although research indicates that parent training can lead to gains in parents' implementation of intervention techniques, the differential effectiveness of various delivery formats, training procedures, and training materials on parental learning is less clear; nonetheless, a number of training models appear to be effective.

Peer- and Sibling-Mediated Interventions

While children with ASD typically show broad difficulties with social interaction, interaction with similar-aged peers is often even more challenging than interaction with adults (e.g. Stone and Caro-Martinez 1990). Given that children with ASD tend to have particular difficulty interacting with similar-aged children, a number of interventions have aimed to involve siblings or peers directly in interventions to promote socialization in children with ASD. Peer- and sibling-mediated intervention may confer several advantages over adult-delivered intervention. First, socially competent peers or siblings can serve as models for appropriate social behavior. Second, social behaviors learned with peers or siblings may be more likely to generalize to other peer interaction situations than skills learned only with adults. Finally, involving peers or siblings directly in interventions for children with ASD may help children form closer relationships or friendships with the involved peers or siblings.

A large body of research has examined the use of peer-mediated interventions for supporting socialization in children with ASD. These interventions range widely in the amount of structure and support given to the interaction partners to promote positive interactions between children with ASD and their typically-developing siblings and peers. Overall, peer-mediated approaches have been among the most well-researched interventions for promoting socialization in children with ASD (McConnell 2002; Rogers 2000). Peer-mediated intervention approaches have been categorized as "emerging and effective" in a recent review of single-subject design research (Odom et al. 2003) and McConnell (2002) includes the use of peer-mediated strategies as a recommendation for educational practice. Social skills interventions that are implemented with the aid of typically-developing peers lead to better generalization and maintenance of skills than interventions implemented by adults alone (Rogers 2000). However, in many of these interventions, generalization of skills to untrained peers has been limited (McConnell 2002); therefore, children with ASD may have difficulty maintaining social gains after leaving a classroom environment in which a successful peer-mediated intervention has been implemented. A number of different intervention strategies involving peers and siblings as intervention agents will be described below.

Inclusion

The 1997 Reauthorized Individuals with Disabilities Education Act (IDEA) stipulates that individuals with disabilities, including those with ASD, should be educated in the "least restrictive environment" suitable for their educational needs. This enables students with ASD to have maximal access to normalized settings and typically developing peers, and to be "included" in classrooms with typically-developing peers. Given this provision, inclusion of children with ASD in classrooms with typically-developing students is a goal for many students with ASD. While typically developing students may be able to serve as models for appropriate social behavior and potential friends for children with ASD, simply placing children with ASD in classrooms with typically developing peers does not guarantee that students with ASD will improve their social interaction skills or form meaningful friendships (Mesibov and Shea 1996). In addition, placing children with ASD in regular classroom settings without additional support may be difficult or impossible for students with greater support needs. Therefore, recent models of inclusion advocate that educational placement in a typical classroom should be accompanied by careful educational planning and the use of a number of empirically supported intervention techniques (including the peer-mediated intervention strategies described below) in order to be most beneficial to children with ASD (Harrower and Dunlap 2001; Simpson et al. 2003).

Arranging the Environment to Promote Interaction

One way of supporting socialization between children with ASD and typically developing peers in an integrated classroom setting is by arranging the classroom situation to promote interactions between children with ASD and their typically developing peers. A classroom environment with structured activities which lend themselves to cooperation among peers, facilitated by adults, may increase the chance of successful social interactions between children with ASD and typically developing peers. For example, the integrated playgroup model typically includes a consistent schedule and routine with play activities appropriate to the developmental level of the children with ASD (Wolfberg and Schuler 1993). In addition, a small number of familiar typically developing peers are involved, and an adult closely monitors the play interactions and encourages the children to become involved in joint activities. Integrated playgroups using these components have led to increased interaction between children with ASD and peers as well as increases in appropriate play behavior in children with ASD (Roeyers 1996; Wolfberg and Schuler 1993).

Peer Buddies/Tutors

Some peer-mediated intervention programs have provided additional impetus for children with ASD to interact directly with their typically developing peers by assigning typically developing peers to serve as "peer buddies" or "peer tutors" for children with ASD (e.g. Garrison-Harrell et al. 1997; Haring and Breen 1992; Kamps et al. 1997). In the peer buddy model, typically developing students are paired with students with ASD to serve as social supports for these students. Typically developing students are educated about the student with whom they are paired (e.g. taught how to use an augmentative communication system, taught to engage in or support specific social interaction behaviors) and may also be reinforced by teachers for engaging in positive interactions with their peer buddies. A related intervention model, a peer network model, pairs a number of students with the student with ASD, rather than using 1:1 pairs. This provides the student with ASD an opportunity to increase his social engagement with a larger number of peers. This approach has been found to be successful for increasing peer acceptance of students with ASD and frequency and duration of social interactions between the students with ASD and trained peers (Garrison-Harrell et al. 1997; Kamps et al. 1997) in young school-aged children. Haring and Breen (1992) reported similar results of a peer network approach when used with two 13-year-old boys with disabilities.

While peer buddy and peer network interventions pair students with the specific goal of promoting social interactions, peer tutoring interventions involve typically developing students as educational supports for children with ASD. In the peer tutoring model, typically developing students are taught to serve as academic tutors (e.g. in reading or math) for students with ASD. Typically developing students are taught specific tutoring skills and then paired with students with ASD. Peer tutoring interventions led not only to improved academic performance for the students with ASD, but also to increased social interactions during free time for these students, when compared to teacher-led programs (Dugan et al. 1995; Kamps et al. 1994, 1999). Peer tutoring has also been used to teach adaptive skills to lower-functioning students with ASD, with improved responding of students with ASD to typical peers reported over time, in addition to mastery of targeted adaptive behaviors (Blew et al. 1985). These studies suggest that pairing students with ASD with typically developing students can lead to social interaction gains for students with ASD, whether or not social skills are specifically targeted in the relationship.

Teaching Peers/Siblings to Initiate Interactions

While the previously described interactions have set up situations in specific ways in the hopes of facilitating social interaction between children with ASD and typical peers (e.g., by arranging the setting in specific ways or pairing children with ASD with typical peers), a number of interactions have directly taught peers skills specifically targeted at successfully initiating social interactions with students with ASD. A number of studies have demonstrated increases in the social interactions of young children with ASD when peers are trained to initiate interactions using "play organizers" such as helping, sharing, giving affection, and praise (e.g. Goldstein et al. 1992). These interventions have demonstrated robust changes in social interactions of children with ASD, including generalization to untrained peers. Generalization and maintenance have been strongest when multiple peers are trained in the intervention and peers are taught to self-monitor after adult prompting and reinforcement is faded (Rogers 2000 for review). These same interventions have also been used successfully to improve interactions between children with ASD and their siblings, with parents serving as teachers for the typically developing siblings (Strain and Danko 1995; Strain et al. 1994).

Teaching Peers/Siblings to Deliver Simple Treatments to Build Skills

A final class of peer- and sibling-mediated interventions has adapted skill-building treatments such as Pivotal Response Training and Incidental Teaching for use by typically developing peers and siblings. These treatments have been effective at increasing child skills (e.g. language, joint attention, play skills) when delivered by adults. Therefore, having peers or siblings deliver these treatment components may potentially confer the double advantage of building specific skills in the child with ASD while also promoting peer and sibling socialization skills. Interventions that have been adapted for use in peer- and sibling-mediated components consisted of skills such as modeling, prompting, and reinforcement in naturalistic settings and have been used with children as young as preschool-aged. McGee et al. (1992) taught preschool-aged children in an inclusive classroom to use incidental teaching with their peers with ASD. Incidental teaching consists of using preferred play materials to create opportunities to prompt and reinforce language use. McGee et al. (1992) found increases in reciprocal social behavior, social initiations, and peer acceptance following the use of peer-mediated incidental teaching. Peers have also successfully used Pivotal Response Training techniques, including modeling, shaping, and reinforcement, to improve social interactions in school-aged children with ASD (Pierce and Schreibman 1997).

Similar intervention procedures have also been used with siblings of children with ASD. Typically-developing siblings have been able to learn a number of interventions that include skills such as modeling, prompting, and reinforcement of appropriate play and language behaviors in their siblings with ASD. Coe et al. (1991) taught school-aged siblings to prompt and praise their siblings' appropriate social behaviors, resulting in an increase in appropriate social interaction behaviors in the siblings with ASD. Walton and Ingersoll (in press) taught siblings to use Reciprocal Imitation Training, a naturalistic behavioral intervention targeting social imitation, leading to qualitative changes in play interactions between the siblings. Tsao and Odom (2006) taught siblings a more complex intervention. In a series of ten lessons, siblings were taught skills such as staying in proximity to their sibling with ASD, creating opportunities for social interaction, giving clear directions, and providing feedback. This intervention led to increases in social interaction as well as joint attention skills for the children with ASD.

These studies suggest that peers and siblings of children with ASD can learn relatively complex intervention packages often used by adult therapists to increase social skills in children with ASD. These interventions lead to skill gains for the children with ASD and facilitate social interactions between the typically developing children and their peers or siblings with ASD.

Summary

In conclusion, a number of techniques involving peers or siblings as intervention agents have been successful at promoting socialization with same-aged play partners in children with ASD. While merely placing children with ASD in the same classrooms as typically developing peers may not be enough to facilitate successful peer interactions, a number of peer-mediated interventions can be implemented to increase successful socialization among these children. Interventions that can successfully promote socialization in children with ASD include organizing and facilitating a supportive environment for peer interaction, pairing typically developing peers with children with ASD as peer buddies or tutors, teaching peers and siblings to initiate interactions with children with ASD, and teaching peers or siblings to deliver more complex intervention packages for children with ASD. It is clear that involving typically developing children in socialization interventions for children with ASD aids in facilitating successful interactions among peers that are more likely to generalize to new settings and maintain over time.

Direct Instruction in Social Skills

A number of interventions have been developed to directly teach a range of appropriate social skills to children with ASD. Direct social skills interventions have been used with children from earliest diagnosis through adolescence; thus the type of skills targeted and the specific instructional techniques used differ depending on the age and ability of the child. The most common techniques include naturalistic interventions, Social Stories, technological interventions (video-based or computer-based instruction), social skills groups, scripting, prompting, or priming procedures (as part of interventions using applied behavior analysis or pivotal response treatments), and self- monitoring (Bellini and Peters 2008; Reichow and Volkmar 2010). This section will focus on naturalistic interventions, video-based instruction, Social Stories, and social skills groups as they have garnered the most empirical support (Bellini and Peters 2008; Reichow and Volkmar 2010).

Naturalistic Interventions

A number of naturalistic interventions have been used to directly teach early social-communication skills—such as joint attention, joint engagement, and social imitation—to young children with ASD. These approaches, which embed teaching within child-chosen play activities, utilize the same intervention techniques as the parent-mediated naturalistic behavioral and developmental interventions described above; however, intervention is provided directly by a trained therapist rather than a caregiver.

A number of single-subject designs (e.g. Ingersoll and Schreibman 2006; Whalen and Schreibman 2003) and several recent randomized controlled trials (Ingersoll 2010b; Kasari et al. 2006) have shown that direct instruction using naturalistic interventions can improve early social skills in young children with ASD. For example, one randomized study examined the effect of adding a 6-week joint attention intervention or symbolic play intervention to a comprehensive program in 58 preschoolers with ASD (Kasari et al. 2006). Children in the treatment groups received 30 min per day of a joint attention or symbolic play intervention as part of an existing intervention program, while children in the control group received the existing program alone (the program did not specifically target early social communication skills). After 6 weeks, the children in the joint attention group used more joint attention and the children in the symbolic play group used more symbolic play acts than the children in the other groups. In addition, the children in both treatment groups had greater gains in language skills 1 year later (Kasari et al. 2008), suggesting that targeting early nonverbal social communication skills may promote the long term development of verbal skills in children with ASD. Another recent study examined the effect of an intervention targeting social imitation in toddlers and preschoolers with ASD (Ingersoll 2010b). Children in the treatment group received 3 h per week of treatment for 10 weeks while children in the control group received treatment as usual in the community. At post treatment, children in the treatment group had significantly greater gains in spontaneous social imitation skills than children in the control group. In a follow-up of the participants at 2–3 months post treatment, children in the treatment group made significantly greater gains in the initiation of joint attention during a structured assessment and on a parent-report measure of social-emotional functioning than the control group (Ingersoll 2012), suggesting that teaching social imitation using a naturalistic treatment approach can lead to broader improvements in social functioning.

Video-Based Instruction

In recent years, video-based instruction has been used extensively to target social skills in individuals with ASD. Video-based instruction takes advantage of the fact that many children with ASD are stronger visual than auditory learners and find video and related technology very reinforcing (Kroeger et al. 2007). Video-based instruction comprises three techniques: video modeling, video self-modeling, and point-of-view modeling. In video modeling, the participant watches a video in which the target skill is modeled immediately prior to engaging in the relevant social situation. The instructor typically provides prompting and reinforcement to increase attention towards the relevant stimuli, and then the participant is given the opportunity to imitate the model demonstrated in the video (Bellini and Akullian 2007, Graetz et al. 2006; Shukla-Mehta et al. 2010; Sigafoos et al. 2007). Video self-monitoring is similar, except that the video is a recording of the actual participant appropriately displaying the target behavior (Hitchcock et al. 2003; Shukla-Mehta et al. 2010). Point-of-view modeling records the components of the environment and activity from the point-of-view of the participant. The video captures each step of the target skill at the eye level of the participant, allowing the individual viewing the recording to have a clear visual representation of what they are supposed to do to accomplish each part of a task (Shukla-Mehta et al. 2010).

A number of studies have supported the efficacy of video-based instruction for increasing a range of social skills in children with ASD (e.g. Kroeger et al. 2007; Nikopoulos and Keenan 2004). In fact, a recent meta analysis of video-based instruction recommended that it be considered an evidence-based practice for the treatment of social skills in ASD (Shukla-Mehta et al. 2010). Several studies have attempted to identify specific elements of video-based instruction that enhance learning by comparing different models (self vs. other, peer vs. adult) or presentation formats (e.g. playing whole video or one step at a time; e.g. Charlop-Christy et al. 2000; Gena et al. 2005). These studies have not found specific elements to be consistently more effective across participants (Shukla-Mehta et al. 2010); however, there is evidence that video models result in more rapid rates of skill acquisition than live models for children with ASD (Charlop-Christy et al. 2000).

Social Stories

Another common approach to direct instruction in social skills is the use of Social Stories. Social Stories are written instructions presented in a story format that are aimed at teaching a child a particular social (or behavioral) concept. The stories are intended to be individualized to the social or behavioral needs of the child, and multiple stories are often used to instruct on a wide variety of skills (Karkhaneh et al. 2010; Reynhout and Carter 2006). Social Stories are composed of text with specific sentence structures, which may be complete or partial, with partial sentences used to encourage children with ASD to anticipate upcoming situations or specific responses (Reynhout and Carter 2006). However, strict adherence to the recommended construction is not always used and does not seem to negatively impact the efficacy of the intervention (Quirmbach et al. 2009; Reynhout and Carter 2006). Like video-based instruction, Social Stories are typically read immediately prior to engaging in the relevant social situation. However, homework, such as reading the story at home or practicing the behaviors described in the text, is also used (Reynhout and Carter 2006). Some Social Story interventions have included additional prompting and reinforcement by the instructor for engaging in the appropriate social behavior (e.g. Kuoch and Mirenda 2003).

Research on the effect of Social Stories on social skills in children with ASD has found inconsistent results, with some studies finding large positive effects whereas others with minimal benefit (see Ali and Frederickson 2006 for review). Variations in outcomes across studies are likely due to the complexity of social skills targeted, other components of the intervention (e.g. prompting and reinforcement), and the skill level of the participants. In the largest study examining the effectiveness of Social Stories (Quirmbach et al. 2009), 45 children with high-functioning autism (ages 7–14) were randomly assigned to a standard Social Story designed to increase game playing skills, a directive sentences only Social Story focused on increasing game play, or control story (Social Story unrelated to game play). Compared to the control group, children in the experimental groups exhibited significant improvement in game playing skills (e.g. asking another person to play a game and accepting their choice of games), as well as generalization of skills to other games. These gains were maintained after 1 week. However, one third of the participants (those with a verbal IQ below 68) did not improve their game playing skills through the intervention. These findings, along with others (e.g. Feinberg 2001), suggest that Social Stories are more likely to be effective for children with ASD whose verbal IQ is in the borderline range or above.

Social Skills Groups

Another approach that has often been used to teach social skills to children with ASD is social skills groups. This approach has been primarily used with school-aged children and adolescents with high-functioning autism or Asperger's Syndrome who have language abilities in the average range. Groups typically include 4–8 children with ASD and 1–2 instructors (e.g. Tse et al. 2007), and are often implemented in a clinic or other "pull-out" setting (Reichow and Volkmar 2010). The number of and content of sessions vary, but most groups are conducted once a week for at least

3 months and cover topics such as recognition and use nonverbal social behaviors, conversation skills, emotion recognition, effective coping, and friendship skills.

Across the literature there is general support for the use of social skills groups for youth with high-functioning ASD and social skills groups are one of the few intervention formats for social skills training that meet criteria set forth by Reichow and colleagues (2008) to be considered an evidence-based program. However, some studies report weak effects, inconsistent results, and poor maintenance of skills (Krasny et al. 2003; Reichow and Volkmar 2010; White et al. 2007). Most of studies that have found positive effects have examined changes in skills directly addressed by the intervention (e.g. improvement in emotion recognition skills). However, they have either not examined or failed to find generalized improvement in more global social skills (e.g. teacher report) or peer interaction skills outside of the group (White et al. 2007). These findings suggest that social skills groups may be limited in their ability to produce broader changes in social functioning, especially when it comes to peer relationships. However, several randomized controlled trials of the PEERS program, have found significant treatment effects on peer interaction skills for children and adolescents with ASD (Gantman et al. 2012; Laugeson et al. 2012). This intervention involves a concurrent parent training group that teaches parents how to help their children carry over their skills to other environments. Thus, parent-assisted social skills intervention implemented in a group format may significantly enhance social outcomes for high-functioning students with ASD.

Future Directions

There is emerging evidence to support the efficacy of a wide variety of interventions for improving social interaction and related skills with peers and adults for children with ASD. Although the evidence is promising, additional research is needed on the ability of these approaches to produce skill gains that generalize to new situations and interaction partners and maintain over time. Generalization appears to be most challenging for interventions that provide direct instruction to children with ASD in specific skills outside of the context in which they are expected to use them (e.g. social skills groups).

An important next step is to conduct direct comparisons between approaches to determine the most effective ways to teach specific types of social behaviors. Thus far, only one randomized controlled trial has directly compared the ability of different intervention approaches to improve peer-related social skills in children with ASD. Kasari and colleagues (2012) compared direct child instruction, peer training, and a combined approach, to a no treatment control in 60 school-aged children with high-functioning ASD included in regular education settings. Intervention (target child instruction or peer instruction) was conducted twice a week in 20 min sessions for 6 weeks. Primary social outcomes involved social network salience and peer engagement during a playground observation. The findings indicated that the peer-mediated approach led to better social outcomes than direct child instruction for both primary outcomes, and that gains maintained at a 12 week follow-up. The children in the combined intervention had the greatest improvements in social network salience, suggesting that a combined approach which teaches both peers and the target child skills may have stronger effects.

There is also a need for the development and evaluation of interventions that can increase socialization in individuals with ASD who have significant intellectual disabilities and/or who remain nonverbal (Rogers 2000; Walton and Ingersoll in press). To date, most social skills interventions for school-age children and adolescents with ASD have been developed for those who are high-functioning or who have at least adequate verbal skills. This may be because these individuals are more likely to be educated in regular education settings and thus, the need for improving peer interaction skills may be viewed as more pressing. However, research indicates that the development of social relationships is an important aspect of quality of life for individuals with ASD across the spectrum (Plimley 2007) and thus it is important to develop approaches that can improve socialization in individuals with ASD who are typically underrepresented in the social skills literature.

In sum, there are a number of promising approaches for increasing socialization in children with ASD. Further research that can identify the optimal approaches for teaching specific types of social behaviors for children at different ages and ability levels is needed.

References

Ali, S., & Frederickson, N. (2006). Investigating the evidence base of social stories. *Educational Psychology in Practice, 22,* 355–377.

Bellini, S., & Akullian, J. (2007). A meta-analysis of video modeling and video self-modeling interventions for children and adolescents with autism spectrum disorders. *Exceptional Children, 73,* 264–287.

Bellini, S., & Peters, J. (2008). Social skills training for youth with autism spectrum disorders. *Child and Adolescent Psychiatric Clinics of North America, 17,* 857–873.

Blew, P. A., Schwartz, I. S., & Luce, S. C. (1985). Teaching functional community skills to autistic children using nonhandicapped peer tutors. *Journal of Applied Behavior Analysis, 18,* 337–342.

Brookman-Frazee, L., Vismara, L., Drahota, A., Stahmer, A., & Openden, D. (2009). Parent Training interventions for children with autism spectrum disorders. In J. Matson (Ed.), *Applied Behavior Analysis for Children with Autism Spectrum Disorders: A Handbook* (pp. 237–257). New York: Springer.

Charlop-Christy, M. H., Le, L., & Freeman, K. A. (2000). A comparison of video modeling with in vivo modeling for teaching children with autism. *Journal of Autism and Developmental Disorders, 30,* 537–552.

Coe, D. A., Matson, J. L., Craigie, C. J., & Gossen, M. A. (1991). Play skills of autistic children: assessment and instruction. *Child and Family Behavior Therapy, 13,* 13–40.

Dugan, E. P., Kamps, D. M., Leonard, B. R., Watkins, N., Rheinberger, A., & Stackhaus, J. (1995). Effects of cooperative learning groups during social studies for students with autism and fourth-grade peers. *Journal of Applied Behavior Analysis, 28,* 175–188.

Estes, A., Munson, J., Dawson, G., Koehler, E., Zhou, X., & Abbott, R. (2009). Parenting stress and psychological functioning among mothers of preschool children with autism and developmental delay. *Autism, 13,* 375–387.

Feinberg, M. J. (2001). Using social stories to teach specific social skills to individuals diagnosed with autism (Doctoral dissertation, California School of Professional Psychology, San Diego). Dissertation Abstracts International.

Gantman, A., Kapp, S., Orenski, K., & Laugeson, E. (2012). Social skills training for young adults with high-functioning autism spectrum disorders: a randomized controlled pilot study. *Journal of Autism and Developmental Disorders, 42,* 1094–1103.

Garrison-Harrell, L., Kamps, D., & Kravits, T. (1997). The effects of peer networks on social-communicative behaviors for students with autism. *Focus on Autism & Other Developmental Disabilities, 12,* 241–254.

Gena, A., Couloura, S., & Kymissis, E. (2005). Modifying the affective behavior of preschoolers with autism using in-vivo or video modeling and reinforcement contingencies. *Journal of Autism & Developmental Disorders, 35,* 545–556.

Goldstein, H., Kaczmarek, L., Pennington, R., & Shafer, K. (1992). Peer-mediated intervention: Attending to, commenting on, and acknowledging the behavior of preschoolers with autism. *Journal of Applied Behavior Analysis, 25,* 289–305.

Graetz, J., Mastropieri, M., & Scruggs, T. (2006). Show time: Using video self-modeling to decrease inappropriate behavior. *Teaching Exceptional Children, 38,* 43–48.

Green, J., Charman, T., McConachie, H., Aldred, C., Slonims, V., Howlin, P., Le Couteur, A., Leadbitter, K., Hudry, K., Byford, S., Barrett, B., Temple, K., Macdonald, W., & Pickles, A. (2010). Parent-mediated communication-focused treatment in children with autism (PACT): A randomized controlled trial. *Lancet, 375,* 2152–2160.

Gutstein, S. (2001). *Solving the Relationship Puzzle.* Arlington: Future Horizons.

Haring, T. G., & Breen, C. G. (1992). A peer-mediated social network intervention to enhance the social integration of persons with moderate and severe disabilities. *Journal of Applied Behavior Analysis, 25,* 319–333.

Harrower, J., & Dunlap, G. (2001). Including children with autism in general education classrooms: a review of effective strategies. *Behavior Modification, 25,* 762–784.

Hitchcock, C., Dowrick, P., & Prater, M. (2003). Video self-modeling intervention in a school-based setting: A review. *Remedial and Special Education, 24*(1), 136–145.

Howlin, P., Goode, S., Hutton, J., & Rutter, M. (2004). Adult outcome for children with autism. *Journal of Child Psychology and Psychiatry, 45,* 212–229.

Ingersoll, B. (2012). Brief report: Effect of a focused imitation intervention on social functioning in children with autism. *Journal of Autism and Developmental Disorders, 42,* 1768–1773.

Ingersoll, B. (2010a). Teaching social communication: A comparison of naturalistic behavioral and developmental, social-pragmatic approaches for children with autism spectrum disorders. *Journal of Positive Behavior Interventions, 12,* 33–43.

Ingersoll, B. (2010b). Brief report: pilot randomized controlled trial of reciprocal imitation training for teaching elicited and spontaneous imitation to children with autism. *Journal of Autism and Developmental Disorders, 40,* 1154–1160.

Ingersoll, B. (2011) Recent advances in early identification and treatment of autism. *Current Directions in Psychological Science, 20,* 335–339.

Ingersoll, B., & Dvortcsak, A (2006). Including parent training in the early childhood special education curriculum for children with autism spectrum disorders. *Journal of Positive Behavior Interventions, 8,* 79–87.

Ingersoll, B., & Dvorcsak, A. (2010). *Teaching social-communication: A practitioner's guide to parent training for children with autism.* New York: Guilford Press.

Ingersoll, B., & Gergans, S. (2007). The effect of a parent-implemented imitation intervention on spontaneous imitation skills in young children with autism. *Research in Developmental Disabilities, 28,* 163–175.

Ingersoll, B., & Schreibman, L. (2006). Teaching reciprocal imitation skills to young children with autism using a naturalistic behavioral approach: Effects on language, pretend play, and joint attention. *Journal of Autism and Developmental Disorders, 36,* 487–505.

Ingersoll, B., & Wainer, A. (in press). *Pilot study of a school-based parent training program for preschoolers with ASD.* Autism.

Kaiser, A. P., Hancock, T. B., & Nietfeld, J. P. (2000). The effects of parent-implemented enhanced milieu teaching on the social communication of children who have autism. *Early Education and Development, 11,* 423–446.

Kamps, D. M., Barbetta, P. M., Leonard, B. R., & Delquadri, J. (1994). Classwide peer tutoring: An integration strategy to improve reading skills and promote peer interactions among students with autism and general education peers. *Journal of Applied Behavior Analysis, 27,* 49–61.

Kamps, D. M., Potucek, J., Lopez, A. G., Kravits, T., & Kemmerer, K. (1997). The use of peer networks across multiple settings to improve social interaction for students with autism. *Journal of Behavioral Education, 7,* 335–357.

Kamps, D. M., Dugan, E., Potucek, J., & Collins, A. (1999). Effects of cross-age peer tutoring networks among students with autism and general education students. *Journal of Behavioral Education, 9,* 97–115.

Karkhaneh, M., Clark, B., Ospina, M.B., Seida, J.C., Smith, V., & Hartling, L. (2010). Social Stories™ to improve social skills in children with autism spectrum disorder: A systematic review. *Autism, 14,* 641–662.

Kasari, C., Feeman, S., & Paparella, T. (2006). Joint attention and symbolic play in young children with autism: a randomized controlled intervention study. *Journal of Child Psychology and Psychiatry, 47,* 611–620.

Kasari, C., Paparella, T. Feeman, S., & Jahromi, L. (2008). Language outcome in autism: randomized comparison of joint attention and play interventions. *Journal of Consulting and Clinical Psychology, 76,* 125–137.

Kasari, C., Rotheram-Fuller, E., Locke, J., & Gulsrud, A. (2012). Making the connection: randomized controlled trial of social skills at school for children with autism spectrum disorders. *Journal of Child Psychology and Psychiatry, 53,* 431–439.

Koegel, R. L., Schreibman, L., Britten, K. R., Burke, J. C., & O'Neill, R. E. (1982). A comparison of parent training to direct child treatment. In R. L. Koegel, A. Rincover, & A. Egel (Eds.), *Educating and understanding autistic children* (pp. 260–279). San Diego: College Hill.

Koegel, R. L., O'Dell, M. C., & Koegel, L. K. (1987). A natural language teaching paradigm for nonverbal autistic children. *Journal of Autism and Developmental Disorders, 17,* 187–200.

Krasny, L., Williams, B., Provencal, S., & Ozonoff, S. (2003). Social skills interventions for the autism spectrum: essential ingredients and a model curriculum. *Child and Adolescent Psychiatric Clinics of North America, 12,* 107–122.

Kroeger, K., Schultz, J., & Newsom, C. (2007). A Comparison of Two Group-Delivered Social Skills Programs for Young Children with Autism, *Journal of Autism and Developmental Disorders, 37,* 808–817.

Kuoch, H., & Mirenda, P. (2003). Social story interventions for young children with autism spectrum disorders. *Focus on Autism and Other Developmental Disorders, 18,* 219–227.

Laski, K. E., Charlop, M. H., & Schreibman, L. (1988). Training parents to use the Natural Language Paradigm to increase their autistic children's speech. *Journal of Applied Behavior Analysis, 21,* 391–400.

Laugeson, E., Frankel, F., Gantman, A., Dillon, A., & Mogil, C. (2012). Evidence-based social skills training for adolescents with autism spectrum disorders: the UCLA PEERS Program. *Journal of Autism and Developmental Disorders, 42,* 1025–1036.

Mahoney, G., Kaiser, A., Girolametto, L., MacDonald, J., Robinson, C., Safford, P., & Spiker, D. (1999). Parent education in early intervention: a call for a renewed focus. *Topics in Early Childhood Special Education, 19,* 131–140.

Mahoney, G., & Perales, F. (2003). Using relationship-focused intervention to enhance the social-emotional functioning of young children with autism spectrum disorders. *Topics in Early Childhood Special Education, 23,* 77–89

McConachie, H., & Diggle, T. (2007). Parent implemented early intervention for young children with autism spectrum disorder: A systematic review. *Journal of Evaluation in Clinical Practice, 13,* 120–129.

McConachie, H., Randle, V., Hammal, D., & LeCouteur, A. (2005). A controlled trial of a training course for parents of children with suspected autism spectrum disorder. *The Journal of Pediatrics, 147,* 335–340.

McConnell, S. R. (2002). Interventions to facilitate social interaction for young children with Autism: Review of available research and recommendations for educational intervention and future research. *Journal of Autism and Developmental Disorders, 32,* 351–373.

McGee, G. G., Almeida, M. C., Sulzer-Azaroff, B., & Feldman, R. S. (1992). Promoting reciprocal interactions via peer incidental teaching. *Journal of Applied Behavior Analysis, 25,* 117–126.

Mesibov, G., & Shea, V. (1996). Full inclusion and students with autism. *Journal of Autism and Developmental Disorders, 26,* 337–346.

National Research Council. (2001). Educating children with autism. Committee on Educational Interventions for Children with Autism. In C. Lord, & J. P. McGee (Eds), *Division of Behavioral and Social Sciences and Education*. Washington, DC: National Academy Press.

Nefdt, N., Koegel, R., Singer, G., & Gerber, M. (2009). The use of a self-directed learning program to provide introductory training in pivotal response treatment to parents of children with autism. *Journal of Positive Behavior Interventions, 12,* 23–32.

Nikopoulos, C. K., & Keenan, M. (2004). Effects of video modeling on training and generalisation of social initiation and reciprocal play by children with autism. *European Journal of Behaviour Analysis, 5,* 1–13.

Odom, S., Brown, W., Frey, T., Karasu, N., Smith-Canter, L., & Strain, P. (2003). Evidence-based practices for young children with autism: contributions for single-subject design research. *Focus on Autism and Other Developmental Disabilities, 18,* 166–175.

Orsmond, G., Krauss, M., & Seltzer, M. (2004). Peer relationships and social and recreational activities among adolescents and adults with autism. *Journal of Autism and Developmental Disorders, 34,* 245–256.

Pierce, K., & Schreibman, L. (1997). Multiple peer use of pivotal response training to increase social behaviors of classmates with autism: Results from trained and untrained peers. *Journal of Applied Behavior Analysis, 30,* 157–160.

Plimley, L. (2007). A review of quality of life issues and people with autism spectrum disorders. *British Journal of Learning Disabilities, 35,* 205–213.

Quintero, N., & McIntyre, L. L. (2010). Sibling adjustment and maternal well-being: An examination of families with and without a child with an autism spectrum disorder. *Focus on Autism and Other Developmental Disabilities, 25,* 37–46.

Quirmbach, L., Lincoln, A., Feinber-Gizzo, M., Ingersoll, B., & Andrews, S. (2009). Social Stories: Mechanisms of Effectiveness in Increasing Game Play Skills in Children Diagnosed with Autism Spectrum Disorder Using a Pretest Posttest Repeated Measures Randomized Control Group Design. *Journal of Autism and Develeopmental Disorders, 39,* 299–321.

Reichow, B. & Volkmar, F. (2010). Social Skills Interventions for Individuals with Autism: Evaluation for Evidence-Based Practices within a Best Evidence Synthesis Framework. *Journal of Autism and Developmental Disorders, 40,* 149–166.

Reichow, B., Volkmar, F., & Cicchetti, D. (2008). Development of the evaluative method for evaluating and determining evidence-based practices in autism. *Journal of Autism and Developmental Disorders, 38,* 1311–1319.

Reynhout, G., & Carter, M. (2006). Social Stories for Children with Disabilities. *Journal of Autism and Developmental Disorders, 36,* 445–469.

Roeyers, H. (1996). The influence of nonhandicapped peers on the social interactions of children with a pervasive developmental disorder. *Journal of Autism and Developmental Disorders, 26,* 303–320.

Rogers, S. (1999). Intervention for young children with autism: from research to practice. *Infants & Young Children, 12,* 1–16.

Rogers, S. J. (2000). Interventions that facilitate socialization in children with autism. *Journal of Autism and Developmental Disorders, 30,* 399–409.

Rogers, J., & Dawson, G. (2009). *Early Start Denver Model for Young Children with Autism: Promoting Language, Learning, and Engagement*. New York: Guilford.

Seltzer, M., Shattuck, P., Abbeduto, L., & Greenberg, J. (2004). Trajectory of development in adolescents and adults with autism. *Mental Retardation and Developmental Disabilities Research Reviews, 10,* 234–247.

Scattone, D. (2007). Social skills interventions for children with autism. *Psychology in the Schools, 44,* 717–726.

Schreibman, L., Kaneko, W. M., & Koegel, R. L. (1991). Positive affect of parents of autistic children: A comparison across two teaching techniques. *Behavior Therapy, 22,* 479–490.

Shukla-Mehta, S., Miller, T., & Callahan, K. (2010) Evaluating the effectiveness of video instruction on social and communication skills training for children with Autism Spectrum Disorders: A review of the literature. *Focus on Autism and Other Developmental Disabilities, 25,* 23–36.

Sigafoos, J., O'Reilly, M., & de la Cruz, B. (2007). *How To Use Video Modeling and Video Prompting*. Austin: Pro-Ed

Sigman, M., Mundy, P., Sherman, T., & Ungerer, J. (1986). Social interactions of autistic, mentally retarded and normal children and their caregivers. *Journal of Child Psychology and Psychiatry, 27,* 647–656.

Simpson, R., de Boer-Ott, S., Smith-Myles, B. (2003). Inclusion of learning with autism spectrum disorders in general education settings. *Topics in Language Disorders, 23,* 116–133.

Strain, P., & Schwartz, I. (2001). ABA and the developmenta of meaningful social relationships for young children with autism. *Focus on Autism and Other Developmental Disabilities, 16,* 120–128.

Strain, P. S., & Danko, C. D. (1995). Caregivers' encouragement of positive interaction between preschoolers with autism and their siblings. *Journal of Emotional and Behavioral Disorders, 3,* 2–12.

Strain, P. S., Kohler, F. W., Storey, K., & Danko, C. D. (1994). Teaching preschoolers with autism to self-monitor their social interactions: An analysis of results in home and school settings. *Journal of Emotional and Behavioral Disorders, 2,* 78–88.

Stone, W., & Caro-Martinez, L. (1990). Naturalistic observations of spontaneous communication in autistic children. *Journal of Autism and Developmental Disorders, 20,* 437–453.

Sussman, F. (1999). *More than Words: The Hanen Program for Parents of Children with Autism Spectrum Disorder*. Toronto: The Hanen Centre.

Symon, J. (2005). Expanding interventions for children with autism: parents as trainers. *Journal of Positive Behavior Interventions, 7,* 159–173.

Tomasello, M. (1995). Joint attention as social cognition. In C. Moore, & P. J. Dunham (Eds.), *Joint attention: its origins and role in development* (pp. 103–130). Hillsdale: Lawrence Erlbaum.

Tonge, B., Brereton, A., Kiomall, M., Mackinnon, A., King, N., & Rinehart, N. (2006). Effects on parental mental health of an education and skills training program for parents of young children with autism: A randomized controlled trial. *Journal of the American Academy of Child and Adolescent Psychiatry, 45,* 561–569.

Tsao, L. -L., & Odom, S. L. (2006). Sibling-mediated social interaction intervention for young children with autism. *Topics in Early Childhood Special Education, 26,* 106–123.

Tse, J., Strulovitch, J., Tagalakis, V., Meng, L., & Fombonne, E. (2007). Social skills training for adolescents with Asperger syndrome and high functioning autism. *Journal of Autism and Developmental Disorders, 37,* 1960–1968.

Vismara, L., Colombi, C., & Rogers, S. (2009). Can one hour per week of therapy lead to lasting changes in young children with autism? *Autism, 13,* 93–115.

Walton, K., & Ingersoll, B. (2012). Evaluation of a sibling-mediated imitation intervention for young children with autism. *Journal of Positive Behavior Interventions, 14,* 241–253.

Walton, K., & Ingersoll, B. (in press). Improving social skills in adolescents and adults with autism and severe to profound intellectual disability: a review of the literature. *Journal of Autism and Developmental Disorders.*

Wetherby, A., Woods, J., Allen, L., Cleary, J., Dickinson, H., & Lord, C. (2004). Early indicators of autism spectrum disorders in the second year of life. *Journal of Autism and Developmental Disorders, 34,* 473–493.

Whalen, C., & Schreibman, L. (2003). Joint attention training for children with autism using behavior modification procedures. *Journal of Child Psychology and Psychiatry, 44,* 456–468.

White, S., Keonig, K., & Scahill, L. (2007). Social Skills Development in Children with Autism Spectrum Disorders: A Review of the Intervention Research. *J Autism Dev Disord, 37,* 1858–1868.

Wolfberg, P. J., & Schuler, A. L. (1993). Integrated play groups: A model for promoting the social and cognitive dimensions of play in children with autism. *Journal of Autism and Developmental Disorders, 23,* 467–489.

Zwaigenbaum, L., Bryson, S., Rogers, T., Roberts, W., Brian, J., & Szatmari, P. (2005). Behavioral manifestations of autism in the first year of life. *International Journal of Developmental Neuroscience, 23,* 143–152.

Chapter 11
Social Emotional Reciprocity

Sara Whitcomb, Verity L. Rodrigues and Kenneth W. Merrell

Introduction

The purpose of this chapter is to provide an overview of strategic interventions, focusing on social-emotional reciprocity skills, which can be implemented with children with High Functioning Autism (HFA) and Asperger's Syndrome (AS). Authors will first describe some of the social-emotional characteristics of these children and then will outline the potential and concerning mental health and behavioral outcomes that may occur if systematic intervention is not provided. Through a discussion of emerging research in this area, authors will delineate features of effective interventions that address social-emotional reciprocity deficits in children with HFA and AS. An overview of the *Strong Kids* programs, *Strong Kids-E*, *Strong Kids-M* (Merrell et al. 2007a, b), *Strong Teens* (Merrell et al. 2007) *Strong Start: Pre-K* (Merrell et al. 2009), and *Strong Start: K-2* (Merrell et al. 2007), one particular systematic social-emotional learning program, will be provided along with specific examples of how this curriculum may be used with this particular population. Ideas for using data to monitor the effectiveness of interventions such as *Strong Kids* will be shared. Finally, authors will conclude with a discussion of the challenges pertaining to this area of research and future directions specifically for social-emotional intervention research with HFA and AS.

V. L. Rodrigues (✉)
Division of Developmental and Behavioral Pediatrics, Cincinnati Children's Hospital Medical Center, 3333 Burnet Avenue, Cincinnati, 45229 OH, USA
e-mail: verityrodrigues@gmail.com

S. Whitcomb · K. W. Merrell
University of Massachusetts, Amherst, 360 Hills South, UMASS, 111 Thatcher Rd., Amherst, 01003-9361 MA, USA
e-mail: swhitcomb@educ.umass.edu

S. Goldstein, J. A. Naglieri (eds.), *Interventions for Autism Spectrum Disorders*, DOI 10.1007/978-1-4614-5301-7_11,

Definition and Etiology of ASD and Asperger's Syndrome

According to the text revision of the *Diagnostic and Statistical Manual of Mental Disorders* (DSM-IV-TR; American Psychiatric Association 2000), Autistic Disorder and Asperger's Disorder fall under the global category of Pervasive Developmental Disorders. Autistic Disorder is considered a spectrum disorder, consisting of behavioral characteristics that range in intensity across diagnosed individuals. In fact, a group of professionals working on the next edition of the DSM has proposed to subsume Asperger's Disorder under the category of Autistic Disorder, given that the characteristics of this disorder appear to be a higher functioning version of autism (American Psychiatric Association 2011). While there is much controversy on this issue, there is overlap in characteristics defining these currently separate disorders, and there are also some significant differences worth discussing. For example, children diagnosed with Autistic Disorder often have clinically significant delays in cognitive development or in the development of age-appropriate adaptive behavior and significant impairments in communication, whereas children diagnosed with Asperger's Disorder do not exhibit clinically significant delays in these areas (American Psychiatric Association 2000). Children diagnosed with Autistic Disorder often will engage in restrictive and repetitive behaviors characterized by the presence of motor mannerisms and may demonstrate marked distress with changes in routines. While children with Asperger's Disorder also typically are agitated by routine changes and display clumsy motor skills, their repetitive behaviors are often characterized by preoccupation with special interest topics, where children will spend a significant amount of time gathering information and facts about those topics. Regarding social interaction, children diagnosed with lower functioning Autistic Disorder tend to exhibit patterns of isolation and aversions to social interaction; however, children diagnosed with high functioning Autistic Disorder or Asperger's Disorder may demonstrate motivation or interest in social interaction, but often lack the skills to initiate or engage in social interactions (White 2007; Stichter et al. 2010). Within the current chapter, authors will focus on social-emotional reciprocity in children diagnosed with Pervasive Developmental Disorders, primarily high functioning Autistic Disorder and Asperger's Disorder, as the development of social-emotional skills within these two diagnoses follows a similar trajectory. The following section will focus specifically on this topic. From this point onward, HFA will be used to describe High Functioning Autism and AS will be used to describe Asperger's Syndrome.

Social-Emotional Development Specific to HFA and AS

One of the critical diagnostic features of HFA and AS is a severe and sustained impairment in social-emotional development and functioning. School-aged children with HFA and AS exhibit social skill or performance deficits that affect their abilities to make and sustain friendships and that negatively impact their overall quality of life (Stichter et al. 2010). Youth with HFA and AS often demonstrate difficulties with social-emotional reciprocity, a complex skill requiring competence across several core social-emotional learning domains, including self-awareness, social awareness, self-management, and relationship skills. Many researchers consider social-emotional reciprocity to be linked to having a theory of mind (Baron-Cohen 2001). Children described as having a theory of mind are those that understand the mental states of themselves and others. This means that they can identify their feelings and accurately infer what others may be feeling (Baron-Cohen 2001).

Children with HFA and AS may demonstrate difficulties with theory of mind tasks such as conveying and recognizing a range of facial expressions and emotions, particularly complex emotions, such as surprise and embarrassment, in themselves and others (Stichter et al. 2010). For example, in a study comparing typically functioning adolescents and those with HFA, Wallace et al. (2011) found that participants with HFA were more likely to recognize basic emotions only when they were expressed through intense facial expression. Typically functioning adolescents, on the other hand, were able to more accurately identify subtle versions of emotional expression. Adolescents with HFA were also particularly limited in their ability to recognize sadness in this study.

Grossman et al. (2000) conducted a study with 13 children with AS, during which they asked participants to identify basic emotions with and without picture labels. Participants were able to recognize basic emotion pictures when they were not labeled; however, when researchers purposefully mislabeled emotions (e.g., labeled a happy picture as angry), they found that participants relied primarily on the language cues provided and inaccurately identified emotions. This suggested that participants were relying on compensatory skills (verbal skills), which could also be the case when they are faced with complex social interactions. These emotion recognition deficiencies greatly impact a child's ability to understand the social nuances of language, and subsequently form connections with peers and adults.

In addition to emotion recognition difficulties, children with HFA and AS most often have social pragmatic deficits (Baron-Cohen 2001). This means that they have difficulty in adapting topics of conversation for particular listeners. For example, children with AS often engage in one-sided conversations, where they may share information about a particular topic without paying attention to their listeners' prior knowledge of the topic, level of interest, etc. They may also fail to recognize when their listeners make attempts to shift the direction of the conversation. Additionally, children with HFA and AS may not have an awareness of what constitutes polite language and may fail to learn how to adapt language for particular populations or particular contexts (Baron-Cohen 2001; Linnand Myles 2004).

Children with HFA and AS may also have difficulties utilizing nonverbal communication strategies, such as eye contact and body posture, further impacting their ability to manage reciprocal social interactions (Crooke et al. 2008). The common inability of children with HFA and AS to understand and recognize that others have different thoughts, intentions, and feelings from their own, directly and negatively impacts their ability to engage in social-emotional reciprocity. These deficits, mixed with cognitive rigidity, poor impulse control, and difficulty with both self-monitoring and social problem solving can be very problematic for this population (Stichter et al. 2010).

Because the above-stated social-emotional difficulties are often experienced by children with HFA and AS, initiating and responding to reciprocal social interactions is challenging. This, in turn, decreases the number of opportunities these children have to practice social skills with their peers, further contributing to social skill and performance deficits. As children enter late elementary and middle school, the social environments become more complex, further exacerbating the social-emotional deficiencies of students with HFA and AS. Without intervention supports targeting social-emotional functioning, early adolescents with HFA and AS are at risk for developing subsequent mental health problems such as depression, and adults with AS are at increased risk for attempting suicide (Barnhill 2004).

The following sections will discuss features of effective interventions for addressing social-emotional reciprocity in children with HFA and AS, school-wide social-emotional programming that can support children with HFA and AS, the *Strong Kids* program as an example of a targeted intervention, and a case example of how *Strong Kids* might also be used as a indicated intervention for this population of students.

Features of Effective Interventions

While a number of clinical strategies have been implemented for years, research on efficacious interventions that address the social-emotional reciprocity deficits of children with HFA and AS is still emerging. The first report from the National Standards Project, an impressive initiative of the National Autism Center, was recently printed (Wilczynski 2009). This project aimed to identify the amount of evidence supporting common educational and behavioral interventions implemented with children with autism and to outline which interventions are most appropriate for children of varying ages and levels of functioning. This project involved several expert panelists, article reviewers, and conceptual model reviewers. After an extensive literature search, 775 articles were included for review, and practices used within articles were identified as having an established, emerging, unestablished, or ineffective/harmful evidence base.

While many different theoretical perspectives were represented in the articles reviewed, interventions utilizing features of applied behavior analysis were most often identified as producing positive behavioral change and were identified as having an established evidence base. Applied behavior analysis is a systematic, data-based approach to observing and changing behavior by arranging features of the environment and directly teaching and reinforcing socially adaptive skills (Baer et al. 1987). Interventions identified as established were antecedent interventions, behavioral interventions in general, Comprehensive Behavioral Treatment for Young Children (CBTYC), Joint Attention Intervention, modeling, naturalistic teaching strategies, Peer Training Package, Pivotal Response Treatment (PRT), schedules, self-management, and story-based interventions (Wilczynski 2009).

Interventions from the National Standards Project that were identified as most effective for students ages 6–18 with HFA or AS were those that incorporated modeling or story-based intervention (Wilczynski 2009). Fifty studies reviewed included modeling strategies. Modeling strategies are those in which a teacher or a peer specifically demonstrates target skills. Modeling is most often paired with both prompting and reinforcement procedures. For example, a teacher or counselor might model how to greet another person through role-playing a social scenario with the target child. She might show how to wave hello and practice conversation starters such as "How are you?" and "What are you up to?" Within a social context, such as the classroom or recess, she might provide the child with a verbal or visual prompt to cue him/her to greet another child. Reinforcement for successfully greeting another may include social praise, tangible rewards, or simply a returned greeting.

Story-based interventions stem from a theory-of-mind perspective and include using brief, carefully worded stories or scripts to teach a targeted skill and the appropriate context or situation for using that skill. Twenty-one articles using story-based interventions were reviewed (Wilczynski 2009). Most common story-based interventions are those involving social stories or comic strip conversations (see Gray 1994, 2010).

In addition to the National Standards Project, there are other published studies in social skills training that offer promising intervention practices for children with autism. Williams White et al. (2007) reviewed several studies using social skills training (SST) with children with autism. Researchers reviewed studies of interventions at various stages of development and stages of research, including single case (technique fine-tuning), manual development, randomized clinical trials, and effectiveness research. Although results of studies were somewhat variable, some suggested promising practices emerged. These also included use of story-based interventions, modeling, and differential reinforcement to increase social initiation and social responding and to reduce challenging behaviors. Studies that effectively promoted generalization of social skills were those that included peers, multiple trainers, parents, and training across multiple settings.

Rao et al. (2008) reviewed social skills interventions specifically for children with AS and HFA. Studies reviewed were a combination of single-case studies and group designs. Many of the studies showed an increase in targeted social skills (e.g., greetings, eye contact), some showed increases in emotion knowledge, and the few that showed convincing, positive results regarding generalization of skills included intervention with systematic practice opportunities with typically functioning peers in alternate environments. Few studies that included global ratings of social skills via teacher or parent report resulted in positive outcomes. These data suggest that (a) the behaviors targeted for social skills training did not change significantly following some of the interventions, (b) the behavioral rating measures being used (e.g., SSRS; Gresham and Elliott 1990) did not target the skill deficits specific to children with HFA or AS, or (c) these measures were not sensitive to positive behavioral change that did occur. Authors of this review suggest that there is a need for a refined definition of what constitutes "social skills" for this population and measurement approaches that will accurately assess behavioral change.

One specific concept that is more recently being systematically addressed with children with HFA or AS is Social Thinking. Social Thinking is an approach to teaching children about the nuances of social communication, such as nonverbal communication cues, perspective taking, and emotional awareness (Winner et al. 2011). Crooke et al. (2008) used a Social Thinking intervention in a single case study with six children with AS or HFA. Interventionists specifically worked to make abstract concepts concrete by providing visual cues to enhance language-based social strategies. They also systematically taught self-awareness and perspective taking and included specific activities to promote generalization of skills. Overall, researchers directly observed increases in expected verbal behavior and decreases in unexpected verbal behavior. Examples of expected verbal behaviors included on-topic comments and responses children used to maintain conversation and verbal initiation comments that served to invite another into conversation. Unexpected verbal behaviors were rude comments, unrelated comments, and perseverative comments. Subjects also engaged in more "listening with eyes" following the intervention, suggesting an increase in nonverbal communication skills. Finally, most subjects experienced a decrease in unexpected nonverbal behaviors, such as moving body parts or using objects in ways inconsistent with their intended use.

Cognitive-behavioral interventions are similar to Social Thinking approaches and are more commonly being used with children with HFA or AS. Traditionally, cognitive behavioral therapy (CBT) consists of skill building instruction. Skills targeted typically include cognitive restructuring, relaxation training, and coping strategies. CBT also includes systematic practice of such skills in uncomfortable or anxiety-provoking situations (Becker 2001; Sze and Wood 2007). Bauminger (2002) conducted a study utilizing a CBT approach in children with HFA aged 8–17 years. Adapted versions of Spivack and Shure's (1974) *Interpersonal Problem-Solving Model* and of Margalit and Weisel's (1990) *I Found a Solution* programs were used. Skills training included a focus on social-interpersonal problem solving. This training included systematic instruction on perceiving nonverbal social cues and emotion recognition, appropriate behavioral enactment based on reading cues, and anticipation of consequences of behavioral decisions. The intervention was implemented in a range of settings with teachers, peers, and parents serving as interventionists. Results indicated that children were able to generate more adaptive solutions to social problems, use more appropriate nonverbal social behavior, and recognize more complex emotions in others, and were rated by teachers as more cooperative and assertive following intervention implementation.

Social-emotional reciprocity is a multidimensional construct that taps one's self-awareness of emotion, thought, and behavior as well as perception of the emotions, thoughts, and behaviors of others. Social-emotional reciprocity also includes one's ability to anticipate consequences of verbal and nonverbal behaviors and to effectively problem-solve when unanticipated situations arise. Though research on building social-emotional reciprocity in children with HFA and AS is still emerging, several themes regarding specific skills to target and promising approaches for targeting such skills have become apparent.

Promising approaches for increasing social-emotional reciprocity are becoming clearer. Uses of modeling and story-based interventions to increase skills are effective methods (Wilczynski 2009), and systematic instruction and coordinated practice of skills across settings and situations is necessary (Bauminger 2002; Crooke et al. 2008; Rao et al. 2008; Williams White et al. 2007). Krasny et al. (2003) additionally outline specific ingredients necessary to consider when developing social skill interventions intended for delivery in a group format. They suggest implementing strategies that will help to make abstract concepts (e.g., emotion recognition) concrete. Interventions that are structured and predictable and provide concrete support for acquisition of social language is important as is providing students with a range of examples of key skills. The range and sequence of examples used to demonstrate instances and non instances of new concepts is critical; for example, effectively designed lessons build upon simpler skills that students have already mastered. They also include examples and non examples of concepts that are both maximally and minimally different from one another so that students can accurately understand the scope of the concept being presented (Watkins and Slocum 2004). Delivery of lessons is important too, and children with HFA or AS are more likely to access information if concepts are stated simply, if interventionists do frequent checks for understanding, and if perseverative language is redirected (Barnhill 2004).

To create a comfortable atmosphere to learn skills, Krasny et al. (2003) suggest that interventionists work to build student self-esteem and develop a reinforcing environment. This includes identifying individual student strengths and providing social praise and encouragement consistently. To shape perspective-taking skills, interventionists should include activities that prompt students to focus on the others in the group (e.g., partner activities) and include opportunities outside of group time that allow students to generalize skills.

Social Emotional Learning Efforts

The examples and features of effective intervention, aiming to enhance the social emotional reciprocity of children with HFA or AS, naturally overlap with social-emotional learning efforts (SEL) that are being propelled forth in schools today. SEL innovations provide a framework for schools aiming to prevent student mental health problems and negative outcomes and build social and emotional competencies. SEL includes systematic and cohesive instruction designed to teach social and emotional skills to children and adolescents. The aim of SEL is to promote wellness and to intervene with mental health and behavioral issues that have already emerged (Greenberg et al. 2003). SEL programs typically address broad-based social competencies, such as self-awareness, self-management, social awareness, relationship management, and responsible decision-making (Denham and Weissberg 2004; Greenberg et al. 2003).

For a SEL program to be most effective, it must address students' developmental needs across multiple years; it must include a direct intervention component; and practice of relevant skills must be systematically embedded over time and across settings. For these programs to be acceptable in schools, they must have a documented evidence-base, be reasonable to implement, and be visible to and involve families and community members (Denham and Weissberg 2004; Elias et al. 2003; Greenberg et al. 2003).

SEL programs focus on individual skill development and specific contexts of which students are a part (e.g., home, school, community). These programs involve direct instruction of skills as well as purposeful infusion of skills throughout school days and across settings. SEL programs are not meant to be fragmented, short-term initiatives, rather they are multiyear innovations that are threaded throughout classroom/school practices and are systematically monitored (Greenberg et al. 2003; Denham and Weissberg 2004; Hemmeter et al. 2006). Currently, there are several SEL programs that have been developed and researched. Though few SEL curricula have been researched with extensive replication efforts, those that have been studied have resulted in increased social competence, academic engagement, and school adjustment as well as decreased aggressive behavior among students (Greenberg et al. 2003; Joseph and Strain 2003; Lopes and Salovey 2003; Payton et al. 2008). Results have also suggested improved classroom instruction and management among teachers (Lopes and Salovey 2003; Payton et al. 2008). In fact, in a technical report recently published by Payton et al. (2008), 180 published studies on universal SEL interventions were summarized. Mean effect sizes measuring the impact of program use on conduct problems/emotional distress and social-emotional skill development were 0.23 and 0.60, respectively.

As SEL efforts are becoming more common in schools, it is critical to consider how to strategically, efficiently, and cost-effectively meet the social-emotional learning needs of students with HFA or AS. This can be done by adapting and intensifying a universally applied curriculum in a way that considers features of effective intervention for this population. In the next section, authors will reference specific examples from the *Strong Kids* SEL curriculum to demonstrate this point.

Strong Kids Example

Strong Kids is a curriculum series designed to teach SEL skills, promote resilience, and increase coping strategies for children in preschool through 12th grade. This inexpensive series was designed to be practical. It is easy to implement and brief; each curriculum guide consists of 10–12 developmentally appropriate lessons. *Strong Kids* was developed based on research of children's social-emotional development and effective instructional design. According to Merrell (2010), approximately 13–15 studies have been conducted to date on the *Strong Kids* series. These studies have been conducted in a range of settings (e.g., general education, special education, alternative placements) with a range of age groups (prekindergarten through high school). Several studies have shown that use of the *Strong Kids* programs is associated with significant increases in students' knowledge of important social-emotional

Table 11.1 *Strong Start K-2* lessons

Lesson 1	The feelings exercise group
Lessons 2 and 3	Understanding your feelings
Lesson 4	When you're angry
Lesson 5	When you're happy
Lesson 6	When you're worried
Lesson 7	Understanding other people's feelings
Lesson 8	Being a good friend
Lesson 9	Solving people problems
Lesson 10	Finishing up!

concepts and that the program has strong treatment integrity and social validity. Studies have also shown that use of the programs can positively impact self-reports and teacher ratings of positive peer relationships and social-emotional competencies (Harlacher and Merrell 2010; Gueldner and Merrell 2007).

Strong Kids specifically aims to prevent the development of internalizing problems such as depression, anxiety, and social withdrawal through systematic promotion of emotion resiliency and social-emotional reciprocity skills. *Strong Start Pre-K* and *Strong Start K-2* lessons focus on building awareness of emotions in self and others. Children are encouraged to recognize physical and situational cues to help identify particular emotions. Children are also taught skills for appropriately handling uncomfortable emotions such as worry and anger, for navigating interpersonal conflict, and for being an empathic friend. *Strong Kids* and *Strong Teens* lessons are appropriate for older elementary students and adolescents, respectively, and additionally focus on cognitive-behavioral strategies such as identifying and changing negative thought patterns to build optimism and empathy skills. Relaxation training is incorporated to teach students how to handle stress, and goal-setting strategies are provided to help with increasing activity levels and healthy social behaviors. Table 11.1 provides a list of each of the lessons in *Strong Start K-2*.

Strong Kids lessons were designed according to principles of effective instruction. According to Kame'enui and Simmons (1990), effective instruction is that which emphasizes both the design and delivery of content. *Strong Kids* lessons are semi-scripted and were designed to carefully consider the precise wording implementers may use to communicate new concepts. Limiting implementer wording overall ensures that students acquire an understanding of the intended vocabulary associated with the content of the lesson without confusion (Becker 2001; Watkins and Slocum 2004). Meticulous attention was paid to the range and sequence of examples used to demonstrate instances and non instances of new concepts. Consecutive lessons are increasingly complex and build upon simpler skills that students have already mastered. With each lesson, visual and/or verbal cues are provided to secure student understanding of concepts and to use later as a prompt for skill practice. Additionally, *Strong Start* lessons include parent newsletters that include both visual and verbal cues from the lessons presented. This increases practice opportunities for children in a context other than school and promotes generalization of skills.

While effective instructional design is a critical element in the facilitation of student learning, delivery of *Strong Kids* lessons is an equally important consideration.

Implementers, who are able to efficiently deliver content, are those who maintain a brisk pace, ensure multiple opportunities for students to respond, and provide immediate and corrective feedback when necessary (Becker 2001; Brophy and Good 1986; Kame'enui and Simmons 1990; Watkins and Slocum 2004). *Strong Kids* includes a sequence of modeling, rehearsing, and role-playing of new skills, which has previously been found to enhance student learning (Joseph and Strain 2003), and implementers who share relevant examples from their own lives are more likely to maintain student engagement (Doll et al. 2004). Finally, *Strong Kids* lessons include "tips for transfer" that are specific strategies for integrating the use of skills learned over time and across contexts. This is essential in order for students to build fluency in choosing appropriate social and emotional responses across a range of contexts and situations (Gresham 2002).

Clearly, the content and design of *Strong Kids* lessons includes several of the features of effective intervention outlined in this chapter for children with HFA and AS. *Strong Kids* is intended to be flexible enough in instructional design and implementation to allow implementers to adapt and/or intensify materials to meet the needs of specific children. For example, *Strong Kids* supplies examples and non examples of each of the skills taught; however, implementers are encouraged to adapt these so that they are more relevant to the children with whom they are working. Children with HFA or AS may benefit from exposure to examples and non examples of key skills that directly relate to issues happening in their own lives. In our own clinical work, we have often built examples of cognitive thinking errors around personal experiences of the particular students/clients with whom we are working and we have also practiced "ok" and "not ok" ways for handling anxiety-provoking situations based on client scenarios.

Many of the lessons in *Strong Kids* include opportunities for adults and peers to model social-emotional skills and simple social scripts. For students with HFA or AS, it is critical that each new behavior is explicitly modeled. This enables students to "see" the skill being practiced and provides a more concrete way for students to access difficult cognitive skills. For example, in *Strong Start*, children learn the *ABC's of Happy Thinking*. This includes helping children to identify when they have (A) a problem that gives them (B) bad feelings and to (C) comfort themselves in a way that makes them feel better. Comforting oneself might include happy self-talk. The first author of this chapter consulted with a teacher who used a relevant example from a student's life to teach her this strategy. This student with AS had a particularly difficult time when she did not win games that she was playing with others. Her teacher first helped her to identify the problem, namely losing, which resulted in a "bad" feeling, frustration. This student learned to engage in self-talk to help herself feel better. At the end of the game she learned to say, "That's ok, maybe next time I will win. That will be great!"

In addition to simple social scripts, more elaborate Social Stories, a specific type of story-based intervention, can also increase understanding for students with AS or HFA. Social Stories can be built on strategies presented in *Strong Kids*. A story was written to incorporate the *ABC's of Happy Thinking* and scripts for losing gracefully for the student mentioned above. This Social Story was very useful to review prior to every attempt at an interactive game. A Power Card could also have been useful in this instance. Power Cards are similar to social stories, in that they provide written and/or visual cues regarding appropriate behavior (see Linn and Myles 2004). Power Cards typically are written to incorporate favorite or preferred characters, which engage in the behavior that is expected of the student. In this case, a Power Card featuring Sesame Street's Elmo, as he practiced successful interactions during game playing, would have been helpful.

Video modeling can also be a powerful method for enhancing students' use of skills presented in *Strong Kids*. This is a particularly helpful strategy for children with HFA or AS and entails video recording individuals as they utilize the newly taught social-emotional skill, such as perspective taking (Charlop-Christy and Daneshvar 2003). Children then watch the video and are able to see themselves successfully using the skill and can learn to point out key features of the skill. Video recording the student who was learning to lose gracefully at board games would likely have been a potent teaching method.

Implementation of *Strong Kids* with children with AS or HFA, who may have interfering behaviors, could also include explicit behavior management programming. Having clear behavioral expectations and even visual cues to remind children of expectations for *Strong Kids* time may be helpful. Sometimes, systematic reinforcement procedures are also useful. This may include giving students points or stickers when they appropriately participate and meet behavioral expectations. One strategy that the first author has used with small groups of younger children is to incorporate "Henry Bear" as a behavior management tool. Henry is a character who is integrated into the *Strong Start Pre-K* and *Strong Start K-2* curriculum. Henry helps to communicate concepts and serves as a puppet/mascot for the lessons. Implementers are encouraged to actually use a stuffed animal to represent Henry. Students generally show great enthusiasm toward Henry and learn to associate *Strong Start* skills with Henry. During lesson implementation, the first author has allowed children, who are appropriately managing themselves and/or positively contributing to the lesson, to hold Henry. After a few minutes with Henry, children are then asked to look around at their group and decide who else is demonstrating appropriate behaviors and should have a chance to hold Henry. This strategy not only acknowledges students who are displaying appropriate behavior but also encourages students to study the behavior of others.

As was noted earlier in the chapter, giving children opportunities to practice skills learned in a range of situations and settings with a variety of individuals is critical. These opportunities are naturally built into the *Strong Kids* curriculum, but increased opportunities for practice is often helpful for children with AS or HFA. For example, each *Strong Start Pre-K* and *Strong Start K-2* lesson includes lists of children's literature relevant to the lesson theme. Implementers are encouraged to read one book per lesson and focus discussion of the book on the lesson's theme. The goal is to help children practice identifying the emotions of characters and discussing how characters might engage in particular *Strong Start* strategies to solve problems at hand. One teacher, with whom the first author consulted, taught *Strong Start* to a small group of K-2 students with AS and HFA. While she only taught one lesson per week, each day she worked to systematically incorporate learning activities that reinforced that lesson's content. She read books from the literature list and facilitated discussion every day. Additionally, this teacher incorporated art activities and games daily to ensure that students were getting exposure to content through a variety of activities.

Ensuring that adults, other than those implementing the curriculum, are involved in skill practice is helpful. Parents, teachers, special subject teachers (e.g., art, music, physical education), speech-language pathologists, school psychologists, guidance counselors, recess monitors, etc. can all take part in prompting students to use skills learned. It is particularly useful if these adults have access to the language and visual cues presented in the curriculum. If all staff cue students to use the *Stop, Count, Breathe in, Breathe out* strategy when they are angry, for example, the likelihood that students will internalize and independently use the strategy increases.

Case Examples

Below are specific examples of cases of individuals with whom authors have worked. Both individuals were diagnosed with AS and struggled with emotion recognition, appropriate social interaction, and symptoms of anxiety. These cases were chosen on the basis of their behavioral similarities, different developmental levels, and exposure to the *Strong Kids* curriculum.

Ali At the time of intervention, Ali was a kindergarten student. She was a very bright Caucasian girl and was beginning to read and understand basic math. Ali's fine motor skills were not fully developed, and writing was very frustrating for her. Additionally, Ali performed best when classroom routines were structured and behavioral expectations were made explicit. Children were naturally drawn to Ali, and at times, she was able to appropriately engage in pretend play with others. During structured, competitive games or when presented with frustrating academic tasks or changes in routine, Ali would often shout out expletives. This was clearly an unacceptable behavior that needed immediate intervention. In addition to the implementation of antecedent strategies (e.g., breaking tasks into manageable chunks) and reinforcement (e.g., visual token board) and extinction procedures, Ali's resource teacher implemented *Strong Start*. Because of the intensity and frequency of Ali's behavior, Ali's teacher intensified aspects of the curriculum. For example, she used a large pocket chart to display pictures of basic emotions offered in the curriculum. She and Ali also accessed the Internet and found several more pictures of more complex emotions (e.g., frustrated, embarrassed). Each picture was labeled. Ali's teacher continually referred Ali to these pictures to help her identify emotions during calm and emotionally charged situations. As Ali progressed through *Strong Start*, she and her teacher developed more visual cues for the pocket chart that were examples of coping strategies and social problem-solving strategies. When Ali experienced strong, uncomfortable emotions, she learned to go to the chart and fill in sentence starter that was placed there. It read, "I feel____________. I will use ____________strategy to help myself feel better." Consistent prompting to use the chart, paired with reinforcement for using the chart was helpful. Ali also benefited from the Social Stories and social scripts that emphasized *Strong Start* strategies (noted above).

Stuart Stuart was in the eighth grade when he was first exposed to the *Strong Kids, Grades 6–8* curriculum. Stuart attended a school for performing arts and was a budding actor. He engaged in individual therapy with the first author. Stuart was highly verbal and had a great sense of humor. At school, teachers reported that Stuart often appeared disorganized, lost assignments, and forget due dates. Teachers also expressed concern about Stuart's humor; he often told jokes inappropriate to the immediate context or individuals surrounding him. Stuart also engaged in several behaviors indicative of social anxiety. He was candid about being afraid to approach kids and often formed rigid, negative perceptions of others and engaged in socially inappropriate behaviors when faced with social interaction opportunities. At times, Stuart reported that he would run in the opposite direction of peers with whom he did not want to have contact. When he did have contact with peers or teachers and felt embarrassed about the comments he made, he would usually state, "Where is the window? I want to jump" or "My suicide is your option." Clearly, these were alarming behaviors grounded in social skill deficits and anxiety.

In addition to working with the school to develop crisis intervention plans and to develop clear expectations for Stuart regarding his use of "self-harming" language, the therapist presented Stuart with content from *Strong Kids* lessons. First, Stuart worked on identifying uncomfortable feelings of varying intensity using an "emotion thermometer" visual. Then, Stuart and the first author identified examples and non examples of appropriately handling uncomfortable emotions that were based on scenarios that were presented by Stuart, his teachers, and his parents. Often, Stuart and the first author would role-play these scenarios multiple times so that Stuart could practice new socially adaptive coping strategies. Finally, Stuart was also provided with visual cues to help him think about what type of "thinking error" he might engage in during certain social scenarios. He was taught to practice how to evaluate the evidence that suggested his thinking error might not be true. These strategies were communicated to parents and school staff, so that practice of skills could also happen in the contexts where they were most relevant. Over time, Stuart began to demonstrate progress in evaluating his social behavior.

Conclusion

The purpose of this chapter was to outline the specific deficits in social-emotional reciprocity that are often seen in populations with HFA or AS. Authors additionally identified emerging research outlining features of effective intervention that address these deficits and gave case examples of *Strong Kids*, a SEL program that incorporates many of these intervention features. The research and clinical work supporting *Strong Kids* is promising; however, clearly, more research needs to be conducted to systematically evaluate its effectiveness with children with AS and HFA.

Future research might also address how schools can use SEL programming within an RTI model to meet the needs of children with AS and HFA. Research evaluating the effectiveness of intensifying/adapting a universally applied curriculum would be useful. This approach could potentially boost generalization of social-emotional skills, especially if all school staff and children are exposed to similar language and concepts, with increased practice opportunities and targeted or individualized support provided to children with AS and HFA. Research addressing this service delivery model as well as behavioral assessment techniques that will help to identify students in need of targeted support and systematically monitor the progress of these students over time is needed.

Over the years, researchers and professionals have learned a great deal about addressing the unique needs of children with HFA and AS. Adaptive skill in social-emotional reciprocity is critical and will ultimately generate more positive outcomes for this population.

References

American Psychiatric Association. (2000). *Diagnostic and statistical manual of mental disorders* (4th ed., text rev.). Washington: Author.

American Psychiatric Association (2011). Retrieved from http://www.dsm5.org/Proposed-Revisions/Pages/proposedrevision.aspx?rid=97.

Baer, D. M., Wolf, M. M., Risley, T. R. (1987). Some still current dimensions of applied behavior analysis. *Journal of Applied Behavior Analysis, 20*, 313–327.

Barnhill, G. P. (2004). Asperger syndrome: A guide for secondary school principals. *Principal Leadership Magazine*, *5*(3)

Baron-Cohen, S. (2001). Theory of mind in normal development and autism. *Prisme, 34*, 174–183.

Bauminger, N. (2002). The facilitation of social-emotional understanding and social interaction in high-functioning children with autism: Intervention outcomes. *Journal of autism and developmental disorders*, *32*(4), 283–98. Retrieved from http://www.ncbi.nlm.nih.gov/pubmed/12199133.

Becker, W. C. (2001). Teaching reading and language to the disadvantaged: What we have learned from research. *Journal of Direct Instruction, 1*(1), 31–52.

Brophy, J., & Good, T. (1986). Teacher behavior and student achievement. In M. C. Wittrock (Ed.), *Handbook of Research on Teaching*, (3rd ed., pp. 328–375). New York: MacMillan.

Charlop-Christy, M. H., & Daneshvar, S. (2003). Using video modeling to teach perspective taking to children with autism. *Journal of Positive Behavior Interventions*, *5*(1), 12–21.

Coie, J. D., Miller-Jackson, S., Bagwell, C. (2000). Prevention science. In A. J. Sameroff, M. Lewis, & S. M. Miller (Eds.), *Handbook of developmental psychopathology* (pp. 93–108). New York: Kluwer Academic/Plenum Publishers.

Cowan, E. (1994). The enhancement of psychological wellness: Challenges and opportunities. *American journal of community psychology, 22*(2), 149–179, doi: 10.1007/BF02506861.

Crooke, P. J., Hendrix, R. E., Rachman, J. Y. (2008) Brief report: Measuring the effectiveness of teaching social thinking to children with Asperger syndrome (AS) and high functioning autism (HFA). *Journal of autism and developmental disorders*, *38*(3), 581–91. doi: 1007/s10803-007-0466-1.

Denham, S. A., & Weissberg, R. P. (2004). Social-emotional learning in early childhood: What we know and where to go from here. In E. Chesebrough, P. King, T. P. Gullota, & M. Bloom (Eds.), *A blueprint for the promotion of prosocial behavior in early childhood* (pp. 13–50). New York: Kluwer Academic/Plenum Publishers.

Doll, B., Zucker, S., Brehm, K. (2004). *Resilient classrooms: Creating healthy environments for learning*. New York: Guilford Press.

Downs, A., & Smith, T. (2004). Emotional understanding, cooperation, and social behavior in high-functioning children with autism. *Journal of autism and developmental disorders, 34*(6), 625–35. Retrieved from http://www.ncbi.nlm.nih.gov/pubmed/15679183.

Elias, M. J., Zins, J. E., Graczyk, P. A., Weissberg, R. P. (2003). Implementation, sustainability, and scaling up of social-emotional and academic innovations in public schools. *School Psychology Review, 32*(3), 303–319.

Fairbanks, S., Sugai, G., Guardino, D., Lathrop, M. (2007). Response to intervention: Examining classroom behavior support in second grade. *Exceptional Children, 73*(3), 288–310.

Greenberg, M. T., Weissberg, R. P., Utne O'Brien, M. T., Zins, J. E., Fredericks, L., Resnik, H., et al. (2003). Enhancing school-based prevention and youth development through coordinated social, emotional, and academic learning. *American Psychologist, 58*, 466–474.

Gresham, F. M. (2002). Teaching social skills to high-risk children and youth: Preventive and remedial strategies. In M. R. Shinn, H. M. Walker, & G. Stoner (Eds.), *Interventions for academic and behavior problems II: Preventive and remedial approaches* (pp. 403–432). Bethesda: National Association of School Psychologists.

Gresham, F. (2005). Response to intervention: An alternative means of identifying students as emotionally disturbed. *Education and treatment of children, 28*(4), 328–344.

Grossman, J. B., Klin, A., Carter, A. S., Volkmar, F. R. (2000). Verbal bias in recognition of facial emotions in children with asperger syndrome. *Journal of child psychology and psychiatry, 41*(3), 369–379.

Gueldner, B. A., & Merrell, K. W. (2007). Interventions for students with internalizing behavioral deficits. In M. A. Bray & T. J. Kehle (Eds.), *The Oxford handbook of school psychology*. New York: Oxford University Press.

Harlacher, J., & Merrell, K. W. (2010). Social emotional learning as a universal level of support: Evaluating the follow up effect of Strong Kids on social and emotional outcomes. *Journal of Applied School Psychology, 26*(3), 212–229.

Hemmeter, M., Ostrosky, M., Fox, L. (2006). Social and emotional foundations for early learning: A conceptual model for intervention. *School Psychology Review*, 35 (4), 583–601.

Horner, R. H., Sugai, G., Todd, A. W., Lewis-Palmer, T. (2005). School-wide positive behavior support: An alternative approach to discipline in schools. In L. Bambara, & L. Kern (Eds.), *Individualized supports for students with problem behavior: Designing positive behavior plans*, (pp. 359–390), New York: Guilford Press.

Joseph, G. E., & Strain, P. S. (2003). Comprehensive evidence-based social-emotional curricula for young children: An analysis of efficacious adoption potential. *Topics in early childhood special education, 23*(2), 65–76.

Kame'enui, E. J., & Simmons, D. C. (1990). Designing instructional strategies: The prevention of academic learning problems. Upper Saddle River: Merrill.

Krasny, L, Williams, B. J, Provencal, S., Ozonoff, S. (2003). Social skills interventions for the autism spectrum: Essential ingredients and a model curriculum. *Child and Adolescent Psychiatric Clinics of North America, 12*, 107–122.

Linn, A., & Myles, B. S. (2004). Asperger syndrome and six strategies for success. *Beyond Behavior, 14*(1), p. 7. (Council for Children with Behavioral Disorders. Council for Exceptional Children, 1110 North Glebe Road, Arlington, VA 22201-5704. Tel: 612-276-0140; Fax: 612–276-0142; Web site: http://www.ccbd.net/beyondbehavior/index.cfm? categoryID=D646D293-C09 F-1. Retrieved April 15, 2011, from http://eric.ed.gov/ ERICWebPortal/recordDetail?accno=EJ854586.)

Merrell, K. W. (2010). Linking prevention science and social-emotional learning: The oregon resiliency project. *Psychology in the schools, 47*(1), 55–70, doi: 10.1002/pits 20451.

Merrell, K. W., & Buchanan, R. (2006). Intervention selection in school-based practice: Using public health models to enhance systems capacity in schools. *School psychology review, 35*(2), 167–180.

Merrell, K. W., Carrizales, D. C., Feuerborn, L., Gueldner, B. A., Tran, O. K. (2007). *Strong Kids-E: A social and emotional learning curriculum for students in grades* (pp.9–12). Baltimore: Paul H. Brookes.

Merrell, K. W., Carrizales, D. C., Feuerborn, L., Gueldner, B. A., Tran, O. K. (2007a). *Strong Kids-M: A social and emotional learning curriculum for students in grades (pp.*3–5). Baltimore: Paul H. Brookes.

Merrell, K. W., Carrizales, D. C., Feuerborn, L., Gueldner, B. A., Tran, O. K. (2007b). *Strong Teens: A social and emotional learning curriculum for students in grades* (pp. 6–8). Baltimore: Paul H. Brookes.

Merrell, K. W., Parisi, D. M., Whitcomb, S. G. (2007). *Strong Start: A social and emotional learning curriculum for students in grades K-2.* Baltimore: Paul H. Brookes.

Merrell, K. W., Whitcomb, S. A., Parisi, D. M. (2009). *Strong Start Pre-K: A social and emotional learning curriculum for student in pre-k.* Baltimore: Paul H. Brookes.

Nelson, J. R., Hurley, K. D., Epstein, M. H. Stage, S., Buckley, J. (2009). The child outcomes of a behavior model. *Exceptional children, 76*(1), 7–30.

Payton, J., Weissberg, R. P., Durlak, J. A., Dymnicki, A. B., Taylor, R. D., Schellinger, K. B., Pachan, M. (2008). *The positive impact of social and emotional learning for kindergarten through eighth-grade students: Findings from three scientific reviews.* Chicago: Collaborative for Academic, Social, and Emotional Learning.

Rao, P. A, Beidel, D. C., Murray, M. J. (2008). Social skills interventions for children with Asperger's Syndrome or High-Functioning Autism: A review and recommendations. *Journal of autism and developmental disorders, 38*(2), 353–361. doi: 1007/s10803-007-0402–4.

Sansosti, F. J., & Powell-Smith, K. (2008). Using computer-presented social stories and video models to increase the social communication skills of children with high-functioning autism spectrum disorders. *Journal of Positive Behavior Interventions, 10*(3), 162–178. doi: 10.1177/1098300708316259.

Solomon, M., Miller, M., Taylor, S. L., Hinshaw, S. P., Carter, C. S. (2011). Autism symptoms and internalizing psychopathology in girls and boys with Autism Spectrum Disorders. *Journal of autism and developmental disorders.* doi: 10.1007/s10803-011-1215-z.

Stichter, J. P., Herzog, M. J., Visovsky, K., Schmidt, C., Randolph, J., Schultz, T., et al. (2010). Social competence intervention for youth with Asperger Syndrome and High-functioning Autism: An initial investigation. *Journal of autism and developmental disorders.* doi:1007/s10803-010-0959-1.

Sze, K. M., & Wood, J. J. (2007). Cognitive behavioral treatment of comorbid anxiety disorders and social difficulties in children with high-functioning autism: A case report. *Journal of Contemporary Psychotherapy, 37*(3), 133–143. doi: 10.1007/s10879-007-9048-y.

Wallace, G. L., Case, L. K., Harms, M. B., Silvers, J. A, Kenworthy, L., Martin, A. (2011). Diminished sensitivity to sad facial expressions in high functioning autism spectrum disorders is associated with symptomatology and adaptive functioning. *Journal of autism and developmental disorders.* doi:1007/s10803-010-1170-0.

Watkins, C. L., Slocum, T. A. (2004). The components of direct instruction. *Journal of Direct Instruction, 3* (2), 75–110.

Wilczynski, S. M. (2009). *The national autism center's national standards project: Findings and conclusions.* Randolph: National Autism Center.

Williams White, S., Keonig, K., Scahill, L. (2007). Social skills development in children with autism spectrum disorders: a review of the intervention research. *Journal of autism and developmental disorders, 37*(10), 1858–1868. doi: 10.1007/s10803-006-0320-x.

Winner, M. G., Crooke, P., Madrigal, S. (2011). Social Communication Learning Styles as a Guide to Treatment and Prognosis: The Social Thinking-Social Communication Profile™ * A Practice-Informed Theory.

Chapter 12
Repetitive Behaviors and Sensory Features: Evidence-Based Intervention Strategies

Brian A. Boyd and Linn Wakeford

There is a history of clinical and first-person accounts reflecting the impact of repetitive behaviors and sensory features on the daily lives and occupations of individuals with autism. In Kanner's (1943) original account, he remarks on the odd, repetitive patterns of behavior displayed by case number one, Donald T., the first known individual to be diagnosed with autism, stating, "Most of his actions were repetitions carried out in exactly the same way in which they had been performed originally. If he spun a block, he most always started with the same face uppermost. When he threaded buttons he arranged them in a certain sequence that had no pattern to it but happened to be the order used by the father when he first had shown them to Donald" (p. 219). In her autobiography of childhood autism, Grandin (1996) recollects difficulties modulating responses to sensory stimuli across visual, auditory, and tactile modalities that subsequently interfered with overall social and adaptive development. She describes several examples of extreme sensory responsiveness: "The pain that racked my head when the fog horn sounded was excruciating. Even with my hands over my ears the hurtful sound assaulted them to the point that I'd throw myself down on the deck and scream" (p. 22). She adds paradoxically, "Intensely preoccupied with the movement of the spinning coin or lid, I saw nothing or heard nothing. People around me were transparent. And no sound intruded on my fixation. It was as if I were deaf. Even a sudden loud noise didn't startle me from my world" (p. 23). Although repetitive behaviors and sensory features are quite salient symptoms of autism, there has been debate about whether or not they represent distinct phenomena, and thus, whether differential treatment approaches should be used.

B. A. Boyd (✉)
Division of Occupational Science and Occupational Therapy,
University of North Carolina at Chapel Hill, Bondurant Hall, CB#7122,
Chapel Hill, NC 27599-7205, USA
e-mail: brian_boyd@med.unc.edu

L. Wakeford
Division of Occupational Science and Occupational Therapy,
University of North Carolina at Chapel Hill, Bondurant Hall Suite 2050,
CB#7122, Chapel Hill, NC 27599-7122, USA

S. Goldstein, J. A. Naglieri (eds.), *Interventions for Autism Spectrum Disorders*,

DOI 10.1007/978-1-4614-5301-7_12,

Phenomenology of Repetitive Behaviors

Restricted, repetitive behaviors in autism refer to an assemblage of behaviors defined by their topographical similarity across contexts, inappropriateness, behavioral rigidity, and repetition. In the *Diagnostic and Statistical Manual of Mental Disorders–Fourth Edition* (American Psychiatric Association 2000), criteria for repetitive behavior can be met by a person exhibiting at least one of the following: "(a) encompassing preoccupation with one or more stereotyped and restricted patterns of interest that is abnormal either in intensity or focus; (b) apparently inflexible adherence to specific, nonfunctional routines or rituals; (c) stereotyped and repetitive motor mannerisms (e.g., hand or finger flapping or complex whole-body movements); or (d) persistent preoccupation with parts of objects." This symptom domain has been conceptually and empirically grouped into at least two categories—"lower order" and "higher order" behaviors (Szatmari et al. 2006; Turner 1999). Lower order motor actions [i.e., stereotyped movements, repetitive manipulation of objects, and repetitive forms of self-injurious behaviors (SIBs)] are characterized by repetition of movement, and "higher order" behaviors (i.e., compulsions, rituals and routines, insistence on sameness, and circumscribed interests) are characterized by a rigid adherence to some rule or mental set (e.g., needing to have things "just so") (Turner 1999). What becomes clear on examination of these diagnostic criteria and individual behaviors is that they are very broad, ranging from repetitive movements of the body to more cognitively mediated symptoms such as intense interests or hobbies. Although no single type of repetitive behavior may be specific to autism, previous studies have found that repetitive behaviors in autism are characterized by a pattern of elevated occurrence and co-occurrence of these behaviors (Bodfish 2010; Bodfish et al. 2000).

Phenomenology of Sensory Features

Previous research has demonstrated that children with autism demonstrate unusual responses to sensory stimuli to a greater degree than their peers with other types of developmental disabilities or typical development (Baranek et al. 2006; Rogers et al. 2003; Watling et al. 2001). Although these unusual behaviors have been categorized in different ways, one current empirically supported conceptualization focuses on three sensory features in autism: hyporesponsiveness, hyperresponsiveness, and sensory seeking (Ashburner et al. 2008; Ben-Sasson et al. 2009; Boyd et al. 2010; Liss et al. 2006). Hyporesponsiveness is characterized by an absence of the expected response to a stimulus (e.g., failing to orient to a novel sound in the environment), a delayed response, or a higher response threshold (e.g., only orienting to a novel sound when it becomes more intense). Hyperresponsiveness is characterized by an exaggerated behavioral reaction, aversive response, or effort to avoid a sensory stimulus. Sensory seeking behaviors are actions that perpetuate or intensify a sensory experience, such as staring intensely at flickering lights or sniffing objects.

These patterns are not mutually exclusive and may co-occur in individual children across sensory modalities (Baranek et al. 2006; Liss et al. 2006).

Relationship Between Sensory Features and Repetitive Behaviors

Repetitive behaviors comprise one faction of the triad of clinical symptoms that characterize autism spectrum disorder (ASD), often presenting concurrently with social and communication symptoms. Higher order behaviors, specifically the presence of restricted or narrow interests, odd object attachments or unusual object preoccupations (e.g., fascination with ceiling fans), are thought to be more unique to autism in comparison to lower order types of repetitive behaviors (e.g., self-injury; Lam et al. 2008). In contrast to repetitive behaviors, sensory features in autism are considered secondary or associated symptoms of the disorder. Aberrant sensory features are presumed to be less specific and universal in autism than the triad of core features, although there is some evidence that the hyporesponsive sensory feature is more associated with autism (Baranek et al. 2006).

In three prior studies, researchers reported associations between sensory features and repetitive behaviors in autism (Boyd et al. 2009, 2010; Gabriel et al. 2008). Gabriel et al. (2008) used parent report measures to examine the association between these atypical behaviors in a sample of 70 children and adolescents with ASDs. The researchers found consistently high levels of sensory features and repetitive behaviors in a subgroup of the sample. Similarly, Boyd et al. (2009, 2010) found the same relationship in a group of school-aged children (6–17 years of age) with higher functioning autism. These studies demonstrated that sensory symptoms and repetitive behaviors often co-occurred in autism. However, both studies only used parent report measures of sensory and repetitive behaviors. Observational methods are needed to validate these clinical phenomena and their interrelationships. In a latter study, Boyd et al. (2010) used a combination of parent report and direct behavioral observation measures to examine the relationship between children's sensory features and repetitive behaviors ($N = 109$). The researchers found that the *hyperresponsiveness* sensory feature was most associated with the expression of repetitive behavior in autism. Examining the relationships between the expression of specific types of sensory symptoms and repetitive behaviors provides a more comprehensive understanding of the behavioral phenotype in autism, and better informs clinical practice and the selection of therapeutic interventions.

Role of Context in the Expression of Repetitive Behaviors and Sensory Features

Based on research, it appears well established that brain abnormalities (Langen et al. 2010; Tommerdahl et al. 2008) as well as genetic factors (Hus et al. 2006; Lam et al. 2008; Tadevosyan-Leyfer et al. 2003) are involved in the expression of repetitive behaviors and sensory features in autism. However, there is also research that points to the importance of environmental (Ashburner et al. 2008) and family context (Bagby et al. 2012; Smith et al. 2008) in the expression of these behaviors in individuals with autism. For example, Ashburner et al. (2008) found that for children with autism, difficulties with sensory processing (e.g., inability to filter auditory information) were a more significant predictor of school academic achievement than IQ scores. Smith et al. (2008) found that the parents of individuals with autism can impact their expression of repetitive behaviors into the adolescent and adult years, with mother–child dyads having a higher relationship quality, more warmth, and praise associated with reductions in these symptoms over time. Thus, assessment of and interventions for repetitive behaviors and sensory features in autism must take into account the transactional effects between the child's environment, including individuals in that environment, and any manifestation of these behaviors.

Ecological, Transactional, and Dynamic Systems Theories Though modeled somewhat differently, ecological (Bronfenbrenner 1992), transactional (Law et al. 1996), and dynamic systems (Smith and Thelen 2003) theories all recognize an ongoing interaction among the child and its environment, and highlight the importance of context as an influence on performance. Therefore, these theories may provide a working model to guide assessment and intervention practices. Each of these theories allows for a holistic view of situations made difficult due to engagement in repetitive behaviors or sensory processing differences, including the effect on parents, siblings and others, and may lead to interventions that seek to change aspects of the environment (including social contexts), aspects of the task, and/or behaviors of the child in order to create an optimal fit, and ultimately, successful engagement. In addition, use of these broader perspectives on participation allows the interventionist to address specific needs of parents and other caregivers using modification, behavioral, and/or education interventions.

Interventions for Repetitive Behaviors

There are different topographies and types of repetitive behaviors expressed in autism, and they often require differential intervention approaches. The field of applied behaviors analysis has informed most of the evidence base on interventions for repetitive behaviors (Boyd et al. 2012). Presently, there is more evidence to support the use of practices to treat lower order behaviors (i.e., self-injury and stereotypy) but less evidence to guide the selection of intervention practices for higher order behaviors (e.g., insistence on sameness). Therefore, the evidence presented for higher order behaviors can be thought of as *promising* practices. Any selection of intervention practices for repetitive behaviors should still be guided by thorough assessment of these behaviors and individualized to the child and its family. Finally, the selection of evidence-based practices should be guided by a combination of the research base and practitioners' use of their professional judgment about context and values (their own and those of the family) in the application of such practices (cf. Buysse and Wesley 2006).

Assessment of Repetitive Behaviors

Methodologies used in the identification and measurement of repetitive behavior and its severity primarily fall into three categories: observational measures, standardized assessments, and informant report. These approaches can involve identification of the repetitive behavior and its frequency, duration, and intensity. Direct behavioral observation often involves coding the child's behavior in real time, and is used quite often in the identification of problem behaviors. One of the issues with direct observation is that it can be hard to capture behavior that is context-bound, meaning that the child may only display the behavior in specific contexts (e.g., home and not school) and under certain environmental circumstances (e.g., only when watching a favorite TV show). Even with stereotypical motor movements, Schultz and Berkson (1995) found direct observation to be only 33 % consistent with teacher report. By using video, more continuous data can be collected and behaviors can be reexamined; however, the limitation is that coding of videos is time consuming and often not practical for clinicians. Standardized assessments often use direct observation or video to rate the child's response to a specific situation or task (e.g., *Autism Diagnostic Observation Schedule*; Lord et al. 2000), but these measures tend to focus on determining the sheer presence of the repetitive behavior rather than the specific type and severity. Rating scales such as the *Repetitive Behaviors Scale—Revised* (Bodfish et al. 1999) and *Pervasive Developmental Disorder Child Yale-Brown Obsessive Compulsive Scale* (Scahill et al. 2006) provide greater specificity with regard to the topography and severity of RRB; however, they often require subjective rating from an informant. It is recommended that a multimethod (e.g., observational and rating scales) and multiinformant (e.g., clinician and parent) approach be used to assess repetitive behaviors in autism and obtain a better understanding of the role of environmental context in the expression of these behaviors.

Theoretical and Conceptual Basis for Repetitive Behavior Interventions

There are at least three distinct theoretical or conceptual models that can inform or have already informed intervention practices for repetitive behaviors in autism. As mentioned previously, the field of applied behavior analysis (ABA) has informed the bulk of the intervention literature for repetitive behaviors. However, research on environmental deprivation and cognitive models of repetitive behavior also can inform intervention selection. These theoretical and conceptual models are briefly described.

Behaviorism One of the most prominent theoretical or conceptual basis for behavioral intervention research is the science of behavior (Skinner 1975), specifically, ABA (Baer et al. 1968). One of the central tenets of ABA that has rapidly evolved over the last 30 years is functional analysis (Iwata et al. 1982, 1994). The basis of functional analysis is to conduct descriptive and preferably experimental assessments of the individual's problem behavior to identify the reason(s) why (i.e., the function or maintaining consequence) the individual engages in the behavior. Prototypically, the function of challenging behavior can be subdivided into two overarching categories, either the individual engages in the behavior for social purposes (i.e., to obtain attention or tangible objects, or to escape environmental demands) or nonsocial purposes (e.g., to obtain or escape internal sensory consequences). These categories have heavily informed intervention research because developed treatments often involve the concept of functional equivalence (Carr and Durand 1985), or teaching the individual a more appropriate response to obtain the same desired outcome provided by engaging in the problem behavior.

Environmental Deprivation Another area of behavioral and developmental psychology that has informed repetitive behavior intervention research is the early work on environmental deprivation. This area of research showed that animals (Lewis et al. 2007; Davenport et al. 1966; Mason and Berkson 1975) and humans (Berkson and Tupa 2000) engage in more stereotypic behavior in the absence of a stimulating environment. Therefore, incorporating into children's environment more opportunities for social engagement or appropriate engagement with developmentally appropriate toys and objects should reduce their need to engage in repetitive or other maladaptive behavior.

Cognitive Models One of the more well-known cognitive models of repetitive behavior in autism is the executive dysfunction account (Bodfish 2010). This model conceptualizes symptoms of restricted and repetitive behaviors to reflect the impaired ability to adapt flexibly to changing environmental contingencies (Turner 1999). Executive functions refer to a range of abilities, including behavioral inhibition, planning, working memory, and mental flexibility. These abilities require the integration of a variety of basic abilities (e.g., language and working memory) to achieve higher order goal attainment and appropriate emotional responses (Zelazo et al. 1997). Numerous studies have documented impaired executive function abilities in ASDs (Ozonoff et al. 1991; Ozonoff and Jensen 1999), and some have found that executive function deficits correlate with clinical ratings of repetitive behavior severity (Lopez et al. 2005). However, not all studies of executive functioning indicate deficits in autism (e.g., Bogte et al. 2008). These seemingly contradictory results may reflect the fact that executive function is not a unitary construct, and neither are repetitive behaviors. Further, there are relatively fewer treatments that have targeted such underlying cognitive processes in autism to determine whether this results in changes in observable behaviors (see Stichter et al. 2010, for an example).

Treatment of Lower Order Repetitive Behaviors

The category of lower order repetitive behaviors is comprised of two types of behaviors—stereotypy and self-injury. The majority of the intervention research has focused on the treatment of behaviors.

Stereotypies and Self-injury Stereotypic behavior is prototypically defined as repetitious behavior that serves no clear extrinsic purpose or goal. SIB or self-harming behavior refers to a complex set of behaviors that can vary by characteristics such as function, site of bodily injury, underlying mechanism, and whether or not it is repetitive in nature (Schroeder et al. 2001; Symons and Thompson 1997). One of the more common intervention strategies that has been used to treat stereotypies and/or SIB in autism and other developmental disabilities includes physically or verbally blocking (e.g., saying, "no") the individual from engaging in the behavior. This treatment approach is referred to as *response interruption and redirection or response blocking* (Ahearn et al. 2007; Koegel et al. 1974; Liu-Gitz and Banda 2010). The cautionary note here is that alternative appropriate behaviors often need to be taught in combination with the use of this behavior modification strategy to prevent other problematic behaviors from surfacing.

Perhaps surprisingly, one of the more replicated findings in the intervention literature is the effect of *physical exercise* on the stereotypic behavior of individuals with autism (see Lang et al. 2010). The intervention often involves the individual engaging in a vigorous exercise routine (e.g., jogging, roller skating) prior to participating in a subsequent task or activity that has been associated with stereotyped behavior (Kern et al. 1984). It is not fully understood why engaging in physical exercise leads to subsequent, even if fleeting, reductions in repetitive behaviors. Lang et al. (2010) proposed two reasons—first, subsequent reductions in repetitive behavior may be an artifact of fatigue; and secondly, that engaging in physical exercise may provide the individual access to the same intrinsic reinforcer as engaging in stereotypic behavior. As Lang et al. point out, it is likely that the first hypothesis can be ruled out because excessive fatigue is counterintuitive to the concurrent increases in appropriate behaviors that have been found following vigorous exercise routines (Kern et al. 1982; Powers et al. 1992). Another possible explanation for the effects of physical exercise on stereotypy is arousal theory. It has long been postulated that individuals with developmental disabilities, including autism, engage in stereotypic behavior to attenuate or intensify their arousal levels, depending upon the environmental circumstances (Turner 1999). Perhaps engaging in physical exercise decreases the need to engage in stereotypy or SIB to modulate one's level of arousal. Still, as Rogers and Ozonoff (2005) point out, the evidence is mixed on the role arousal plays in the sensory or repetitive behaviors of individuals with ASD.

Finally, *environmental enrichment* has been used to decrease stereotypic behavior. This class of interventions involves providing the individual free access to appropriate, competing sources of reinforcement, such as preferred objects (Rapp and Vollmer 2005). In comparison to environmental enrichment, *skill enrichment* entails teaching the individual more adaptive skills (e.g., social initiation skills); with the thought being that an increase in appropriate skills will offset the need to engage in behaviors that do not serve a clear purpose or goal. Through a series of single-case design studies, Loftin et al. (2005, 2008) demonstrated that the use of peer-mediated intervention strategies, direct social skill instruction for the child with ASD, the use of self-monitoring strategies, or some combination thereof, led to increases in children's social interactions with peers and concomitant decreases in stereotypic behavior (Lee et al. 2007; Loftin 2005; Loftin et al. 2008).

Treatment of Higher Order Behaviors

Higher order behaviors include the repetitive behaviors of obsessions and compulsions, circumscribed interests, and the child's insistence on sameness. As with lower order repetitive behaviors, an ABA perspective has informed much of the intervention research on higher order repetitive behaviors. One exception to this is the intervention research on obsessive and compulsive behavior in individuals with autism, which can trace some of its roots to cognitive-behavioral therapy (CBT).

Obsessions and Compulsions A specific form of CBT termed "exposure and response prevention" (ERP) is an evidence-based treatment for both children and adults with Obsessive-Compulsive Disorder (Abramowitz et al. 2003; Huppert and Franklin 2005). The *exposure* component of ERP typically has involved the repeated, gradual exposure of the client to environmental stimuli associated with symptoms of anxiety and the subsequent expression of compulsive behaviors (Rapoport and Inoff-Germain 2000). The *response prevention* component has involved the individual's self-inhibition of the compulsive act that typically follows the obsessive thought.

In two published case studies, CBT was used to treat "repetitive behavior-like" symptoms of individuals with ASD (Lehmkuhl et al. 2008; Reaven and Hepburn 2003). Both studies involved traditional elements of CBT/ ERP—(a) psychoeducation session(s) with caregivers or children to help reframe their thinking about why the individual engages in obsessive-compulsive behaviors; (b) the development of a stress hierarchy that involves listing symptoms of OCD from least to most distressing to identify the individual's "transition zone" (i.e., the area where the individual has had some success in inhibiting OCD symptoms); and (c) homework assignments that involve the individual practicing ERP techniques outside of the clinic sessions (March and Mulle 1998). In addition, modifications to traditional CBT techniques were included to accommodate symptoms of autism; for instance, the use of written schedules to denote the sequence of activities that would occur during the therapy session. Currently, it appears that CBT/ ERP could be a promising treatment for individuals with ASD who have a comorbid diagnosis of OCD. However, given the cognitive components (e.g., cognitive reframing) involved in CBT it appears more applicable to individuals with intact cognitive abilities, thus, the application of CBT to individuals with autism who have cooccurring intellectual or language disabilities is indeed an area for future research.

Circumscribed Interests Circumscribed or restricted interests have been defined as interests that are unusual in their narrowness of focus and duration of time and/or intensity the individual spends pursing the interest (e.g., fascination with certain TV shows or characters) (Nadig et al. 2010). Circumscribed interests are a unique category of repetitive behavior because not only may they be specific to individuals with ASD (Lam et al. 2008), but also for parents and clinicians they may reflect "islands of ability" for their children (Mercier et al. 2000); therefore, there may not be an interest in decreasing or eliminating the individual's pursuit of these interests. It is interesting that the research on interventions for circumscribed interests somewhat reflects this perspective. For example, circumscribed interests have been included in cooperative games to increase the social behaviors of children with autism during interactions with peers (Baker 2000; Baker et al. 1998; Boyd et al. 2007) or siblings (Baker 2000). Boyd et al. compared the frequency of social initiations and duration of social interactions for three preschool-aged children with autism when engaged in a game with a typical peer that included their circumscribed interest (e.g., "Thomas the train" toys) versus a neutrally preferred toy, and found higher amounts of social engagement when the child's interest was included in the game. Further, Vismara and Lyons (2007) used circumscribed interests to improve the joint attention skills of three nonverbal children with autism. From the research, it appears that circumscribed interests could potentially be used to motivate children with autism by including them in games or academic tasks to promote social engagement and cognitive development.

Routines and Insistence on Sameness Behaviors This category of higher order behaviors is quite broad, and includes behaviors such as children noticing subtle changes in their environment, insisting their parents drive the same route in the car each time, and repetitiously acting out the same play scenario. Given such a range of behaviors it would be difficult to discuss all of the possible intervention strategies; therefore, we focus on an intervention technique that could perhaps be applied across a variety of behaviors that comprise this category—*differential reinforcement of variability* (DRV). This is a specific type of differential reinforcement, a common behavior intervention strategy, which involves reinforcing the individual for varying his behavior (Miller and Neuringer 2000; Neuringer 2004), with the reinforcement being linked to how novel the behavior is. As a practical example, if David, a 3-year-old child with autism, insists on arranging his toys in a single file line, first he may be reinforced for moving one of the toys out of line; next he may be reinforced for actually playing with one toy instead of including it in the line, and so forth. The basic premise behind this behavioral approach is that engaging in novel behavior is incompatible with engaging in perserverative responding (Neuringer 2004). Boyd et al. (2012) recently reported on the effectiveness of DRV, combined with response interruption, to decrease the repetitive behaviors and increase the appropriate behaviors of five preschool-aged children with autism. It is also important to point out that other intervention techniques, such as the use of visual schedules or video-based technologies have been used quite successfully to help children with autism tolerate changes to their routine or expand their repetitive play behaviors (Hine and Wolery 2006; Odom et al. 2003).

Summary and Limitations of Intervention Research for Repetitive Behaviors

The field of ABA has made significant and lasting contributions to the evidence base for the treatment of repetitive behavior in autism. Although the science of behavior provides a wealth of knowledge, there are limitations with the current state of the evidence. The primary limitation is that most of the research has focused on lower order behaviors, such as stereotypies or self-injury, thus, less is known about the effectiveness of these strategies or other therapeutic approaches to treat higher order repetitive behaviors.

Intervention for Sensory Features

As noted in previous sections, sensory features associated with autism may include hyperresponsivity, hyporesponsivity, and sensory seeking behaviors, and many children present with mixed patterns of sensory processing. In order to optimize intervention, one must understand the effect of sensory processing on behavior, conduct a thorough and appropriate assessment, use a valid theoretical model to guide intervention planning, and use intervention strategies that are evidence-based, family-centered, and can be implemented within everyday environments and routines.

Assessment of Sensory Features

Assessment of sensory processing patterns is based on a combination of skilled observations and the report of parents and/or other caregivers who know the child well. Skilled observations of the child's responses to a variety of sensory experiences may take place in natural and/or clinical settings, but should include a combination of the two whenever possible. In addition, observations should occur in more than one instance, if possible, in order to discern whether the child's responses reflect true patterns of sensory processing or are the result of isolated or specific circumstances. Observations should include not only the behavior of the child, but also the sensory, physical, social, and temporal aspects of the environment and of the activities in which the child is engaged during that observation period. There is currently no standardized observational tool for use in natural environments, but clinical observational measures include the *Test of Sensory Function in Infants* (DeGangi and Greenspan 1989) and the *Sensory Processing Assessment* (Baranek 1999; Baranek et al. 2007).

The report of parents and other adult caregivers who know the child well offers a historical perspective on responses to various sensory experiences, and contributes significantly in determining the sensory processing patterns of the child. Standardized caregiver report measures such as the *Sensory Profile* (Dunn 1999), the *Infant-Toddler Sensory Profile* (Dunn 2002), the *Sensory Processing Measure* (Kuhaneck et al. 2007), the *Sensory Processing Measure—Home Form* (Parham and Ecker 2007), and the *Sensory Experiences Questionnaire* (Baranek et al. 2006) are often used in addition to the skilled observations of an occupational therapist to assess a child's patterns of sensory processing. This thorough assessment process is important not only to gather information about the child's sensory processing differences, but also to ascertain when those sensory processing differences *are not* the cause of a particular child's behaviors. For instance, without thorough assessment, assumptions may be made that a child reacts aversively to get its hair cut because of the tactile sensations on his head and around his face, when in fact it is actually a combination of other aspects of that routine, rather than sensations inherent in haircutting, that are difficult for him to handle.

Theoretical and Conceptual Models of Sensory Features

There are a variety of theoretical or conceptual models that have been used to guide the planning and implementation of intervention to address sensory processing differences in children with autism. These models support a common outcome—the optimal fit among the child, his or her environment, and the routine or activity in which the child is engaged. However, the models propose different agents of change, which significantly influences the course of intervention, which may be aimed at remediation, modification, or education. For instance, models that propose to change the child's intrinsic abilities to process various types of sensation as a way to create this optimal fit will support a remediative approach to intervention, focusing strategies on the child, rather than on the environment or the activity. Several representative theories are described briefly below.

Coping Theory Typically applied in situations that demand psychosocial interventions, coping theory addresses the ability of an individual to return to an emotional equilibrium after a new or challenging event has occurred, so that engagement in an activity can begin or continue (Olsen 1999). Intervention based on this theory may support the development of the child's ability to meet challenges presented by sensory differences in a positive manner, and to develop resilience in the face of those challenges (Baranek et al. 2008). This intervention may make use of changes in or additions to the environment in order to help create the optimal fit.

Sensory Integration (SI) Theory Originally developed by A. Jean Ayres beginning in the early 1960's, SI theory is based on assumptions about the ways in which sensation is processed and organized within the central nervous system, and then integrated to help produce an adaptive behavioral response. Ayres' SI treatment approach, based on this theory, uses specific and intentional combinations of sensory input, implemented by a therapist in the context of the child's play, in a manner that is theorized to enhance neural processing. Enhanced neural processing is assumed to lead to more adaptive behaviors. This remediative approach is controversial, in part because of lack of empirical support for the efficacy of the intervention, and in part because it has spurred the development of a number of sensory-based interventions that also lack a supportive body of evidence (Baranek 2002).

Sensory Processing Theories More contemporary theories of sensory processing, such as those explicated by Dunn (1997), Dunn et al. (2002), and Baranek (2001), acknowledge the transactional nature of child–environment–activity interactions, with particular focus on the ways in which individual patterns of sensory processing influence this transaction. Interventions based on these theories lead to individualized approaches that may include adapting activities, modifying environments, encouraging child participation, and supporting parents and other caregivers through collaboration and education; the goal of the intervention is to minimize the influence of sensory processing differences and maximize successful performance of daily life activities.

Intervention Strategies

The strategies discussed in this section are largely consistent with the use of the contemporary theories of sensory processing noted above, as well as the use of motor learning and coping theories. The one exception is a brief discussion of Ayres' SI treatment in the section on remediative strategies. In addition, the strategies discussed below can be implemented in a manner that is congruent with family-centered practices and use of daily activities and routines, and natural environments. Although many of these strategies have empirical support for their use to address the needs of children with autism, and all have been tested in early childhood contexts (Wolery 1994), their application specifically to children with sensory processing differences is largely untested. Therefore, it is recommended that not only should the use of these strategies be individualized, but also that formal or informal means of data collection be included in implementation planning, so that the efficacy of the strategies and satisfaction with changes in child participation can be measured regularly.

Educational Strategies

The collaborative process of intervention related to sensory processing differences should include not only the inclusion of parents in the assessment and planning process, but also the exchange of various types of information. For the interventionist, this should include helping parents and other caregivers to understand the ways in which children process sensory information, the behavioral results of those patterns of sensory processing, and connecting those behaviors with the difficulties in daily life activities reported by parents and other caregivers. This may allow parents to better understand and interpret the behaviors exhibited by their child, and lead to broader perspectives that will support intervention planning.

In addition to using educational approaches to help parents understand their child's behaviors better, therapists have recently had some preliminary success with teaching parents simple ways to change how they interact with their child with sensory processing differences. High quality parent–child interactions may be a protective factor for young children with sensory processing disorders, and the parent-mediated intervention tested by Jaegermann and Klein (2010) sought to support the mother–child interaction that may be disrupted due to sensory-related behaviors and/or parent interpretation of those behaviors. The results of this study indicated that the quality of mother–toddler interactions increased significantly for dyads in the Mediational Intervention for Sensitizing Caregivers intervention ($n = 30$) in comparison to dyads in an alternative intervention designed to improve the child's sensory processing ($n = 28$) and in comparison to a control group ($n = 28$). Although these results suggest that going beyond simply educating parents about sensory processing differences in young children may be effective in supporting improved parent–child interactions, the investigators did not report whether or not any changes occurred in the children's responses to sensory experiences across experimental groups.

Remediative Strategies

Strategies designed to remediate the effects of sensory processing differences often include the use of sensorimotor activities and/or the teaching of new skills, with the goal of making relatively permanent changes in the inherent capacities (e.g., tactile processing) and behaviors of the child. Although intervention using remediative strategies may include opportunities for generalization or may be implemented in natural environments, this type of intervention more often occurs in clinic or one-to-one settings. General teaching strategies that support learning of new skills and remediation of deficits resulting from difficulty in processing sensory information may include modeling, prompting and time-delay, feedback (including sensory input), practice and repetition, chaining, and scaffolding. These strategies may be used in various combinations over time to help a child learn a new skill or behavior (Wolery 1994).

Other types of remediative approaches, such as Ayres' SI treatment, may be implemented in specialized clinic environments, using specific types of equipment (swings, therapy balls, etc.). This allows the therapist to control the type, frequency, duration, intensity, novelty, and complexity of sensations experienced by the child, and to do so in the context of play. The immediate goal of this type of intervention is to enhance and optimize the neurological capacity of the child to use sensory inputs effectively, with assumptions that this will lead to changes in adaptive behaviors. However, as noted previously, SI treatment has been criticized for lacking empirical support and for inconsistencies with current understandings of neurological principles. Following developments in SI, related intervention approaches have evolved, including the use of a "sensory diet." The sensory diet is based on the idea that an individually designed set of sensory activities integrated across the child's day can be helpful to meet the child's sensory needs. For example, jumping on a mini-trampoline may be used to increase arousal prior to performing homework activities. Other sensory programs (e.g., Alert Program) use cognitive and behavioral strategies for older or higher functioning children to further support self-regulatory behaviors. Again, empirical support for these approaches is very limited, despite anecdotal reports by some parents and therapists. Other controversial remediation methods aimed at improving processing in a specific sensory modality include the Wilbarger Protocol (brushing and joint compressions), Auditory Integration Training, Prism Lenses, and the Hug Machine.

Although some remediative strategies can be certainly implemented by adults other than a therapist or teacher, many tend to use a specialized knowledge base and to be comprised of techniques or methods that must be implemented with high levels of fidelity. While these strategies may at times be useful and appropriate, they do make use of a more "expert" than collaborative model for working with families and intervention teams, and make assumptions about the potential for intermittent interactions with the therapist to have generalized affects in daily life situations.

Modification Strategies

Modification strategies target the environment and/or the activity in order to create a more optimal fit among child, task, and environment. These strategies lend themselves well to implementation in natural settings, activities, and routines, and typically are relatively easy for parents, teachers, and others to understand and implement. For children with autism, these strategies must be implemented with consideration for factors other than just sensory processing differences. These factors include the demands of the environment for social interaction, the other intervention goals that may be addressed during the activity, and the emotional and physical safety of the child. For example, 6-year-old Ethan, who demonstrates moderate hyporesponsivity to movement and moderate hyperresponsivity to sound, typically sits on a bench in the playground and interacts minimally with others. Modifying outdoor play by having him choose from several pictures of playground activities and classmates before going out on the playground may enhance his awareness of the play environment, support his engagement, and increase his peer interactions. However, the intervention team must consider the total demand of the situation, i.e., Ethan's ability to manage both more social demands and more sensory demands as a result of his engagement in a peer-play activity. The team may decide to start with choosing an activity from among the photos, and allow Ethan some time to get used to being more attentive to his environment via more motor activity, and the likelihood that noise levels will increase as he engages more proximally with peers. Once his responses to this new level of participation have evened out, the team may implement the use of pictures to choose a playmate in addition to an activity.

Environment and task modifications can be put in place in various combinations in order to meet the sensory needs of the child and enhance the possibilities for sustained and successful engagement in a variety of activities. For instance, for a child who is hyperresponsive to some tactile sensations, play-doh could first be explored while in a closed Ziploc bag, and a variety of tools may be provided as an alternative to using fingers in fingerpaints. The goal in this case is to help the child stay engaged in the activity while minimizing the likelihood that the child will become overwhelmed by the sensations inherent in the activity. For a child with sensory seeking behaviors, activities with more intense sensory qualities may be offered (e.g., running errands, moving chairs, washing tables, etc.) at key times during the school day in order to provide needed stimulation in a socially acceptable manner (Baranek et al. 2008). For the child with hyporesponsiveness, the sensory qualities of the task or environment may be enhanced to assure that the child orients to what is happening or is able to maintain engagement. For instance, rather than having this child sit at a table drawing a picture on an $8.5 \times 11''$ piece of paper, the art teacher may put a large sheet of paper on the wall, offer brightly colored paints, and offer a variety of textured tools for painting (toothbrush, halved fruit, plastic fork, etc.).

Environmental modifications may include setting up a "home base," arranging the environment to make needed activities available or to minimize distractions, and making intentional decisions about the proximity of peers and adults. Home base refers to a location apart from the child's routine environment that allows him or her to plan, regroup, or recover (Dunn et al. 2002). The use of a home base is neither intended to be punitive (i.e., time out) nor to be an escape from participation, but rather is intended to support the child in recovering from stressful situations in a positive manner. Arranging aspects of the built and natural environment can allow for various types of sensory experiences, such as the placement of stepping stones beside the driveway and up to the front door of the house, such that the child can jump from one to another rather than simply walking up a smooth path, or the placement of pillows and throw blankets on the sofa to allow a child to "cocoon" herself or himself when sibling-play gets too loud. In one study of modifications to the environment, Duker and Rasing (1989) found that redesigning a classroom environment increased on-task behaviors and decreased the incidence of self-stimulation and inactivity for three adolescent or young adult males with autism.

Social environments can also influence a child's sensory experiences and thus the intentional arrangement of adults or peers may be helpful modifications of the environment. For example, a child with sensory hyporesponsiveness may be given several partners to dance with at the beginning of circle time in order to increase her arousal level and general responsiveness. In contrast, the child with hyperresponsiveness may need a reduction in the number of peers (and, therefore, the likelihood of noise and unexpected touch) while playing in the block area of the classroom. Adaptations to the temporal context may be necessary when a child's patterns of sensory processing, sleep or wake cycles, and hunger sensations do not fit neatly with existing routines and expectations. While generally supporting flexibility and the development of coping mechanisms, caregivers may find that changing the order in which one or two daily events occur also increases the ability of the child to participate in those events.

Task modifications may include use of priming techniques, visual supports, and social stories, among others. These strategies allow the child with autism to be prepared for the sensory processing demands that may occur during particular events and for contingency plans and coping strategies to be developed as needed. Priming (Dunn et al. 2002) may be used to familiarize the child with upcoming activities, with no demand for performance and no attempts at "teaching" by the adult. Exposure, exploration, and accommodation are the goals of this strategy. This method adapts the process of task initiation, thus providing greater predictability and time for the child to "process" the future demands of the activity. Several research studies have demonstrated the benefits of priming for decreasing problem behaviors and increasing prosocial behaviors in preschoolers with autism (Koegel et al. 2003; Sawyer et al. 2005), but there is no specific empirical evidence for the use of priming to address sensory processing difficulties.

Visual supports may help a child to generate ideas for play activities, prepare for a sequence of events, make transitions easier, and provide more predictability and control over aversive features in the environment. They may take a variety of forms, including pictures (drawings or photographs) and objects, and are used to assist the child in the prediction, understanding, and response aspects of managing daily events (Bryan and Gast 2000; Dunn et al. 2002), and may include the sensory qualities inherent in those events. Social Stories™ (http://www.thegraycenter.org/social-stories), initially designed to support the social interactions of children with autism (Gray and Garand 1993; Kuoch and Mirenda 2003), have been adapted in a variety of ways (Brownell 2002; Sandt 2008) including as a means to address sensory processing difficulties (Baltazar and Bax 2004; Marr et al. 2007).

The use of musical interventions as a means of modifying tasks has been demonstrated to be useful for children with autism (Brownell 2002; Kern et al. 2007; Register and Humpal 2007), though the use of music specifically to address sensory processing differences has not been investigated. Musical interventions that are comprised of individualized lyrics or melody are typically designed by a music therapist, but using a familiar tune and modifying the lyrics, or using a previously existing tune and lyrics are strategies that can be implemented in a variety of settings by various caregivers. For instance, choosing a child's favorite song and timing the singing of it to match exactly how long it takes to wash her hair will allow the child to learn (likely over several trials) and predict how long the aversive sensations that go with hair washing will last, making the situation more tolerable overall. She knows that when the song is over, so is hair washing, and then she can return to the rest of the bathing experiences that she enjoys. Conversely, for the child who is hyporesponsive, singing, rapping or chanting the directions for the next activity may get his attention more readily than would the usual method of simply saying them.

Summary and Limitations of Intervention Research for Sensory Features

Intervention designed around the use of modification strategies is usually generalizable across environments and implementers, and strategies are easily combined as an intervention "package." Modification strategies also present with more empirical support than do educational and remediative strategies. However, despite the research evidence that exists related to modification strategies, many of these have not been tested specifically in the context of addressing sensory processing differences. There are educational and remediative strategies that are being studied and have promising results, and though both these types of strategies may be useful at times, alone or in combination with other types of strategies, both rely on a more "expert," rather than collaborative model than does a modification approach.

Recommendations for Practice

The current state of the research on the phenomenology of, and interventions for, repetitive behaviors and sensory processing differences in autism lead to at least three substantive recommendations for clinical and educational practice. First, is the importance of assessment to inform the selection of treatments for repetitive behaviors and sensory processing differences. Even though repetitive behaviors may provide the individual nonsocial or intrinsic forms of reinforcement, such information is still useful in the selection of treatment strategies. For example, if the actual function (i.e., reason "why") of the behavior cannot be identified, then environmental and adaptive skill enrichment approaches may prove beneficial. Further, it appears that assessment of repetitive behaviors must go further than identifying types and functions of these behaviors but attempt to understand the degree to which these behaviors contribute to overall patterns of inflexibility and interfere with the development of other adaptive skills. In terms of sensory processing differences, assessment of the child's patterns of sensory processing and the analysis of the sensory experiences present within a specific context or activity is crucial to understanding the lack of fit that exists among child, task, and environment. Thus, thorough assessment of repetitive behavior and/or sensory processing differences can inform intervention selection.

Second, early intervention could be essential to the treatment of repetitive behaviors and sensory processing differences in autism. It is known that these behaviors manifest in the early childhood years in autism and continue, to some degree, into adulthood, thus, there is the potential to counteract the negative developmental sequelae associated with these behaviors through early intervention. Again, at issue, is that current evidence-based practices related to repetitive behaviors mainly are effective at reducing lower order and not higher order forms of repetitive behaviors, and many of the interventions that may be applied to sensory processing differences do not have empirical support specific to sensory processing.

Finally, there is evidence to suggest that repetitive behaviors and sensory processing differences substantially impact the well-being and health of the family (Bishop et al. 2007; Lounds et al. 2007; Bagby et al. 2012), and not just the child. Thus, it is important to provide parents the education and training on how to effectively address behaviors resulting from repetitive patterns of behavior and sensory processing differences that manifest in their everyday lives.

References

Abramowitz, J. S., Foa, E. B., & Franklin, M. E. (2003). Exposure and ritual prevention for obsessive-compulsive disorder: Effects of intensive versus twice-weekly sessions. *Journal of Consulting and Clinical Psychology, 2,* 394–398.

Ahearn, W. H, Clark, K. M, MacDonald, R. P. F, & Chung, B. (2007). Assessing and treating vocal stereotypy in children with autism. *Journal of Applied Behavior Analysis, 40,* 263–275.

American Psychiatric Association. (2000). *Diagnostic and statistical manual of mental disorders.* (4th ed., text rev.). Washington, DC: American Psychiatric Association.

Ashburner, J., Ziviani, J., & Rodger, S. (2008). Sensory processing and classroom emotional, behavioral, and educational outcomes in children with autism spectrum disorders. *American Journal of Occupational Therapy, 62,* 564–573.

Baer, D. M., Wolf, M. M., & Risley, T. R. (1968). Some current dimensions of applied behavior analysis. *Journal of Applied Behavior Analysis, 1,* 91–97.

Bagby, M. S., Dickie, V. A., & Baranek, G. T. (2012). How sensory experiences in children with and without autism affect family occupations. *American Journal of Occupational Therapy, 66*(1), 78.

Baker, M. J. (2000). Incorporating the thematic ritualistic behaviors of children with autism into games: Increasing social play interactions with siblings. *Journal of Positive Behavior Interventions, 2*(2), 66–84.

Baker, M. J., Koegel, R. L., & Koegel, L. K. (1998). Increasing the social behavior of young children with autism using their obsessive behaviors. *Journal of the Association for Persons with Severe Handicaps, 23,* 300–308.

Baltazar, A., & Bax, B. E. (2004). Writing social stories for the child with sensory integration dysfunction: An introductory resource and guide for therapists, teachers, and parents. *Sensory Integration Special Interest Section Quarterly, 27,* 1–3.

Baranek, G. T. (1999). *Sensory processing assessment for young children (SPA).* Unpublished manuscript, University of North Carolina at Chapel Hill.

Baranek, G.T., Reinhartsen, D., & Wannamaker, S. (2001). Play: Engaging children with autism. In R. Heubner (Ed.), Sensorimotor interventions in autism. Philadelphia: F.A. Davis.

Baranek, G. T. (2002). Efficacy of sensory-motor interventions for children with autism. *Journal of Autism and Developmental Disorders, 32*(5), 397–422.

Baranek, G. T., David, F. J., Poe, M. D., Stone, W. L., & Watson, L. R. (2006). The sensory experiences questionnaire: Discriminating response patterns in young children with autism, developmental delays, and typical development. *Journal of Child Psychology and Psychiatry, 47*(6), 591–601.

Baranek, G. T., Boyd, B. A., Poe, M. D., David, F. J., & Watson, L. R. (2007). Hyperresponsive sensory patterns in young children with autism, developmental delay, and typical development. *American Journal of Mental Retardation, 112,* 233–245.

Baranek, G. T., Wakeford, C. L., & David, F. J. (2008). Understanding, assessing, and treating sensory-motor Issues in young children with autism. In K. Chawarska, A. Klin, & F. Volkmar (Eds.), *Autism spectrum disorders in infancy and early childhood.* New York: Guilford.

Ben-Sasson, A., Hen, L., Fluss, R., Cermak, S., Engel-Yeger, B., & Gal, E. (2009). A meta-analysis of sensory modulation symptoms in individuals with autism spectrum disorders. *Journal of Autism and Developmental Disorders, 39,* 1–11.

Berkson, G., & Tupa, M. (2000). Early development of stereotypes and self-injurious behaviors. *Journal of Early Intervention, 1,* 1–19.

Bishop, S. L., Richler, J., Cain, A. C., & Lord, C. (2007). Predictors of perceived negative impact in mothers of children with autism spectrum disorder. *American Journal of Mental Retardation, 112*(6), 450–461.

Bodfish, J. W. (2010). Repetitive behaviors in individuals with autism spectrum disorders. In *Autism spectrum disorders.* Cary: Oxford University Press.

Bodfish, J. W., Symons, F. J., & Lewis, M. H. (1999). The repetitive behavior scales (RBS). *Western Carolina Center Research Reports.*

Bodfish, J. W., Symons, F. J., Parker, D. E., & Lewis, M. H. (2000). Varieties of repetitive behavior in autism: Comparisons to mental retardation. *Journal of Autism and Developmental Disorders, 30*(3), 237–243.

Bogte, H., Flamma, B., Van Der Meere, J., & van Engeland, H. (2008). Cognitive flexibility in adults with high functioning autism. *Journal of Clinical and Experimental Neuropsychology, 30*(1), 33–41

Boyd, B. A., Conroy, M. A., Mancil, G. R., Nakao, T., & Alter, P. (2007). Effects of circumscribed interests on the social behaviors of children with autism spectrum disorders. *Journal of Autism and Developmental Disorders, 37,* 1550–1561.

Boyd, B. A., McBee, M., Holtzclaw, T., Baranek, G. T., & Bodfish, J. W. (2009). Relationships among repetitive behaviors, sensory features, and executive functions in high functioning autism. *Research in Autism Spectrum Disorders, 3*(1), 959–996.

Boyd, B. A., Baranek, G. T., Sideris, J., Poe, M., Watson, L. R., Patten, E., & Miller, H. (2010). Sensory features and repetitive behaviors in children with autism and developmental delays. *Autism Research, 3,* 78–87.

Boyd, B. A., McDonough, S. G., & Bodfish, J. W. (2012). Evidence-based behavioral interventions for repetitive behaviors in autism. *Journal of Autism and Developmental Disorders, 42*(6), 1236–1248.

Boyd, B. A., McDonough, S. M., Rupp, B., Khan, F., & Bodfish, J. W. (2012). Effects of a family-implemented treatment on the repetitive behavior of children with autism. *Journal of Autism and Developmental Disorders.* doi:10.10007Is10803–010-1156-y.

Bronfenbrenner, U. (1992). Ecological systems theory. In Urie (Ed.), *Making human beings human: Bioecological perspectives on human development* (pp. 106–173). Thousand Oaks: Sage (Reprinted from original in Bronfenbrenner).

Brownell, M. D. (2002). Musically adapted social stories to modify behaviors in students with autism: Four case studies. *Journal of Music Therapy, 39*(2), 117–44.

Bryan, L. C., & Gast, D. L. (2000). Teaching on-task and on-schedule behaviors to high-functioning children with autism via picture activity schedules. *Journal of Autism and Developmental Disorders, 30*(6), 553–67.

Buysse, V., & Wesley, P. W. (2006). Evidence-based practice: How did it emerge and what does it really mean for the early childhood field? In V. Buysse & P. W. Wesley (Eds.), *Evidence-based practice in the early childhood field* (pp. 1–34). Washington, DC: ZERO TO THREE.

Carr, E. G., & Durand, V. M. (1985). Reducing behavior problems through functional communication training. *Journal of Applied Behavior Analysis, 18*(2), 111–126.

Davenport, R. K. Jr., Menzel, E. W. Jr., & Rogers, C.M. (1966). Effects of severe isolation on "normal" juvenile chimpanzees. *Archives of General Psychiatry, 14,* 134–138.

DeGangi, G., & Greenspan, S. (1989). The development of sensory functions in infants. *Physical and Occupational Therapy in Pediatrics, 8*(4), 21–33.

Duker, P. C., & Rasing, E. (1989). Effects of redesigning the physical environment on self-stimulation and on-task behavior in three autistic-type developmentally disabled individuals. *Journal of Autism and Developmental Disorders, 19*(3), 449–60.

Dunn, W. (1997). The impact of sensory processing abilities on the daily lives of young children and their families: A conceptual model. *Infants and Young Children, 9*(4), 23–35.
Dunn, W. (1999). *The sensory profile*. San Antonio: The Psychological Corporation.
Dunn, W. (2002). *Infant/toddler sensory profile*. San Antonio: The Psychological Corporation.
Dunn, W., Saiter, J., & Rinner, L. (2002). Asperger syndrome and sensory processing: A conceptual model and guidance for intervention planning. *Focus on Autism and Other Developmental Disabilities, 17*(3), 172–185.
Gabriel, R., Agnew, J., Miller, J., Gralla, J., Pan, Z., Goldson, E., et al. (2008). Is there a relationship between restricted, repetitive, stereotyped behaviors and interests and abnormal sensory response in children with autism spectrum disorders? *Research in Autism Spectrum Disorders, 2,* 660–670.
Grandin, T. (1996). *Emergence: Labeled autistic*. New York: Warner Books.
Gray, C. A., & Garand, J. D. (1993). Social stories: Improving responses of students with autism with accurate social information. *Focus on Autistic Behavior, 8*(1), 1–10.
Hine, J. F., & Wolery, M. (2006). Using point-of-view video modeling to teach play to preschoolers with autism. *Topics in Early Childhood Special Education, 26,* 83–93.
Huppert, J. D., & Franklin, M. E. (2005). Cognitive behavioral therapy for obsessive-compulsive disorder: An update. *Current Psychiatric Reports, 7,* 268–273.
Hus, V., Pickles, A., Cook, E., Risi, S., & Lord, C. (2006). Using the autism diagnostic interview-revised to increase phenotypic homogeneity in genetic studies. *Biological Psychiatry, 61,* 438–448.
Iwata, B. A., Dorsey, M., Slifer, K., Bauman, K., & Richman, G. (1982). Toward a functional analysis of self-injury. *Analysis and Intervention in Developmental Disabilities, 2,* 3–20.
Iwata, B. A., Pace, G. M., Dorsey, M. F., Zarcone, J. R., Vollmer, T. R., Smith, R. G., Rodgers, T. A., Lerman, D. C., Shore, B. A., Mazaleski, J. L., Goh, H., Cowdery, G. E., Kalsher, M. J., McCosh, K. C., & Willis, K. D. (1994). The functions of self-injurious behavior: An experimental-epidemiological analysis. *Journal of Applied Behavior Analysis, 27,* 215–240.
Jaegermann, N., & Klein, P. S. (2010). Enhancing mothers' interactions with toddlers who have sensory-processing disorders. *Infant Mental Health Journal, 31,* 291–311.
Kanner, L. (1943). Autistic disturbances of affective contact. *Nervous Child, 2,* 217–250.
Kern, L., Koegel, R. L., Dyer, K., Blew, P. A., & Fenton, L. R. (1982). The effects of physical exercise on self-stimulation and appropriate responding in autistic children. *Journal of Autism and Developmental Disorders, 12*(4), 399–419.
Kern, L., Koegel, R. L., & Dunlap, G. (1984). The influence of vigorous versus mild exercise on autistic stereotyped behaviors. *Journal of Autism and Developmental Disorders, 14*(1), 57–56.
Kern, P., Wakeford, L., & Aldridge, D. (2007). Improving the performance of a young child with autism during self-care tasks using embedded song interventions: A case study. *Music Therapy Perspectives, 25*(1), 43–51.
Koegel, R. L, Firestone, P. B, Kramme, K. W, & Dunlap, G. (1974). Increasing spontaneous play by suppressing self-stimulation in autistic children. *Journal of Applied Behavior Analysis, 7,* 521–528.
Koegel, L. K., Koegel, R. L., Frea, W., & Green-Hopkins, I. (2003). Priming as a method of coordinating educational services for students with autism. *Language, Speech, and Hearing Services in Schools, 34*(3), 228–235.
Kuhaneck, H. M., Henry, D. A., & Glennon, T. J. (2007). *The sensory processing measure: Main classroom and school environments forms*. Los Angeles: Western Psychological Services.
Kuoch, H., & Mirenda, P. (2003). Social story interventions for young children with autism spectrum disorders. *Focus on Autism and Other Developmental Disabilities, 18*(4), 219–227.
Lam, K. S., Bodfish, J. W., & Piven, J. (2008). Evidence for three subtypes of repetitive behaviors in autism that differ in familiarity and association with other symptoms. *Journal of Child Psychology and Psychiatry, 49,* 1193–1200.
Lang, R., Koegel, L. K., Ashbaugh, K., Regester, A., Ence, W., & Smith, W. (2010). Physical exercise and individuals with autism spectrum disorders: A systematic review. *Research in Autism Spectrum Disorders, 4,* 565–576.

Langen, M., Durston, S., Staal, W. G., Palmen, S., & van England, H. (2010). Caudate nucleus is enlarged in high-functioning medication-naïve subjects with autism. *Biological Psychiatry, 62,* 262–266.

Law, M., Cooper, B., Strong, S., Stewart, D., Rigby, P., & Letts, L. (1996). The person-environment-occupation model: A transactive approach to occupational performance. *Canadian Journal of Occupational Therapy, 63,* 9–23.

Lee, S., Odom, S. L., & Loftin, R. (2007). Social engagement with peers and stereotypic behavior of children with autism. *Journal of Positive Behavior Interventions, 9*(2), 67–79.

Lehmkuhl, H. D., Storch, E. A., Bodfish, J. W., & Geffken, G. R. (2008). Brief report: Exposure and response prevention for obsessive compulsive disorder in a 12-year-old with autism. *Journal of Autism and Developmental Disorders, 38,* 977–981.

Lewis, M. H., Tanimura, Y., Lee, L. W., & Bodfish, J. W. (2007). Animal models of restricted repetitive behavior in autism. *Behavior Brain Research, 176*(1), 66–74.

Liss, M., Saulnier, C., Fein, D., & Kinsbourne, M. (2006). Sensory and attention abnormalities in autism spectrum disorders. *Autism, 10,* 155–172.

Liu-Gitz, L., & Banda, D. (2010). A replication of the RIRD strategy to decrease the vocal stereotypy in a student with autism. *Behavioral Interventions, 25*(1), 77–87.

Loftin, R. L. (2005). Self-monitoring treatment package for increasing social initiations and the collateral reduction of stereotypic behavior. (Doctoral dissertation, Indiana University, 2005).

Loftin, R. L., Odom, S. L., & Lantz, J. F. (2008). Social interaction and repetitive motor behaviors. *Journal of Autism and Developmental Disorders, 38,* 1124–1135.

Lopez, B. R., Lincoln, A. J., Ozonoff, S., Lai, Z. (2005). Examining the relationship between executive functions and restricted, repetitive symptoms of autistic disorder. *Journal of Autism and Developmental Disorders, 35*(4), 445–460.

Lord, C., Risi, S., Lambrecht, L., Cook, E. H., Leventhal, B., DiLavore, P. C., Pickles, A., & Rutter, M. (2000). The autism diagnostic observation schedule-generic: A standard measure of social and communication deficits associated with the spectrum of autism. *Journal of Autism and Developmental Disorders, 30,* 205–223.

Lounds, J., Seltzer, M. M., Greenberg, J., & Shattuck, P. (2007). Transition and change in adolescents and young adults with autism: Longitudinal effects on maternal wellbeing. *American Journal on Mental Retardation, 112,* 401–417.

March, J. S., & Mulle, K. (1998). *OCD in children and adolescents: A cognitive-behavioral treatment manual.* New York: Guilford.

Marr, D., Mika, H., Miraglia, J., Roerig, M., & Sinnott, R. (2007). The effect of sensory stories on targeted behaviors in preschool children with autism. *Physical and Occupational Therapy in Pediatrics, 27,* 63–79.

Mason, W. A., & Berkson, G. (1975). Effects of maternal mobility on the development of rocking and other behaviors in rhesus monkeys: A study with artificial mothers. *Developmental Psychobiology, 8,* 197–211.

Mercier, C., Mottron, L., & Belleville, S. (2000). A psychosocial study on restricted interests in high-functioning persons with pervasive developmental disorders. *Autism, 4*(4), 406–425.

Miller, N., & Neuringer, A. (2000). Reinforcing variability in adolescents with autism. *Journal of Applied Behavior Analysis, 33,* 151–165.

Nadig, A., Lee, I., Singh, L., Bosshart, K., & Ozonoff, S. (2010). How does the topic of conversation affect verbal exchange and eye gaze? A comparison between typical development and high-functioning autism. *Neuropsychologia, 48,* 2730–2739.

Neuringer, A. (2004). Reinforced variability in animals and people: Implications for adaptive actions. *American Psychologist, 59*(9), 891–906.

Odom, S. L., Brown, W. H., Frey, T., Karasu, N., Smith-Canter, L., & Strain, P. (2003). Evidence-based practices for young children with autism: Contributions for single-subject design research. *Focus on Autism and Other Developmental Disabilities, 18,* 166–175.

Olsen, L. J. (1999). Psychosocial frame of reference. In P. Kramer & J. Hinojosa (Eds.), *Frames of reference in pediatric occupational therapy* (2nd ed., pp. 323–350). Baltimore: Lippincott, Williams & Wilkins.

Ozonoff, S., & Jensen, J. (1999). Brief report: Specific executive function profiles in three neurodevelopmental disorders. *Journal of Autism and Developmental Disorders, 29*(2), 171–177.

Ozonoff, S., Pennington, B. F., & Rogers, S. J. (1991). Executive function deficits in high-functioning autistic individuals: Relationship to theory of mind. *Journal of Child Psychology and Psychiatry, 32,* 1081–1105.

Parham, L. D., & Ecker, C. (2007). *The sensory processing measure: Home form.* Los Angeles: Western Psychological Services.

Powers, S., Thibadeau, S., & Rose, K. (1992). Antecedent exercise and effects on self-stimulation. *Behavioral Residential Treatment, 7,* 15–22.

Rapoport, J. L., & Inoff-Germain, G. (2000). Practitioner review: Treatment of obsessive-compulsive disorder in children and adolescents. *Journal of Child Psychology and Psychiatry, 41,* 419–431.

Rapp, J. T., & Vollmer, T. R. (2005). Stereotypy I: A review of behavioral assessment and treatment. *Research in Developmental Disabilities, 26,* 527–547.

Reaven, J., & Hepburn, S. (2003). Cognitive-behavioral treatment of obsessive compulsive disorder in a child with Asperger syndrome. *Autism, 7*(2), 145–164.

Register, D., & Humpal, M. (2007). Using musical transitions in early childhood classrooms: Three case examples. *Music Therapy Perspectives, 25,* 25–31.

Rogers, S. J., & Ozonoff, S. (2005). Annotation: What do we know about sensory dysfunction in autism? A critical review of the empirical evidence. *Journal of Child Psychology and Psychiatry, 46*(12), 1255–68.

Rogers, S. J., Hepburn, S., & Wehner, E. (2003). Parent reports of sensory symptoms in toddlers with autism and those with other developmental disorders. *Journal of Autism and Developmental Disorders, 33*(6), 631–42.

Sandt, D. (2008). Social stories for students with autism in physical education. *JOPERD, 79,* 42–45.

Sawyer, L. M., Luiselli, J. K., Ricciardi, J. N., & Gower, J. L. (2005). Teaching a child with autism to share among peers in an integrated preschool classroom: Acquisition, maintenance, and social validation. *Education and Treatment of Children, 28*(1), 1–10.

Scahill, L., McDougle, C. J., Williams, S. K., Dimitropoulos, A., Aman, M. G., McCracken, J. T., et al. (2006). Children's Yale-Brown obsessive compulsive scale modified for pervasive developmental disorders. *Journal of American Academy of Child and Adolescent Psychiatry, 45*(9), 1114–1123.

Schroeder, S. R., Oster-Granite, M. L., Berkson, G., Bodfish, J. W., Breese, G. R., Cataldo, M. F., et al. (2001). Self-injurious behavior: Gene-brain-behavior relationships. *Mental Retardation and Developmental Disabilities Research Reviews, 7,* 3–12.

Schultz, T., & Berkson, G. (1995). Definition of abnormal focused affections and exploration of their relation to abnormal stereotyped behaviors. *American Journal on Mental Retardation, 99*(4), 376–390.

Skinner, B. F. (1975). The steep and thorny way to a science of behavior. *American Psychologist, 30*(1), 42–49.

Smith, L., & Thelen, E. (2003). Development as a dynamic system. *Trends in Cognitive Sciences, 7*(8), 343–348.

Smith, L. E., Greenberg, J. S., Seltzer, M. M., & Hong J. (2008). Symptoms and behavior problems of adolescents and adults with autism: Effects of mother-child relationship quality, warmth, and praise. *American Journal of Mental Retardation, 113*(5), 387–104.

Stichter, J. P., Herzog, M., Visovsky, K., Schmidt, C., Randolph, J., Schultz, T., & Gage, N. (2010). Social competence intervention for youth with Asperger syndrome and high-functioning autism: An initial investigation. *Journal of Autism and Developmental Disorders, 40,* 1067–1079.

Symons, F. J., & Thompson, T. (1997). Self-injurious behaviour and body site preference. *Journal of Intellectual Disability Research, 41,* 456–468.

Szatmari, P., Georgiades, S., Bryson, S., Zwaigenbaum, L., Roberts, W., Mahoney, W., et al. (2006). Investigating the structure of the restricted, repetitive behaviours and interests domain of autism. *Journal of Child Psychology and Psychiatry, 47*(6), 582–590.

Tadevosyan-Leyfer, O., Dowd, M., Mankoski, R., Winklosky, B., Putnam, S., McGrath, L., et al. (2003). A principal components analysis of the autism diagnostic interview-revised. *Journal of the American Academy of Child and Adolescent Psychiatry, 42*(7), 864–72.

Tommerdahl, M., Tannan, V., Holden, J., & Baranek, G. T. (2008). Absence of stimulus-driven synchronization effects on sensory perception in autism: Evidence for local under connectivity? *Behavioral and Brain Functions, 4*(19), 1–9.

Turner, M. (1999) Annotation: Repetitive behavior in autism: A review of psychological research. *Journal of Child Psychology and Psychiatry, 40,* 839–849.

Vismara, L. A., & Lyons, G. L. (2007). Using perseverative interests to elicit joint attention behaviors in young children with autism: Theoretical and clinical implications for understanding autism. *Journal of Positive Behavior Interventions, 9,* 214–228.

Watling, R. L., Deitz, J., & White, O. (2001). Comparison of sensory profile scores of young children with and without autism spectrum disorders. *American Journal of Occupational Therapy, 55*(4), 416–423.

Wolery, M. (1994). Instructional strategies for teaching young children with special needs. In M. Wolery & J. S. Wilkers (Eds.), *Including children with special needs in early childhood programs*. Washington, DC: NAEYC.

Zelazo, P. D., Carter, A., Reznick, J. S., & Frye, D. (1997). Early development of executive function: A problem-solving framework. *Review of General Psychology, 1*(2), 198–226.

Chapter 13
Self-Regulation Strategies for Students with Autism Spectrum Disorder

Robert Reid, Linda Mason and Kristie Asaro-Saddler

Historically the ability to self-regulate behavior has been prized (Harris et al. 2004). In today's schools this ability may be a critical determinant of success in the classroom because it affects both behavioral and academic performance (Harris et al. 2005). The ability to self-regulate is even more relevant for students with disabilities in inclusive classrooms. Self-regulation is a critical determinant of one's ability to function effectively. In this chapter, we discuss the issue of self-regulation in children with autism spectrum disorders (ASD). Note that because self-regulation has been the focus of many researchers across a number of domains there are numerous definitions of self-regulation (Harris et al. 2004). In this chapter we define self-regulation as a "... process whereby students activate and sustain cognitions, behaviors, and affects, which are systematically oriented toward attainment of their goals." (Schunk and Zimmerman 1994, p. 309). We first preview the problem for children with ASD and their needs for receiving interventions to enable them to self-regulate their behavior. We then introduce five types of self-regulation interventions (self-monitoring, self-evaluation, goal setting, self-instruction, and self-reinforcement). Next, we provide examples of research with students with ASD in the areas of social and communication skills and for academic learning skills. Finally, we will discuss the limitations of these studies and implications for teachers and practitioners working with students with ASD.

R. Reid (✉)
Special Education, University of Nebraska, 202L Barkley, Lincoln, NE 68583-0732, USA
e-mail: Rreid2@unl.edu

L. Mason
The Pennsylvania State University, 213 CEDAR, University Park, PA 16802, USA
e-mail: Lhm12@psu.edu

K. Asaro-Saddler
University of Albany, ED 228, Albany, NY 12222, USA
e-mail: ksaddler@albany.edu

S. Goldstein, J. A. Naglieri (eds.), *Interventions for Autism Spectrum Disorders*,
DOI 10.1007/978-1-4614-5301-7_13, © Springer Science+Business Media New York 2013

Self-Regulation and ASD

The Center for Disease Control and Prevention (CDC) estimates that 1 in 110 children born in the United States will be diagnosed with an ASD, resulting in approximately 730,000 children aged between 0 and 21 who currently have an ASD (CDC 2010). These children with ASD are increasingly being served in general education settings (Myles and Simpson 2002), with approximately 90 % of students with ASD aged between 6 and 21 spending at least 40 % of their school day in general education classes (United States Department of Education 2009). One of the difficulties that children with ASD face in the classroom is problems in self-regulation (Gomez and Baird 2005). In essence, self-regulation allows students to control and monitor their own level of performance and attention to a task (Harris et al. 2005). Self-regulated learners are able to set goals, use strategies to complete tasks, evaluate performance, and maintain motivation (Bashir and Singer 2006). Given the defining characteristics and core deficits of children with ASD, it is understandable that they exhibit many deficits in self-regulation and that these deficits persist over time (Bieberich and Morgan 2004; Myles 2005). Problems with executive functions are one likely reason children with ASD often experience difficulties in self-regulation. Children with ASD exhibit deficits in several executive function components, including planning, cognitive flexibility, inhibition, and self-monitoring (see Hill 2004, for a review), which directly impact the ability to self-regulate.

Self-Regulation and Classroom Performance

While the causes of these self-regulation deficits in children with ASD are not fully understood, the impact on classroom performance is unquestionable. A lack of self-regulation is evident in many of the behaviors that children with ASD commonly exhibit. The thinking and behavior of children with ASD often appears rigid and inflexible (Mruzek et al. 2007). They may persist in following exact routines and become anxious over even minor changes in the environment. They often exhibit perseverative behaviors (Hill 2004), which may result from a basic self-regulation deficiency (Adrien et al. 1995). They may focus on one narrow interest or repetitively engage in one stereotyped behavior (Ozonoff et al. 1991). This is the result of poor cognitive flexibility, including the inability to shift attention or multitask (Mackinlay et al. 2006), and difficulty in the ability to regulate motor control and cognitive acts (Hill 2004). The impact of these difficulties can affect a student's ability to complete simple tasks in the classroom, such as following a schedule and completing an assignment.

Language can be a critical factor in self-regulation. Early on in development children learn to use self-statements to help to regulate and guide behaviors. One would expect that using language to moderate behavior would be a problem for children with ASD because difficulty with language is a defining characteristic of ASD (American Psychiatric Association 2000). Researchers have suggested that children with ASD do not use language for self-regulation (Joseph et al. 2005) and that their ability to use self-speech is also impaired (Whitehouse et al. 2006). These deficits would directly impact the ability of students with ASD to regulate problem-solving activities and impair effective communication with others (Winsler et al. 2007).

Regulating emotional responses is difficult for children with ASD as they often can neither recognize their own emotional state nor modulate their emotional responses (Dunn et al. 2002). The inability to recognize their own emotional state may result in aggressive behaviors and behavioral "meltdowns" (Myles and Simpson 2002). Even when students with ASD do recognize their emotions they are often unable to moderate them (Dunn et al. 2002). This in turn can lead to internalizing and externalizing problem behaviors and can result in isolation from classmates (Myles and Simpson 2002). These behaviors may interfere with relationships with the general education teacher, as teacher relationships with children with ASD have been found to be directly correlated to problematic behaviors (Robertson et al. 2003).

The Case for Self-Regulation Interventions for Children with ASD

One reason teachers may experience difficulty with students with ASD may be a lack of knowledge and training in effective intervention techniques (National Research Council 2001; Scheuermann et al. 2003). Another may be found in a lack of acceptance of scientifically based interventions for children with ASD (Simpson 2005). There is now a strong movement advocating the use of scientifically-based approaches to treat children with ASD (Lee et al. 2007b). We suggest that there are several reasons why practitioners should consider using self-regulation interventions with students with ASD.

First, recent reviews of literature exploring the use of self-regulation interventions with children with ASD found these to be a highly effective treatment. Second, these interventions are practical for use in the real-world classroom. They are relatively easy for teachers to implement and are acceptable to classroom teachers (e.g., Ganz and Sigafoos 2005; Reid 1996). This is significant, because few schools have the resources to instruct teachers in practices that require extensive time, effort, and implementation training (Lerman et al. 2004). Self-regulation interventions require little time to implement and less support from teachers after they have been implemented (Apple et al. 2005; Dorminy et al. 2009; Ganz and Sigafoos 2005). This is especially important in inclusive classrooms (Callahan and Rademacher 1999), which is critical given how many students with ASD are currently being served in general education classes (Myles and Simpson 2002).

Perhaps the greatest benefit of self-regulation interventions is that they can be used across many different types of settings, behaviors, and instructional programs (Lee et al. 2007b). Self-regulation interventions have been used effectively in general education classes (Dorminy et al. 2009), resource rooms (Soares et al. 2009), self-contained settings (Holifield et al. 2010), special education schools (Ganz and Sigafoos 2005), and home environments (Strain et al. 1994). Self-regulation interventions are extremely flexible because they address many areas, "without the time consuming process of individually targeting separate behaviors" (Hume et al. 2009, p. 1333). These interventions can be easily integrated into existing classroom programs (Koegel et al. 1999), such as Positive Behavior Support (Lee et al. 2007a) and Discrete Trial Training (Newman et al. 2000). Finally, self-regulation interventions can be easily customized to meet individual student needs (Wilkinson 2008).

A number of strategies can be taught to assist students develop self-regulation capabilities. Commonly used self-regulation strategies include self-monitoring (also called self-assessment or self-recording), self-evaluation (also termed self-management), self-instruction, goal setting, and self-reinforcement. All of these self-regulation strategies have demonstrated effectiveness for a wide range of students with self-regulation difficulties (e.g., LD, ADHD) (Mace et al. 2001; Reid 1996, Reid 1999). Note that although we discuss each strategy separately, in practice these self-regulation strategies are generally more effective when combined. Specific applied examples of each self-regulation intervention will be provided later.

Self-Monitoring

Self-monitoring, the most thoroughly researched self-regulation strategy, is defined as occurring when an individual first self-assesses whether or not a target behavior has occurred, and then self-records the occurrence, frequency, duration, etc of the target behavior (Nelson and Hayes 1981). Self-monitoring may well be one of the most important subprocesses of self-regulation because the feedback provided on the individual's behavior fosters awareness of the behavior (Reid 1996; Shapiro et al. 2002). As Barkley (2006) noted, there cannot be self-regulation without self-awareness. Self-monitoring was originally developed as an assessment procedure for psychologists to use for gathering information from patients in order to evaluate effectiveness of interventions (Kanfer 1977; Shapiro et al. 2002). They soon discovered that merely being aware of and recording specific behaviors resulted in changes in the frequency of those behaviors (Nelson and Hayes 1981). This behavior change, termed "reactivity," led to the use of self-monitoring as an intervention. Procedures for teaching self-monitoring are well established (see Reid and Lienemann 2006).

Step One: Identify the Target Behavior
The first step in teaching self-monitoring is to identify and specify the target behavior—the behavior that the students will self-assess and self-record. An operational definition that precisely delineates the target behavior is created. "On-task," for example, could be specified as the student "looking at the teacher," "doing assigned work," or "raising a hand to ask a question." The target behavior should be:

(a) easy for the student to control, (b) one that the student can already perform, (c) at the appropriate cognitive level for the student, and (d) simple enough to be useful. It is critical that the target behavior be well specified because students must be able to self-assess whether they have actually performed the behavior. Note that self-monitoring is not intended to develop novel behaviors, only to change the frequency, duration or intensity of behaviors students already possess. Teachers should also determine the number of opportunities that students have to the display the behavior (Rafferty 2010); a behavior that may only be performed once or twice a day is not a good target behavior.

Step Two: Collect Baseline Data

Baseline data on the target behavior is collected in the second step. For example, over a period of several days, the teacher might count the number of academic tasks a student completed in an instructional period and then graph the results. Collecting student performance data prior to intervention helps the teacher assess the need for intervention, identify appropriate target behaviors, and establish the extent to which the self-monitoring affects the target behavior.

Step Three: Teach Self-Monitoring

The third step is to teach the students the self-monitoring procedures. Typically this begins with teaching students to accurately discriminate and identify the target behavior (e.g., accurately determine whether they have completed a task or asked for help appropriately). This is an essential step, because for self-monitoring to be effective, students must be able to self-assess whether or not they have performed the target behavior.

After the students can reliably discriminate the target behavior, the student is ready to learn the self-monitoring procedures. There are two commonly used self-monitoring procedures: self-monitoring of attention (SMA) and self-monitoring of performance (SMP). SMA requires students to monitor some aspect(s) of their attention to task (e.g., doing work, asking a question, listening to the teacher). Students are cued to self-assess (i.e. determine if they were paying attention) and self-record (mark a recording sheet appropriately). Figure 13.1 shows an example of a self-recording sheet. The recording is typically done using auditory cues (e.g., a beep) presented at predetermined intervals. SMP requires students to monitor some aspect of a task (e.g., the amount of work completed, the accuracy of work completed) and self-record the results. Self-recording in SMP often uses graphing (see Fig. 13.2 for an example) however, self-recording can be as simple as making a tally mark.

When students have mastered the self-monitoring procedures they are ready to apply them to a task. During this stage the teacher should remind the students to use the procedures and then monitor the students to be sure the procedures are being used correctly and consistently. If students are not using the procedures correctly and/or consistently, booster sessions may be required or it may be necessary to modify procedures. The teacher should also take data on the target behavior to evaluate the effectiveness of self-monitoring. In practice, when self-monitoring is effective there is an immediate and pronounced therapeutic change in the target behavior.

WAS I PAYING ATTENTION?

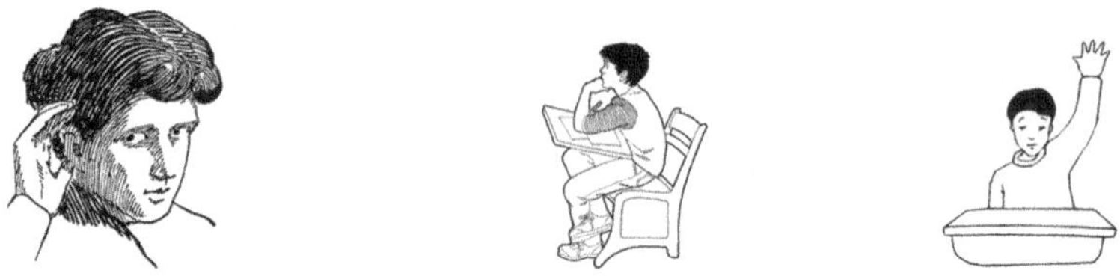

Listening? Working at desk? Asking for help?

Yes	No
☐	☐
☐	☐
☐	☐
☐	☐
☐	☐
☐	☐

Fig. 13.1 Example SMA recording sheet. (Adapted from Mason et al. (in press))

Self-Evaluation

Self-evaluation (also termed self-management) is closely related to self-monitoring and is also well supported by research (Reid et al. 2005). Self-evaluation closely resembles self-monitoring in that it requires students to evaluate their behavior at

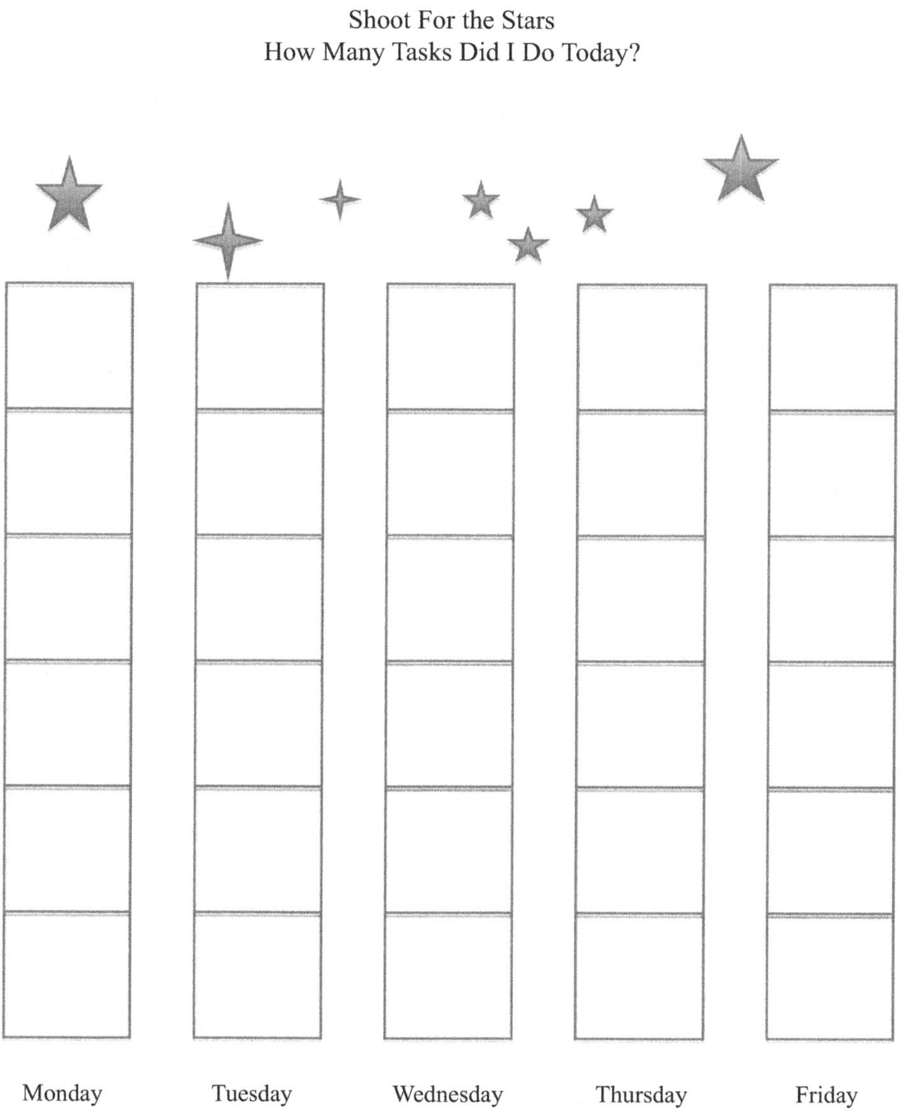

Fig. 13.2 Example SMP graph. (Adapted from Mason et al. (in press))

set intervals (Shapiro and Cole 1994), and in practice self-monitoring is often incorporated in self-evaluation. It differs from self-monitoring in that self-evaluation involves the use of external comparisons, and reinforcers are explicitly incorporated. The first steps in self-evaluation are to identify the target behavior and take baseline data (Shapiro et al. 1998; Wilkinson 2008). The same directives for well-defined, appropriate behaviors noted previously apply here. Next, the teacher should meet with the students to: (a) explain the purpose of the intervention (i.e., it will help them manage their behavior), (b) set performance goals, and (c) establish reinforcers that the students will receive for attaining goals. The teacher then instructs the students in the procedures.

Self-evaluation procedures have included rating behavior on a scale of 1 (did not follow directions or finish work) to 5 (followed all directions and finished all work) for a period, and simpler 'Yes' or 'No' ratings. Regardless of the scale, students are taught to self-record their ratings using a rating sheet when they are cued at pre-determined intervals. Students' ratings are then compared to the evaluation of an external observer such as a teacher, paraprofessional or to a pre-determined goal such as getting 20 math problems correct. The teacher and students meet regularly and discuss performance. This meeting might be daily, or directly following the period in which the students self-evaluated. Students are then awarded points or tokens (which can be redeemed for reinforcers) or reinforcement based on how closely the students rating matched the external evaluation or goal. In the final step, after students are able to consistently and accurately rate their performance and their behavior has improved, the external matching is faded with students self-awarding points or tokens based on their own self-evaluation.

Self-Instruction

Self-instruction strategies involve the use of induced self-statements to enable students to self-regulate behavior (Reid and Lienemann 2006). Quite simply, children are taught how to "talk themselves through" a task or activity. Self-instruction techniques developed from Vygotsky's (1934/1962) discovery that children used overt verbalizations to help control behavior. This self-talk (often termed "private speech") helps children to self-regulate and guide behavior and is a part of the normal developmental process (Harris 1990). Self-instruction techniques imitate the way that language is used to self-regulate behavior. Self-instructions can serve many functions: (1) problem definition—defining the nature and demands of a task; (2) focusing attention and planning—attending to task and generating plans; (3) strategy related—engaging and using a strategy; (4) self-evaluation—error detection and correction; (5) coping—dealing with difficulties or failures; and (6) self-reinforcement—rewarding oneself (Graham et al. 1992).

Teaching students to use self-instruction involves a four-step process (Graham et al. 1992). First, the teacher and students meet and discuss the importance of verbalizations. The teacher stresses that what we say to ourselves can affect our behavior. For example, if we tell ourselves that we will make a mistake, we probably will. Next, the teacher and students jointly develop meaningful, individualized task-appropriate self-statements. This often involves the teacher providing models of self-statements and helping students to develop their own. The best self-statements are ones that are personally meaningful to the students. Third, the teacher and students discuss when and where the self-statements would be useful and practice the use of self-statements. The final step is providing collaborative practice in the use of self-instruction to perform the task. The ultimate goal is for students to progress from the use of modeled, overt self-statements to covert, internalized speech (Harris 1990). Self-instructions are commonly used as a component in strategy instruction interventions (e.g., Graham and Harris 1996).

Goal-Setting

Goal-setting is viewed as a vital aspect of self-regulation (Bandura 1986). Goals serve to structure effort, provide information on progress, and to motivate performance (Schunk 1990). Students who can see their progress toward a goal are more likely to sustain effort (Bandura 1986). Goals may be either absolute (i.e., with a fixed standard such as completing 10 math problems correctly in 2 min) or normative (i.e., doing as well as another student on the math problems). Effective goals have three critical features: specificity, proximity, and difficulty (Bandura 1988). Specificity refers to how well a goal is defined. Goals which are ill defined, such as try your hardest on the test, are not as effective as those which are well specified (e.g., get 80 % correct on the test). Proximity refers to temporal aspects of goals. Proximal goals can be completed relatively quickly (e.g., get 80 % correct on Friday's spelling test), and are generally more effective than distal goals, which can only be completed in the far future (e.g., learn 100 new spelling words by the end of the semester). However, it is possible to use a series of proximal goals to accomplish a distal goal.

Difficulty refers to the degree of challenge a goal poses. Goals that are easily attained usually will not help to enhance or maintain effort (Johnson and Graham 1990). The most effective goals are moderately challenging; they are neither too easy nor too difficult. Note that it is critical for goals to be valued and accepted by the students. If a goal has little or no importance it is unlikely to improve performance or maintain motivation or effort. Attributions (the perceived cause of an outcome) must also be considered (Schunk 2001). Students should see progress toward a goal as being the primary result of their efforts rather than external factors (e.g., luck or outside help). In practice, goal setting is typically used in conjunction with other self regulation strategies. For example, in self-evaluation strategies, the criterion serves as a goal, and self-monitoring serves to provide students with feedback on progress toward the goal.

Self-Reinforcement

Self-reinforcement occurs when a student selects a reinforcer, and then self-awards it after a predetermined criterion is met (e.g., when I finish reading the chapter I get a piece of pie) (Graham et al. 1992). This process resembles the natural process where a child learns that meeting expectations often results in positive reinforcement, while failing to meet them usually results in no response or a negative response (Zimmerman and Schunk 1989). The process teaches children to self-reinforce (or self-punish) their own behavior. In practice, self-reinforcement is typically used as in combination with other strategies. For example, the final step in self-evaluation involves students awarding themselves reinforcement. The initial steps in implementing self-reinforcement (Reid and Lienemann 2006) involve the teacher and students meeting to determine standards for reinforcement and to select reinforcers. Next the teacher teaches the students how to evaluate performance to determine if the criterion for reinforcement has been met. In the last step, the student performs the task, evaluates performance and self-awards reinforcement when the criterion is reached. The notion that individuals can actually engage in self-reinforcement may be seen by some as counter to a strict operant perspective of self-regulation (see Mace et al. 2001, for a detailed critique); regardless, the technique itself is quite effective.

Self-regulation Interventions for Social Skills

Several studies have used self-regulation interventions to teach social skills to children with ASD. Researchers have examined self-regulation in combination with external reinforcement, peer training, and video modeling.

Self-monitoring and reinforcement Self-monitoring plus reinforcement is the most commonly used self-regulation strategy for social skills instructions. Koegel and Koegel (1990) created procedures to teach self-monitoring skills to children with ASD and severe disabilities. They began by identifying functional reinforcers for each child, and by teaching children to discriminate between appropriate and inappropriate behaviors by modeling examples and non-examples, and by scoring, or not scoring a correct response, respectively. Researchers then taught each child how to use a self-monitoring wrist counter. Teaching consisted of providing an example of the desired response (appropriate to the skill being taught), prompts for recording responses on the wrist counter, and immediate reinforcement for a correct response. Children received reinforcement for not self-recording an inappropriate response. Prompts were faded over time, and the length of time between reinforcement increased, until the child was independently able to record instances of appropriate responses.

During the training phase, children were taught to solicit their own reinforcers (self-reinforcement). Children had to first identify when the wrist counter reached the number needed for reinforcment. Researchers reminded the children how many points they needed for a reinforcer and then prompted children to look at their counters. Systematic fading of prompts (i.e. asking the child, "What happens when you earn all of your points?" and non-verbal gestures such as glancing at the wrist counter) occurred until the child was able to self-reinforce with no prompts from the researcher.

Several researchers have used these procedures to teach self-monitoring to children with ASD. Koegel et al. (1992) used procedures with four children (6–11 years old) considered by teachers to be unresponsive to verbal initiations. Self-monitoring increased the number of instances of appropriate responses across clinical, home, school, and community settings. Accuracy of self-recording was also assessed; all four children were able to accurately self-monitor with a range of 72–95 % accuracy. Koegel and Frea (1993) used self-monitoring to improve social communicative skills for two teenage male students with high-functioning ASD. Self-recording procedures varied slightly in that students were given a cued-preset-alarm stopwatch for self-assessing. When the alarm sounded, the students were taught to place a mark in the numbered boxes on a self-monitoring sheet if they exhibited the target behavior during the time interval. After instruction, students performed at or near 100 % for the target behaviors—eye gaze, facial expression, voice volume, and perseveration. Stahmer and Schreibman (1992) utilized the same procedures to teach three children (7–13 years old) appropriate play skills in unsupervised environments. All three children exhibited more than 80 % appropriate play at post-test. Additionally, improvements generalized to unsupervised settings with different toys.

In a series of studies Newman and colleagues investigated whether self-monitoring could improve students with ASD initiations and appropriate conversational responses. First, students were asked to take a token when they had exhibited an appropriate response. During self-monitoring, teachers reduced prompting, asking students if they had earned a token. Prompting was then faded entirely and the students began self-monitoring and reinforcing. In a first study (Newman et al. 1996), three teenage male students with ASD were taught to self-monitor appropriate verbal responses. Students exhibited more appropriate responses during the self-monitoring conditions than the baseline conditions. Interestingly, students tended to under reinforce (i.e., not reinforce themselves for a correct response) rather than over reinforce (reinforce themselves when it was not appropriate).

Similar procedures were used in two other studies that examined self-monitoring with students from preschool to 9 years old. Newman et al. (2000) taught two 6-year-olds and one preschool-aged student to vary verbal responding and to decrease perseverative play. Accuracy of self monitoring was variable for each student, with each student again under-reinforcing. Newman and Ten Eyck (2005) taught three 6–9 year old students with ASD and mild to moderate mental retardation to increase social initiations. After being taught to self-monitor, one student maintained approximately the same rate of response, while the other two participants exhibited a greater number of initiations. Initiations increased even when students were not accurately self-monitoring. Newman et al. (1997) taught three children with ASD (4, 6, and 12 years old) to self-monitor a differential reinforcement of other behaviors (DRO) program to reduce disruptive behaviors (e.g., nail flicking, out of seat). After the DRO program had reduced the disruptive behaviors to low levels, the students were taught to self-reinforce when cued by a timer if they had not engaged in the disruptive behavior during the previous interval. This procedure was effective at maintaining the gains of the DRO program.

Self-monitoring and self-reinforcement was used to help a 12-year-old girl with ASD and moderate mental retardation to reduce inappropriate behaviors (Mancina et al. 2000). After the student was taught to discriminate between quiet and noisy (i.e. inappropriate verbalizations) the student was taught to mark quiet boxes on a self-recording sheet when cued at 5 s intervals via a beep from a timer. For each quiet box checked, the student self-awarded herself an edible reinforcer (e.g., a raisin). The student also self-reinforced (i.e., a sticker, tape player, soda) when she attained a predetermined performance criterion.

Self-regulation with peers Researchers have also utilized a peer mediation component to improve social skills for children with ASD. Loftin et al. (2008) taught three 9–10-years old students with ASD to increase social initiations and decrease repetitive behaviors. Students were taught to socially initiate using three steps: (1) task analysis; (2) sequential teaching of task analyzed skills using modeling, repeated trials, prompts, and reinforcement; and (3) multiple exemplars to train for generalization. Peers were trained to naturally reinforce all initiations made by the students with ASD. All three students with ASD demonstrated an increase in social initiations from baseline to intervention and a decrease in repetitive behaviors. Behavior was maintained when the self-monitoring was removed; both parents and teachers agreed that the self-monitoring procedures were helpful.

Another study used peer mediation and self-monitoring to teach four students (10–13 years old) with ASD and Asperger's Syndrome (AS)-like symptoms to increase requesting, commenting, and sharing (Morrison et al. 2001). Each time a student exhibited the target skill and correctly recorded it by placing a check in a box on a self-monitoring sheet; they were provided with a reinforcer. The peer condition was similar, but in this case the peer checked off the boxes and delivered rewards when the target behavior was exhibited. All students increased instances of requesting, commenting, and sharing in both the self and peer monitoring conditions, and there was little difference between the two conditions. Two of the four students generalized their skills to two additional settings, one student generalized to one other setting, while one participant did not generalize findings to any other setting.

Self-monitoring and video modeling Combining self-monitoring with video modeling is an emerging method for teaching children with ASD social and behavioral skills. Apple et al. (2005) used self-monitoring with video modeling with to teach two boys with AS (5 years 9 months old) and one girl (3 years five months old) diagnosed with ASD to give compliments. Students first were shown a video of the target skill, demonstrated by children. The students returned to their class and peers were directed to engage with the students, giving opportunities to provide compliments. The next instructional phase consisted of: (a) video modeling sessions, (b) the teacher telling the students that if they gave four compliments when they returned to class they would receive a preferred reinforcer (c) instruction in self-monitoring with either a wrist counter or a checklist. In the final phase, after viewing a video, students were told that when two compliments were made, they could obtain a reinforcer. After viewing videos on compliment giving and being taught self-monitoring, all three participants reached criteria of providing at least two compliments to peers.

Self-monitoring plus video modeling was used to teach social initiation to three boys with autism (5–7 years old) who were in the process of transferring from a self-contained to a general education class (Deitchman et al. 2010). After being videotaped prior to instruction, students were provided with video feedback. In this feedback session, students were shown a clip of their interaction. For an appropriate social interaction, the researcher said "good talking" and pointed to a green smiling face. When showing the student a clip of an inappropriate interaction, the researcher said, "not good talking," and pointed to a red frowning face. After five examples were presented in this manner, the researcher then asked the student "Was that good talking or not good talking?" while pointing to the happy and sad faces. If the student responded correctly, he received a penny in his jar. If he did not respond correctly, he was physically redirected to point to the correct picture and the researcher provided specific feedback. All cases of inappropriate social response, whether correctly or incorrectly identified, were followed by a suggestion from the researcher of what the student could have said to make an appropriate response. After training, all three students increased their social initiations. Two students also generalized their initiations to other settings and maintained their initiations after the feedback sessions were discontinued.

Coyle and Cole (2004) used similar procedures with three students (9–11 years old), with ASD. All of these students were described as low functioning and all exhibited pronounced deficiencies in language and adaptive behaviors. Students were shown videos taken of them while they were attending to a task. The instructor also used communication picture cards to help draw attention to appropriate on-task behaviors. Students self-monitored whether or not they were on-task at 30 s intervals by marking a box under a picture of a child working or one not working. They then self-reinforced when they had marked themselves on task. All students' time off-task immediately decreased markedly. For two students time off task was near zero. Self-monitoring also resulted in a decrease in the number of prompts needed to decrease hand flapping and inappropriate verbalizations.

Self-regulation for Learning Tasks

Maintaining focus on a task and completing tasks can be difficult for students with ASD. This in turn can lead to behaviors that are disruptive to the classroom environment (e.g., walking around the room, talking to other students) and academic problems. This is a serious concern because students with ASD typically spend a considerable portion of their time in the general education classroom. Self-regulation procedures have potential to help students with ASD maintain focus on tasks and complete tasks. They may also be useful in supporting academic skills development (Taft and Mason 2010; Whalon et al. 2009).

Self-monitoring for on-task behaviors Callahan and Rademacher (1999) used a combination of self-monitoring, self-evaluation, and goal setting in the general education classroom to increase the time on-task of an 8 year old boy with ASD with average to above average intellectual ability. The student was taught to self-monitor attention, which was defined as (1) in seat, (2) working quietly, and (3) looking at teacher or materials. To self-monitor, the student was cued to self-assess using a taped tone presented at random intervals (from 15 s to 2 min 15 s). The student used a self-recording sheet and marked a smiley face if he was on task or a sad face if he was not. There were ten opportunities to self-monitor in each session, and the student completed three sessions each day. Prior to each session, the student would set a performance goal for the session (e.g., 7 out of 10 smiley faces) and a daily goal (e.g., 21 out of 30 smiley faces). During each session, an aide monitored the student's behavior and completed an identical self-monitoring sheet. After each session, the two sheets were compared. If the number of smiley faces matched exactly, the student received 3 points (which could be redeemed for reinforcers) and received points for meeting or exceeding his daily goal.

Coyle and Cole (2004) used similar procedures with three students, aged 9–11, with ASD. All of these students were described as low functioning and all exhibited pronounced deficiencies in language and adaptive behaviors. The authors used video modeling to teach the self-monitoring procedures. Students were shown videos taken of them while they were attending to a task. The instructor also used communication picture cards to help draw attention to appropriate on-task behaviors. Students self-monitored whether or not they were on-task at 30 s intervals by marking a box under a picture of a child working or one not working. They then self-reinforced when they had marked themselves on task. All students' time off-task immediately decreased markedly. For two students time off task was near zero. The authors also reported that the self-regulation strategy also resulted in a decrease in the number of prompts needed to decrease hand flapping and inappropriate verbalizations.

Students with ASD can also self-monitor their academic performance. Soares et al. (2009), worked with a 13-year-old male student with AS who had serious problems remaining on task without teacher prompting. As a result of this problem the student exhibited out-of-seat behavior and other behaviors disruptive to the classroom (e.g., tantrums, self-injurious behaviors). The student was taught to identify when his work was completed, and then to use a computer to cut-and-paste a Mickey Mouse figure onto a self-monitoring chart. The cut-and-paste served as self-recording. After self-monitoring began, the student more than doubled the number of activities he completed. There was also a therapeutic effect on the students disruptive behavior—the number of tantrums and self-injurious behaviors also decreased markedly during self-monitoring. This study illustrates another useful aspect of self-monitoring; there are often effects on behaviors other than the behavior that students actually self-monitor.

Self-regulation for task completion Takeuchi and Yamamoto (2001) implemented SMA and SMP for reading homework performance across three subject areas: Japanese, social studies, and science with one sixth grade student with ASD. For SMA, a clock alarm, set at 5 min time intervals, prompted the student to self-record whether or not he was concentrating by marking yes or no on a self-recording sheet. In a combined SMA and SMP intervention, the student monitored attention in the timed-condition and recorded the percentage of correct answers to solved problems on a self-graphing sheet. Student performance was measured: (a) task completion time, (b) rest time requested by the student, (c) total session time (task + rest time), (d) academic accuracy, and (e) classroom test scores. Both task completion time and rest time decreased, resulting in a total session time reduction, as an outcome of the intervention. Accuracy also improved with SMA, however, science problem accuracy was only improved with the addition of SMP. Effects generalized to improved classroom test performance in Japanese, social studies, science, and one non-related subject, home economics. Takeuchi and Yamamoto (2001) noted the simplicity of the intervention for both home and school application. Holifield et al. (2010) reported results similar to Takeuchi and Yamamoto (2001) for self-monitoring of reading homework. Additionally they found that: (1) self-monitoring was, "relatively easy to implement and blended well into the typical school procedure" (Holifield et al. 2010, p. 236); (2) self-monitoring attention to task resulted in increased accuracy in performance across academic tasks; and (3) self-monitoring increased independence in completing both homework and class work.

In a another study, two students with ASD, in fifth-grade and third-grade, were provided self-monitoring instruction to improve attention in independent work in their self-contained language arts and mathematics class (Holifield et al. 2010). Students were provided a simple definition of attending to task. Key words such as "count" and "write" were used on a self-monitoring recording sheet. Students were prompted to circle "yes" or "no" in response to verbal cues provided at 5 min intervals over a 20 min period. Prior to instruction, both the students' attention to task in language arts was recorded at a mean of 32 %; levels of accuracy varied with one student obtaining a mean of 72 % and the other 51 %. During self-monitoring, the students' attention to task more than doubled; accuracy increased to means of 93 % and 95 % respectively for language arts and to 90 % and 97 % for mathematics.

Self-regulation for writing Researchers have established, across four studies including eight students with ASD and AS, the effects of self-regulation in combination with strategy instruction in improving written expression performance (Delano 2007a; Delano 2007b; Asaro and Saddler 2009; Asaro-Saddler and Saddler 2010). In each study, Self-Regulated Strategy Development (SRSD) instruction was used (Harris et al. 2008). Four self-regulation procedures are imbedded throughout SRSD instruction: goal setting, self-monitoring, self-instruction, and self-reinforcement. Six instructional stages facilitated student mastery of strategy use: (a) develop preskills and background knowledge, (b) discuss the strategy, (c) model the strategy, (d) memorize the strategy, (e) guided practice, and (f) independent practice (see Table 13.1 for SRSD instruction). In SRSD, responsibility for strategy use and self-regulation of the writing process is gradually shifted from the teacher to the student by scaffolding instruction. Instruction is criterion-based rather than time-based; students demonstrate mastering a particular phase before moving on to the next phase.

The first Delano study (2007a) used SRSD to teach expository essay writing to three adolescents with ASD, with videos for supporting both self-regulation and strategy application. The first video was used to facilitate application of SRSD self-monitoring procedures by creating a "movie about the self-monitoring strategy" (Delano 2007a, p. 347). Each student was video-taped while saying aloud the self-monitoring steps: (1) counting the number of words written, (2) recording the number

Table 13.1 SRSD instructional overview

Develop and activate knowledge needed for writing and self-regulation
Collaboratively read model papers in the genre being addressed (stories, persuasive essays, informative), to develop students' knowledge of genre characteristics and components
Develop students' appreciation of effective writing. Use concrete examples and non-examples to illustrate a paper with few components compared to one with all genre components. Note the paper that is more fun to read!
Explore and discuss both writing and self-regulation strategies to be learned. Begin goal setting by establishing initial goals for writing papers with genre components—papers that are more fun to read. Procedures for self-monitoring can be introduced
Students' knowledge development will be continued through the next two stages, as needed, until all key concepts are learned
Discuss the strategy
Explore students' current writing and self-regulation abilities and their attitudes and beliefs about writing. Pay attention and document what they are saying to themselves as they write
Introduce graphing for self-monitoring genre components. Students' previously written paper may be used for demonstrating self-monitoring by counting the genre components (skip graphing prior performance if the student may react negatively). Goal setting can be developed by establishing the number of genre components or strategy steps to use in writing. Further discuss strategy to be learned by focusing on the purpose and benefits
To foster generalization and maintenance, discuss how and when the strategy and self-regulation procedures can be used in different contexts
Discuss and establish the students' commitment to learn the strategy mnemonic and steps, and self-regulation procedures
Discuss and establish the students' commitment to be collaborative partners with the teacher
Discuss and establish role of student effort in using self-regulation to support strategy use
Model how to use the strategy
Model how to use the strategy and self-regulation procedures for the writing task. Think aloud using positive self-instructions, modeling for the students how to correct negative self-statements
Model self-assessment and self-recording by graphing the components written
Analyze and discuss strategies, self-regulation, and the model's performance. Develop students' personal self-statements using the teachers' self-statements as needed
Continue to foster generalization and maintenance by discussing how and when the strategy and self-regulation procedures can be used in different contexts
Memorize strategy mnemonics and steps
Memorization is typically begun in earlier stages by providing student practice in memorization of strategy steps, mnemonics, and positive self-instructions
Memorization is supported and continued in following stages
Students should have strategy steps and mnemonics memorized, as well as understanding what each means, prior to the Independent Performance stage
Support students' strategy use
Student writing is scaffolded by starting with teachers and students collaboratively writing while using the strategy and self-regulation procedures. Instructional materials such as strategy charts, self-instruction sheets, and graphic organizers are used to prompt and support strategy and self-regulation
Challenging initial goals are established collaboratively. Criterion levels are increased gradually until final goals are met
Instructional material, teacher guidance, and collaboration are faded gradually and individually until the students can compose successfully alone

Table 13.1 (continued)

Goal setting, self-instructions, self-monitoring and self-reinforcement are all being used by this stage. The teacher should monitor students use of these procedures and correct any misuse
Continue to foster generalization and maintenance by discussing how and when the strategy and self-regulation procedures can be used in different contexts
Independent performance
Students are able to use writing strategies and self-regulation strategies independently. Teachers should continue monitor and support the students as needed
Overt self-regulation (e.g., graphing) may be faded
Generalization and maintenance is supported across contexts and time

of words on a bar chart, (3) evaluating achievement of the writing goal, and (4) setting a new goal. The students then reviewed their video at the beginning of each intervention session. A second video was then created for modeling the strategy (TREE: Topic sentence, Reasons—three or more, Explain each reason, Ending) for writing persuasive essays. Students created their own personal modeling video by following the modeling script while talking aloud about the process of planning and writing a persuasive essay. Following SRSD plus video modeling, students' essays improved from pre-instruction levels of 2–3 essay elements to 10–15 essay elements. In months after the intervention, students' writings were above pre-instruction levels however, performance was lower than post-instruction.

In a second study, Delano (2007b) implemented SRSD instruction for teaching Graham and Harris' (2005) writing vocabulary strategy to a 12-year-old boy with AS. The student was first taught to write action words for improving both the interest and the length of a story. The student was taught to brainstorm action words, plan to use action words in a story, encouraged to set goals for increasing the number of action words written, and then revised the story by adding action words. After the student had demonstrated the use and increase of action words in writing a story, the instructional procedure was repeated for describing words. Following this instruction, a third revision goal setting strategy for adding three ideas to the story was taught. Prior to the SRSD intervention for the three strategies, the student wrote no more than 11 words during story writing. Following instruction the students' stories average a total of 84 words in length, including an average of 13.6 action words and 7.6 describing words, and 3 revisions per story. Delano noted that prior to instruction for the third goal setting strategy, the student did not engage in revisions, resulting in low quality scores. This finding suggests that goal setting should be emphasized in instruction.

In two studies, Asaro and Saddler (Asaro and Saddler 2009, Asaro-Saddler and Saddler 2010) implemented SRSD for story writing with POW + WWW, What = 2, How = 2 (Pick my ideas, Organize my notes, Write and say more + Who are the main characters, Where does the story take place, When does the story take place, What do the main characters do, What happens next, How does the story end, How do the main characters feel). Procedures described in Table 13.1 were followed for teaching the strategies. In the first study with three elementary students with ASD, performance improved from 1 to 4 story elements during baseline to 6–7 elements after instruction, and remained at 5–7 elements during maintenance. The authors noted that throughout instruction students struggled with using self-instructions, and recommend that concrete materials, direct instruction, and practice be provided to support learning and maintenance of self-regulation.

In a second study, SRSD for the WWW, What = 2, How = 2 story writing strategy was implemented for a fourth-grade student with ASD. Although the student demonstrated inflexible thinking and resistance in planning throughout instruction, story writing performance did improve in terms of story elements (mean of 3 parts at baseline to 6 at posttest) and story quality (mean of 1.5 at baseline to 4.6 at posttest). The student did learn the strategy mnemonic and strategy steps. In fact, the student developed a personalized bulleted self-monitoring system to self-check strategy steps during and after writing. These authors noted the importance of instructional persistence when working with students with ASD.

In summary, SRSD for writing has demonstrated potential benefits for students with ASD and AS. Modeling, both teacher-led and student-led video self-modeling, and extended, guided practice for goal-setting, self-monitoring, and self-instruction are important in helping students learn, apply, and maintain strategy use. Teacher persistence and flexibility in assisting students develop personal self-regulation procedures to support learning is critical.

Discussion

Self-regulation interventions for students with ASD have been used for a number of social and academic behaviors across a wide age-span, pre- to high-school. Teaching students to self-regulate social and academic skills in classrooms has resulted in improved appropriate verbal responding, social communicative behavior, requesting and sharing, as well as decreased perseveration, repetitive behavior, and disruptive behavior. In addition, students have been taught to stay on-task and complete classroom assignments and homework, and to improve story writing. Furthermore, self-regulation strategies have also been used successfully in both the home and school environments to increase self-sufficiency, organization, and planning.

Implementing self-regulation strategies in the home, for example, can help parents to better deal with behavior problems. For example, Lee et al. (2007a) used self-monitoring and self-reinforcement to help a 17-year-old student with ASD to complete his bed-time routine. The student was taught to self-monitor completion of four behaviors: (1) taking a pill, (2) washing his face, (3) brushing his teeth, and (4) setting his alarm clock. The student used a self-monitoring sheet and was taught to check off each activity as it was completed. The student was then provided with his chosen reinforcement based on his performance. This strategy increased the student's self-sufficiency for the bed time routine and decreased the need for verbal prompting to complete the routine.

A similar benefit of self-regulation interventions is that the procedures used may help promote greater independence by actively involving students in the learning process (Ganz and Sigafoos 2005; Koegel et al. 1999; Lee et al. 2007b). This involvement is desirable, as children with ASD often experience low levels of motivation in school (Koegel et al. 2010) and students with ASD who are more actively involved in their learning often have improved academic outcomes. Additionally, improved self-regulation can increase student engagement and decrease inappropriate behavior (Lee et al. 2008). Perhaps one reason for increased engagement is that self-regulation procedures require students to become more overtly aware of their behaviors, which in turn makes them more responsible for those behaviors and thus may facilitate the changing of those behaviors (Rankin and Reid 1995; Wilkinson 2008). Self-awareness of behavior is a critical component for effective self-regulation (Barkley 2006). This increased self-awareness may result in an elimination of the "power struggle" that occurs with children with ASD when others implement consequences and schedules of reinforcement for them (Myles and Simpson 2002), reducing reliance on teachers for successful outcomes in behavior change (Apple et al. 2005).

Difficulty in planning and organizing is common among children with ASD (Myles and Simpson 2001). These deficits directly impact academics, most notably written composition (Asaro-Saddler and Saddler 2010) and mathematics and problem solving tasks (Myles and Simpson 2001). The use of strategy instruction using the SRSD approach has demonstrated promise in improving academic performance for students with ASD. This approach expressly teaches planning and incorporates self-regulation techniques to help students master and maintain the use of the strategy. Additionally, it is possible that teaching a student a strategy—which consists of a series of actions that can be used to accomplish a task—can also help a student self-regulate behavior (Reid and Harris 1993). Knowing how to attack a task may actually help students to structure and self-regulate their behavior. Including self-regulation interventions for students with ASD, across academic domains, is an emerging and promising area for research and practice.

Implications for Practitioners and Researchers

When teaching students with ASD to use self-regulation interventions, it is critical to include explicit instruction in performing the targeted self-regulated behavior by modeling, guided practice, and/or role play (Morrison et al. 2001). Students with ASD will often require several training sessions in which they are reinforced for identification of the target behavior, to support their skills in accurate discrimination between performance and non-performance of the target behavior. Supplementing instruction with video modeling to reinforce understanding of appropriate and inappropriate responding and to demonstrate a well-done task process has also proven effective for these students (Delano 2007a).

Accurate self-monitoring is a concern for some students with ASD. This is consistent in research with other populations (e.g., LD) where inaccurate self-monitoring is relatively commonplace. Interestingly, there does not appear to be a strong relation between accurate self-monitoring and reactivity. In other words, students' self-monitoring can be extremely inaccurate, yet positive effects on behavior still occur (Reid 1996). The same appears to be true for students with ASD. In practice, inaccurate self-monitoring may not be a concern if reactivity occurs.

Procedures selected to support self-recording, and to make the self-recording process more salient, can vary widely. For example, Morrison et al. (2001) used a paper-and-pencil system in which students first wrote the target behavior on paper and then placed a check on a box each time they performed the target behavior. In another study, the student was required to move a block each time he performed the target behavior, and another place tokens on a laminated poster (Ganz and Sigafoos 2005). Koegel et al. (1992) used a wrist counter, and another study used computer-generated smiley faces which were printed out and pasted on a self-recording sheet (Soares et al. 2009). Using pictures or visual representations of the behaviors that are self-monitored may help students to connect their behavior with target behaviors. For example, Coyle and Cole (2004) used pictures of students working and not working on the self-recording sheet. In addition, students typically were provided reinforcement for correctly performing self-recording procedures.

Goal setting can be used effectively with and without external reinforcement. Ganz and Sigafoos (2005), for example, set a criterion for task completion—one task completed within 5 min—in order for a student to receive reinforcement. After the student was able to consistently meet the criterion, the number of completed tasks needed to achieve the goal was raised. In this study, the student was allowed to choose his reinforcer. In contrast, in Asaro and Saddler's studies (2009; 2010) external reinforcement was not used. Students set performance goals (i.e., to write a story with all seven parts), then used a simple bar graph to self-record the number of story parts they included in their stories. Goal setting is also an important part of self-determination. For example, Fullerton and Coyne (1999) used "life maps" where students graphically depicted their vision for their future to help develop and plan realistic life goals. We would note that the use of self-regulation strategies to assist students with ASD in self-determination appears to be an area that has not been well studied.

Self-instruction strategies have not been used commonly with students with ASD. This may be due at least in part to problems with language for self-regulating behaviors that are common among students with ASD (Joseph et al. 2005). We are not aware of any instances in which self-instruction strategies have been used as the sole self-regulation strategy. Several studies have used self-instructions in combination with other self-regulation strategies (e.g., Asaro and Saddler 2009). There was, however, some resistance to the procedures on the part of the students, and because other self-regulation strategies were used the extent to which self-instructions affected behavior cannot be determined. Despite the lack of research findings, helping students with ASD use language to mediate their behavior seems to be highly desirable. For example, as students with ASD learn to complete higher-level academic tasks such as writing, a self-instruction component would be helpful to support the student in the writing process (Harris et al. 2008).

One of the greatest challenges in educating children with ASD is their difficulty in generalization (Hagiwara 2001–2002). Behaviors are more likely to generalize when teachers use reinforcing consequences that occur naturally and do not need to be specifically facilitated by the teacher (Cowan and Allen 2007). Self-regulation strategies satisfy these requirements. Self-regulation strategies have resulted in generalization of target skills in socialization, and language (Lee et al. 2007b). Combining self-regulation with other interventions such as video modeling and feedback (Deitchman et al. 2010), peer tutoring (Gilberts et al. 2001), or token economies (Southall 2010) may increase the likelihood of the target skill being generalized.

In summary, we would stress that self-regulation interventions for students with ASD have great promise for improving outcomes for these students in real-world classroom. Self-regulation interventions can be relatively easy to implement and are therefore more likely to be implemented by classroom teachers. As noted earlier in the chapter, and confirmed by our study review, self-regulation interventions can be used across many different types of settings, behaviors, and instructional programs (Lee et al. 2007b), and can be easily adapted to meet the special characters of students with ASD (Wilkinson 2008).

References

Adrien, J. L., Martineau, J., Barthelemy, C., Bruneau, N., Garreau, B., & Sauvage, D. (1995). Disorders of regulation of cognitive activity in autistic children. *Journal of Autism and Developmental Disorders, 25,* 249–262.

American Psychiatric Association. (2000). *Diagnostic and statistical manual of mental disorders* (4th ed., text rev.). Washington, DC: Author.

Apple, A. L., Billingsley, F., & Schwartz, I. S. (2005). Effects of video modeling alone and with self-management on compliment-giving behaviors of children with high-functioning ASD. *Journal of Positive Behavior Interventions, 7,* 33–47.

Asaro, K., & Saddler, B. (2009). Effects of planning instruction on a young writer with Asperger syndrome. *Intervention in School and Clinic, 44,* 268–275.

Asaro-Saddler, K., & Saddler, B. (2010). The effects of planning and self-regulation training on the writing performance of young writers with autism spectrum disorders. *Exceptional Children, 77,* 107–124.

Bandura, A. (1986). *Social foundations of thought and action.* Englewood Cliffs: Prentice Hall.

Bandura, A. (1988). Self-regulation of motivation and action through goal systems. In V. Hamilton, G. H. Browder & N. H. Frijda (Eds.), *Cognitive perspectives on emotion and motivation* (pp. 37–61). Dordrecht: Kluwer Academic.

Barkley, R. A. (2006). *Attention-deficit hyperactivity disorder: a handbook for diagnosis and treatment* (3rd ed.). New York: Guilford.

Bashir, A. S., & Singer, B. D. (2006). Assisting students in becoming self-regulated writers. In T. A. Ukrainetz (Ed.), *Contextualized language intervention: scaffolding pre K-12 literacy achievement* (pp. 565–598). Eau Claire: Thinking Publications.

Bieberich, A. A., & Morgan, S. B. (2004). Self-regulation and affective expression during play in children with autism or Down syndrome: a short-term longitudinal study. *Journal of Autism and Developmental Disorders, 34*(4), 439–448.

Callahan, K., & Rademacher, J. (1999). Using self-management strategies to increase the on-task behavior of a student with autism. *Journal of Positive Behavior Interventions, 1*(2), 117–122.

Center for Disease Control and Prevention. (2010). Autism spectrum disorders. http://www.cdc.gov/ncbddd/autism/data.html.

Cowan, R. J., & Allen, K. D. (2007). Using naturalistic procedures to enhance learning in individuals with autism: focus on generalized teaching within the school setting. *Psychology in the Schools, 44,* 701–715.

Coyle, C., & Cole, P. (2004). A videotaped self-modelling and self-monitoring treatment program to decrease off-task behaviour in children with autism. *Journal of Intellectual & Developmental Disability, 29*(1), 3–15.

Deitchman, C., Reeve, S. A., Reeve, K. F., & Prograr, P. R. (2010). Incorporating video feedback into self-management training to promote generalization of social initiations by children with autism. *Education and Treatment of Children, 33,* 475–488.

Delano, M. E. (2007a). Improving written language performance of adolescents with Asperger syndrome. *Journal of Applied Behavior Analysis, 40,* 345–351.

Delano, M. E. (2007b). Use of strategy instruction to improve the story writing skills of a student with Asperger syndrome. *Focus on Autism and Other Developmental Disabilities, 22,* 252–258.

Dorminy, K., Luscre, D., & Gast, D. L. (2009). Teaching organizational skills to children with high functioning autism and Asperger's syndrome. *Education and Training in Autism and Developmental Disabilities, 44,* 538–550.

Dunn, W., Myles, B., & Orr, S. (2002). Sensory processing issues associated with Asperger syndrome: a preliminary investigation. *American Journal of Occupational Therapy, 56,* 97–102.

Fullerton, A., & Coyne, P. (1999). Developing skills and concepts for self-determination in young adults with autism. *Focus on Autism and Other Developmental Disabiliites, 14,* 42–52.

Ganz, J. B., & Sigafoos, J. (2005). Self-monitoring: are young adults with MR and. autism able to utilize cognitive strategies independently? *Education and Training in Developmental Disabilities, 40,* 24–33.

Gilberts, G. H., Agran, M., Hughes, C., Wehmeyer, M. (2001). The effects of peer delivered self-monitoring strategies on the participation of students with severe disabilities in general education classrooms. *Journal of the Association for the Severely Handicapped, 26*(1), 25–36.

Gomez, C. R., & Baird, S. (2005). Identifying early indicators for autism in self-regulation difficulties. *Focus on Autism and Other Developmental Disabilities, 20*(2), 106–116.

Graham, S., & Harris, K. R. (1996). Self-regulation and strategy instruction for students who find writing and learning challenging. In C. M. Levy & S. Randall (Eds.), *The science of writing: theories, methods, individual differences, and applications* (pp. 347–360). Mahwah: Erlbaum.

Graham, S., & Harris, K. R. (2005). *Writing better: teaching writing processes and self-regulation to students with learning difficulties.* Baltimore: Brookes.

Graham, S., Harris, K. R., & Reid, R. (1992). Developing self-regulated learners. *Focus on Exceptional Children, 24,* 1–16.

Hagiwara, T. (2001–2002). Academic assessment of children and youth with Asperger syndrome, pervasive developmental disorder—not otherwise specified, and high functioning autism. *Assessment for Effective Intervention, 27*(1&2), 89–100.

Harris, K. R. (1990). Developing self-regulated learners: the role of private speech and self-instructions. *Educational Psychologist, 25,* 35–49.

Harris, K. R., Reid, R., & Graham, S. (2004). Self-regulation among children with LD and ADHD. In B. Wong (Ed.), *Learning about learning disabilities.* San Diego: Elsevier.

Harris, K. R., Friedlander, B. D., Saddler, B., Frizzelle, R., & Graham, S. (2005). Self-monitoring of attention versus self-monitoring of performance for spelling practice among students with ADHD. *Journal of Special Education, 39,* 145–156.

Harris, K. R., Graham, S., Mason, L. H., & Friedlander, B. (2008). Powerful writing strategies for all students. Baltimore: Brookes.

Hill, E. L. (2004). Evaluating the theory of executive dysfunction in autism. *Developmental Review, 24,* 189–233.

Holifield, C., Goodman, J., Hazelkorn, M., & Heflin, L. J. (2010). Using self-monitoring to increase attending to task and academic accuracy in children with autism. *Focus on Autism and Other Developmental Disabilities, 25,* 230–238.

Hume, K., Loftin, R., & Lantz J. (2009). Increasing independence in autism spectrum disorders: a review of three focused interventions. *Journal of Autism and Developmental Disorders, 39,* 1329–1338.

Johnson, L., & Graham, S. (1990). Goal setting and its application with exceptional learners. *Preventing School Failure, 34,* 4–8.

Joseph, R. M., McGrath, L. M., & Tager-Flusberg, H. (2005). Executive dysfunction and its relation to language ability in verbal school-age children with autism. *Developmental Neuropsychology, 27*(3), 361–378.

Kanfer, F. H. (1977). The many faces of self-control, or behavior modification changes its focus. In R. B. Stuart (Ed.), *Behavioral self-management* (pp. 1–48). New York: Brunner/Mazel.

Koegel, R. L., & Frea, W. D. (1993). Treatment of social behavior in autism through the modification of pivotal social skills. *Journal of Applied Behavior Analysis, 26,* 369–377.

Koegel, R. L., & Koegel, L. K. (1990). Extended reductions in stereotypic behavior of students with autism through a self-management treatment package. *Journal of Applied Behavior Analysis, 24,* 119–127.

Koegel, L. K., Koegel, R. L., Hurley, C., & Frea, W. D. (1992). Improving social skills and disruptive behavior in children with autism through self-management. *Journal of Applied Behavior Analysis, 25,* 341–353.

Koegel, R. L., Koegel, L. K., & Carter, C. M. (1999). Pivotal teaching interactions for children with autism. *School Psychology Review, 28*(4), 576–594.

Koegel, L. K., Singh, A. K., & Koegel, R. L. (2010). Improving motivation for academics in children with autism. *Journal of Autism and Developmental Disorders, 40,* 1057–1066.

Lee, S., Poston, D., & Poston, A. (2007a). Lessons learned through implementing a positive behavior support intervention at home: a case study on self-management with a student with autism and his mother. *Education and Training in Developmental Disabilities, 42,* 418–427.

Lee, S. H., Simpson, R., & Shogren, K. A. (2007b). Effects and implications of self-management for students with autism: a meta-analysis. *Focus on Autism and Other Developmental Disabilities, 22,* 2–13.

Lee, S. H., Wehmeyer, M. L., Palmer, S. B., Soukup, J. H., & Little, T. D. (2008). Self-determination and access to the general education curriculum. *The Journal of Special Education, 42,* 91–107.

Lerman, D. C., Vorndran, C. M., Addison, L., & Kuhn, S. C. (2004). Preparing teachers in evidence-based practices for young children with autism. *School Psychology Review, 33,* 510–526.

Loftin, R. L., Odom, S. L., & Lantz, J. F. (2008). Social interaction and repetitive motor behaviors. *Journal of Autism and Developmental Disorders, 38,* 1124–1135.

Mace, F. C., Belfiore, P. J., & Hutchinson, J. M. (2001). Operant theory and research on self-regulation. In B. Zimmerman, & D. Schunk (Eds.), *Self-regulated learning and academic achievement* (pp. 39–65). Mahwah: Erlbaum.

Mackinlay, R., Charman, T., & Karmiloff-Smith, A. (2006). High functioning children with autism spectrum disorder: a novel test of multitasking. *Brain and Cognition, 61,* 14–24.

Mancina, C., Tankersley, M., Kamps, D., Kravits, T., & Parret, J. (2000). Reducation of inappropriate vocalizations for a child with autism using a self-management treatment program. *Journal of Autism and Developmental Disorder, 30,* 599–606.

Mason, L. H., Harris, K. R., & Graham, S. (in press). Strategies for improving student outcomes in written expression. In M. Tankersley, & B. Cook (Eds.), *Effective practices in special education.* Upper Saddle River: Pearson.

Morrison, L., Kamps, D., Garcia, J., & Parker, D. (2001). Peer mediation and monitoring strategies to improve initiations and social skills for students with autism. *Journal of Positive Behavior Interventions, 3,* 237–250.

Mruzek, D., Cohen, C., & Smith, T. (2007). Contingency contracting with students with autism spectrum disorders in a public school setting. *Journal of Developmental and Physical Disabilities, 19,* 103–114.

Myles, B. S. (2005). Children and youth with Asperger syndrome. Thousand Oaks: Corwin.

Myles, B. S., & Simpson, R. L. (2001) Effective practices for students with Asperger syndrome. *Focus on Exceptional Children, 34*(3), 1–14.

Myles, B. S., & Simpson, R. L. (2002). Asperger syndrome: an overview of characteristics. *Focus on Autism and Other Developmental Disabilities, 17*(3), 132–137.

National Research Council. (2001). *Educating children with autism*. Washington: National Academy Press.

Nelson, R. O., & Hayes, S. C. (1981). Theoretical explanations for reactivity in self-monitoring. *Behavior Modification, 5,* 3–14.

Newman, B., & Ten Eyck, P. (2005) Self-management of initiations by students diagnosed with autism. *The Analysis of Verbal Behavior, 21,* 117–122.

Newman, B., Buffington, D. M., & Hemmes, N. S. (1996). External and self-reinforcement used to increase the appropriate conversation of autistic teenagers. *Education and Training in Mental Retardation and Developmental Disabilities, 31,* 304–309.

Newman, B., Tuntigian, L., Ryan, C. S., & Reinecke, D. R. (1997). Self-management of a DRO procedure by three students with autism. *Behavioral Interventions, 12,* 149–156.

Newman, B., Reinecke, D. R., & Meinberg, D. (2000). Self-management of varied responding in children with autism. *Behavioral Interventions, 15,* 145–151.

Ozonoff, S., Pennington, B. F., & Rogers, S. J. (1991). Executive function deficits in high functioning autistic individuals: relationship to theory of mind. *Journal of Child Psychology and Psychiatry, 32*(7), 1081–1105.

Rafferty, L. (2010). Step-by-step: teaching students to self-monitor. *Teaching Exceptional Children, 43*(2), 50–58.

Rankin, J., & Reid, R. (1995). The SM rap—or here's the rap on self-monitoring. *Intervention in School and Clinic, 30,* 181–188.

Reid, R. (1996). Research in self-monitoring with students with learning disabilities: the present, the prospects, the pitfalls. *Journal of Learning Disabilities, 29,* 317–331.

Reid, R. (1999). Attention deficit hyperactivity disorder: effective methods for the classroom. *Focus on Exceptional Children, 32*(4), 1–20.

Reid, R., & Harris, K. R. (1993). Self-monitoring of attention versus self-monitoring of performance: effects on attention and academic performance. *Exceptional Children, 60,* 29–40.

Reid, R., & Lienemann, T. O. (2006). *Strategy instruction for students with learning disabilities*. New York: Guilford.

Reid, R., Trout, A., & Schartz, M. (2005). Self-regulation interventions for children with attention deficit hyperactivity disorder. *Exceptional Children, 71,* 361–377.

Robertson, K., Chamberlain, B., & Kasari, C. (2003). General education teachers' relationship with included students with autism. *Journal of Autism and Developmental Disorders, 33,* 123–130.

Scheuermann, B., Webber, J., Boutot, E. A., & Goodwin, M. (2003). Problems with personnel preparation in autism spectrum disorders. *Focus on Autism and Other Developmental Disabilities, 18,* 197–206.

Schunk, D. (1990). Goal setting and self-efficacy during self-regulated learning. *Educational Psychologist, 25,* 71–86.

Schunk, D. (2001). Social cognitive theory and self-regulated learning. In B. Zimmerman, & D. Schunk (Eds.), *Self-regulated learning and academic achievement* (pp. 125–151). Mahwah: Erlbaum.

Schunk, D. H., & Zimmerman, B. J. (1994). *Self-regulation of learning and performance: issues and educational applications*. Hillsdale: Erlbaum.

Shapiro, E. S., & Cole, C. L. (1994). *Behavior change in the classroom*. New York: Guilford.

Shapiro, E. S., DuPaul, G. J., & Bradley-Klug, K. L. (1998). Self-management as a strategy to improve the classroom behavior of adolescents with ADHD. *Journal of Learning Disabilities, 31,* 545–555.

Shapiro, E. S., Duman, S. L., Post, E. E., & Levinson, T. S. (2002). Self-monitoring procedures for children and adolescents. In M. R. Shinn, H. M. Walker, & G. Stoner (Eds.), *Interventions for academic and behavioral problems II: Preventive and remedial approaches* (pp. 433–454). Bethesda: NASP Publications.

Simpson, R. L. (2005). Evidence-based practices and students with autism spectrum disorders. *Focus on Autism and Other Developmental Disabilities, 20*(3), 140–149.

Soares, D., Vannest, K., & Harrison, J. (2009). Computer aided self-monitoring to increase academic production and reduce self-injurious behavior in a child with autism. *Behavioral Interventions, 24,* 171–183.

Southall, C. (2010). Self-management across the autism spectrum: How can I use it with my student? *DADD Express, 21*(4), 1–4.

Stahmer, A. C., & Schreibman, L. (1992). Teaching children with autism appropriate play in unsupervised environments using a self-management treatment package. *Journal of Applied Behavior Analysis, 25,* 447–459.

Strain, P. S., Kohler, F. W., Storey, K., & Danko, C. D. (1994). Teaching preschoolers with autism to self-monitor their social interactions: an analysis of results in home and school settings. *Journal of Emotional and Behavioral Disorders, 2,* 78–88.

Takeuchi, K., & Yamamoto, J. (2001). A case study of examining the effects of self-monitoring on improving academic performance by a student with autism. *Japanese Journal of Special Education, 38,* 105–116.

Taft, R., & Mason, L. H. (2010). Examining effect of writing interventions: spotlighting results for students with primary disabilities other than learning disabilities. *Remedial and Special Education*. doi:10.1177/0741932510362242.

Vygotsky, L. S. (1962). *Thought and language.* In E. Hanfmann, & G. Vakar (Eds.), & Trans. Cambridge: MIT Press. (Originally published, 1934)

Whalon, K. J., Al Otaiba, S., & Delano, M. E. (2009). Evidence-based reading instruction for individuals with autism spectrum disorder. *Focus on Autism and Other Developmental Disabilities, 22,* 3–16.

Whitehouse, A. J. O., Maybery, M. T., & Durkin, K. (2006). Inner speech impairments in autism. *Journal of Child Psychology and Psychiatry, 47*(8), 857–865.

Wilkinson, L. A. (2008). Self-management for children with high-functioning autism spectrum disorders. *Intervention in School and Clinic, 43,* 150–157.

Winsler, A., Abar, B., Feder, M. A., Schunn, C. D., & Rubio, D. A. (2007). Private speech and executive functioning among high-functioning children with autistic spectrum disorders. *Journal of Autism and Developmental Disorders, 37,* 1617–1635.

United States Department of Education (2009). Office of special education programs, Individuals with Disabilities Education Act (IDEA) database. https://www.ideadata.org/arc_toc9.asp#partbLRE.

Zimmerman, B. J., & Schunk, D. (1989). *Self-regulated learning and academic achievement: theory, research, and practice*. New York: Springer.

Chapter 14
Interventions to Support Social Communication Skills

Geralyn R. Timler

Four-year-old Ryan likes to push cars at the sand table in his Head Start classroom. His peers have tried to push cars with him but Ryan ignores their words and actions. He frequently plays alone. When he does interact with someone else, it is usually with one of his teachers.

Eight-year-old Katelyn likes to talk about her favorite animals at the zoo. She reports many facts about these animals but her classmates have grown tired of listening to her talk about the same topic repeatedly. Katelyn would like to have more friends at school but she does not know how to start and maintain interesting conversations with her classmates.

Sixteen-year-old Sean is listening to a classmate describe his parents' divorce. It is clear to others in the room that the classmate is extremely upset. When the classmate stops talking, Sean says, "I'm glad my parents are not divorced." The classmate glances at Sean, says, "Thanks dude" in a sarcastic tone of voice and walks away. Sean has no idea that he just offended his classmate.

Ryan, Katelyn, and Sean, like many children with autism spectrum disorders (ASD), have sufficient language abilities to communicate with others. They produce interesting and grammatically correct sentences revealing intact semantic and syntax skills; however, their *pragmatic skills*, or language use during social interactions, are compromised. Moreover, children with ASD show deficits in social-emotional reciprocity and in nonverbal communicative behaviors such as eye contact, body language, and emotion recognition (American Psychiatric Association 2010). Because pragmatic deficits are particularly apparent in peer interactions, the term *social communication deficits* most accurately captures the pervasive challenges that children with ASD confront when attempting to navigate the social world of their typical peers. Social communication skills include the words and actions children use when entering peer groups, maintaining conversations, and resolving conflicts with peers (Timler et al. 2005). Effective execution of social communication skills reflects children's underlying pragmatic knowledge (e.g., what words are most appropriate for greeting someone?), social cognition (e.g., taking the perspective of another to decide what the other person knows and what information must be shared), and social

G. R. Timler (✉)
Speech Pathology and Audiology, Miami University, 2 Bachelor Hall, Oxford, OH 45056, USA
e-mail: timlergr@muohio.edu

S. Goldstein, J. A. Naglieri (eds.), *Interventions for Autism Spectrum Disorders*,
DOI 10.1007/978-1-4614-5301-7_14,

inferencing abilities (e.g., determining the implied meaning of facial expressions and sarcasm; Adams 2008).

The development of social communication begins in the first year of life. Through interactions with responsive caregivers, infants learn to establish joint attention, i.e., infants learn to shift their attention from an object to a caregiver and use eye gaze, gestures, and vocalizations to initiate an interaction or respond to a caregiver. These basic conversation skills—initiating and responding—form the foundation for continued development of social communication skills.

The skills of initiating and responding become more refined during the preschool and school-age years. Children learn to match conversation topics with communication partners (e.g., Is it ok to tell the teacher that reading is boring or a peer that you do not like his shirt?). They also begin to decipher the hidden and sometimes multiple meanings of simple and complex phrases such as "Hi, how are you?" (Is the speaker expecting a short greeting or a detailed retell of your weekend?). When children are engaged in a conversation, they learn to monitor a communication partner's reaction so that they can accommodate a partner who begins to look bored or confused. If a communication partner is sharing a sad event during a conversation, older school-age children read the partner's facial expressions and say something that is appropriately empathetic. If a communication partner makes a sarcastic comment (e.g., "I really liked that movie" when the partner's intonation suggests clearly that he did not), children learn to focus on the implied intention and acknowledge that intention by saying something that shows understanding of the partner's "real" message. Importantly, social communication is more than just the words within social interactions. Children learn to initiate and respond to communication partners in such a way that their voice (e.g., loudness, pitch, tone), eye gaze, facial expressions, and body movements do not draw undue negative attention so that communication partners are able to focus on the intended message rather than how the message was delivered.

Most children master the complexity and subtleties of social communication through interactions with others and without much effort. However, children with ASD need explicit, comprehensive, and systematic interventions to participate effectively in social interactions. This chapter describes intervention strategies and approaches for supporting the social communication skills of children with ASD. The "social" aspect of social communication is underscored by the evidence base, which supports the use of interventions implemented by children's parents, siblings, and peers to develop and facilitate the social interactions of children with ASD. For developmentally young children, the primary goals of social communication interventions focus on facilitating verbal and nonverbal turn-taking skills—responding and initiating—to increase the children's engagement in social interactions with others. For older children, adolescents, and adults, social communication goals include refinement of turn-taking and perspective taking skills so that initiations and responses are appropriate and relevant to specific social communication situations. In the sections that follow, specific intervention strategies and programs are described. As children with ASD require comprehensive interventions, the reader is encouraged to consider implementation of multiple strategies and approaches to optimally support the social communication skills of children with ASD.

Interventions to Support Development of Joint Attention Skills in Toddlers and Preschoolers

Joint attention interventions have been classified as "established" evidence-based treatments for children with ASD by the National Autism Center (2009). Joint attention is defined broadly as two individuals who are sequentially shifting their eye gaze and attention between each other and an activity or object of joint interest (see Yoder and McDuffie 2006 for review of various definitions and types of joint attention). For example, a toddler and an adult might both be looking at a wind-up toy; the toddler then shifts her eye gaze from the toy to the adult and the adult meets her gaze. Responsive adults might interpret the toddler's shift in eye gaze as a nonverbal request to reactivate the toy. Moments of joint attention between the child and adult provide opportunities for supporting young children's initiations (e.g., the child vocalizes to get the adult's attention and then gives the wind-up toy to the adult). Children's responses to adult turns are also supported within joint attention moments (e.g., the adult says "more?" and the toddler looks expectantly at the adult or nods her head or points to the object or vocalizes to acknowledge the adult's question).

By the end of the first year of life, typically developing infants not only use joint attention to request but also will use joint attention to "comment"—vocally or nonverbally—about an activity. For example, a young child might look at a new toy, then look at her mom and smile to share her enthusiasm as if to say, "Did you see that?" Young children with autism do not develop or use "commenting" as early or as frequently as children without ASD (Shumway and Wetherby 2009). As such, the initial goals of joint attention interventions for children with ASD usually focus on increasing children's responses to adults before changes can be expected in children's initiations for requesting and commenting.

The structure of joint attention interventions vary in their approach to teaching and the reinforcement or consequences that are provided in response to a child's behaviors (Kasari et al. 2010; Yoder and McDuffie 2006). Interventions that support the development of children's joint attention skills include discrete trial training, naturalistic behavioral interventions, and relationship-based interventions. Of these three, discrete trial training is the most structured approach. In this approach, adults use specific verbal and physical prompts to elicit a child's behaviors (e.g., modeling, physically manipulating the child's hand into the shape of a point directed at an object). Discrete trial training is usually conducted during tabletop activities that are selected and presented by the adult. The number of opportunities to elicit the child's behaviors is defined prior to the start of the therapy session so that a predetermined number of drills or trials are conducted. Related (e.g., the toy) and unrelated (e.g., stickers or other tokens) reinforcement or consequences are provided when the child performs the targeted behavior correctly. Compared to discrete trial training approaches, the naturalistic behavioral approaches rely less on the structure. The naturalistic behavioral approaches avoid or limit use of physical prompts and emphasize delivery of only natural consequences. These approaches are child-led, in that the adult waits for the child to become engaged in a particular activity before attempting to elicit a response from the child. The adult may use time delay or pause time to elicit the response (e.g., the adult looks expectantly at the child, moving the desired object to a space between the adult's face and the child's face so that the child's glance at the object is simultaneously a glance at the adult's eyes). Other adult behaviors within naturalistic behavioral interventions include modeling of a desired behavior and setting up a verbal routine for the child to complete (e.g., adult says excitedly, "One, two," and waits for the child to say "Three" before pushing the child on a swing). In response to the child's verbal or nonverbal communication attempts (e.g., eye gaze, gestures, and signs), natural consequences are provided such as praise, the object, or the action. Unlike discrete trial approaches, unrelated consequences, such as stickers, are not used. The philosophy for relying on only natural consequences is that these consequences are similar to the consequences that occur in the day-to-day interactions between children and their caregivers. Thus, child behaviors are expected to generalize more quickly to new situations and with new communication partners. A final approach for supporting children's joint attention skills are programs that emphasize relationship building between the child and the adult. In relationship-based interventions, increases in joint attention are not a target of the intervention, but are an expected by product of activities whereby a responsive adult imitates a child's words and actions to support and elicit the child's engagement. Most of the empirical evidence for the efficacy of joint attention interventions has been provided by discrete trial training and naturalistic behavioral approach; support for relationship-based interventions is emerging.

Best practices guidelines for serving children with ASD emphasize parent training as central to early intervention services because services are to be provided in the child's natural environment with familiar communication partners (IDEA 2004; Smith et. al. 2007). Parent implementation of the intervention reduces the need for generalization programming as parent and child interaction is the focus of these interventions (Kasari et al. 2010). A number of studies have demonstrated that parent training successfully increases the joint attention and functional play skills of children with ASD (Girolametto et al. 2007; Kasari et al. 2010; Yoder and McDuffie 2006). Effective parent training for implementation of joint attention interventions includes specific instruction in methods to follow the child's lead so that the child is actively engaged in an activity. Parents then learn strategies, such as modeling and imitation of a child's actions and vocalizations, to expand the child's play and joint attention skills. General guidelines for training parents to implement joint attention interventions are provided in Table 14.1.

In parent-implemented interventions, it is important to carefully match child abilities with child goals so that neither the parent nor the child experiences too much frustration. For example, if a child does not have joint attention at the beginning of the intervention, parents are first taught specific strategies to facilitate and increase

Table 14.1 Guidelines for teaching caregivers how to support children's joint attention skills (Adapted from Girolametto et al. 2007; Kasari et al. 2010; Yoder and McDuffie 2006)

Arrange the environment. Help caregiver to identify a set of objects and activities that are of high interest to the child; ideally these objects and activities should allow for some adult assistance and playfulness. Consider activities that are already preferred by the child (e.g., movement activities such as swinging or rocking or running; play routines that could foster nonverbal and verbal turn-taking such as pushing and stopping cars)
Facilitate child engagement within activities. Assist caregivers to establish turn-taking routines. For example, caregivers should sit near and at the same level as the child to facilitate eye contact. Encourage caregivers to imitate the child's actions and vocalizations to maintain child interest in the activity
Follow child's lead and interests. Teach caregiver to synchronize words and actions within child's focus of attention: Talk about what the child is doing (if child is playing with a car, talk about/act upon the car)
Use expectant waiting to allow child time to initiate a request or comment
When child gestures, vocalizes, or verbalizes, acknowledge the child's communicative turn by providing the words for the gestures or adding to a verbalization that the child has said. For example, if the child hands an object to the adult to "request" that the adult to do something, model the words that the child is trying to communicate with this gesture. If the child produces a word to make a request, add a word or two to this request. For example, the child says "more" and the adult says "more tickle"
Videotape the sessions so that the caregivers can watch and discuss interactions with their child. Provide feedback to the caregiver about the caregiver's words and actions and child's responses to those words and actions

child's responses to the parent. It is equally important to match the parent's enthusiasm for the strategies. Children of parents who are most adept at capitalizing on opportunities for joint attention (i.e., when the child is actively engaged in an activity) make the most gains. Importantly, two specific types of parent utterances are associated with child gains: *follow-in commenting* and *follow-directing* (McDuffie and Yoder 2010). *Follow-in commenting* includes utterances that parents make about what the child is doing (e.g., child is swinging and adult says "swing!") as opposed to comments that redirect the child to do something else. *Follow-directing* is defined as parent utterances that are synchronized with the child's focus of attention but include a request that a child change an ongoing behavior connected with the activity (e.g., Adult says, "Daddy open?" when child is struggling to open a container).

One caveat about the success of joint attention interventions is that the success of these interventions is somewhat dependent on the child's engagement and interest levels. Parents only have opportunities to provide follow-in commenting when the child is exploring, manipulating, or engaging in or with an activity or object. Moreover, the child must attempt to direct the parents' actions before the parent can respond to the child. Children who have higher levels of sustained, productive object engagement will likely have better language outcomes because parents have more opportunities for follow-in talking. Similarly, children who produce more acts of intentional communication will likely have better language outcomes because parents have more opportunities to provide contingent verbal utterances (McDuffie and Yoder 2010).

Interventions to Support Peer Interactions in Preschool and School Settings

Overview

When children enter school, their social communication skills are developed and refined through day-to-day interactions with peers. Effective social communication interventions for preschoolers and school-age children with ASD emphasize strategies for facilitating these important peer interactions, and may include training the peers of children with ASD. Peer training packages or peer-mediated interventions aim to teach and reinforce peers for their attempts to interact with children with ASD. Although peer-mediated interventions provide more opportunities for children to interact, most children with ASD will continue to require direct and specialized interventions to learn and refine specific social communication skills. Evidence-based social communication interventions for children with ASD include published programs such as the Picture Exchange Communication System (Frost and Bondy 1994) and Social Stories^{TM} (Gray 1995, 2000), specific strategies such as video-based instruction and script training, as well as investigator and clinician-designed packaged interventions targeting social skills, social pragmatic skills, and social cognitive skills. "Packaged" interventions incorporate multiple procedures and strategies to teach children one or more social communication skills. A review of these interventions follows.

Peer-Mediated Interventions

Inclusive preschool classrooms offer children with ASD opportunities to learn social communication skills through interactions with typically developing peers. Unfortunately, observations of peer interactions within inclusive classrooms reveal that children with high and low levels of social communication abilities do not usually initiate and sustain interactions with each other. For example, some children with ASD ignore or respond inappropriately to typically developing peers' attempts to engage them in conversation, and in turn, typically developing peers limit their interactions with children with ASD (see reviews by Sainato et al. 2008; Strain et al. 2008).

Peer training packages or peer-mediated interventions are an evidence-based method for increasing the interactions of children with ASD and their typically developing peers (National Autism Center 2009). These interventions train peers to initiate and to persist in their efforts to interact with children with ASD. For example, Thiemann and Goldstein (2004) taught peers five social communication skills to use during interactions with children with ASD: (1) "look, wait, and listen" to allow a child with ASD to initiate an interaction with the peer; (2) "answer questions" to encourage the peer to respond to the child with ASD; (3) "start talking" to initiate an interaction; (4) "say something nice"; and (5) "keep talking" to sustain the interactions. The peers were taught each of these skills through modeling, role-play, and adult feedback. Upon completion of the peer training, each peer was paired with one child with ASD (in peer training interventions, the child with ASD is referred to as the "focus child") during a 10-minute social activity in the classroom. Just before the social activity, the peers reviewed the five social communication skills and a visual feedback system of happy, neutral, and sad faces was introduced to encourage the peers to perform each of the social communication skills. Peers were informed that if they used each skill at least two times during the social activity with their individual focus child, they would receive a prize. The focus children also received a written text intervention comprising phrases that they could say during the social activity (script training is reviewed in a later section of this chapter). Positive changes were demonstrated in the quantity and quality of the interactions including increases in the focus children's initiations, responses, and time spent engaged with peers. Table 14.2 provides guidelines for implementation of peer-mediated interventions in preschool and school settings.

Picture Exchange Communication System (PECS)

PECS is a manualized intervention program for teaching minimally verbal children with ASD to initiate interactions with another individual. Through a series of sequential steps, the child is taught to initiate a request by giving/exchanging a picture symbol of a desired activity to a communication partner. A meta-analysis of PECS intervention studies revealed that PECS was more effective than traditional joint attention interventions for increasing the communicative behaviors of children with limited joint attention skills (Flippin et al. 2010). PECS does not require prerequisite skills such as imitation, gesture, or joint attention. As such, PECS is often introduced as an alternative communication system for children with limited verbal skills and for children who are difficult to engage in social interactions. One important clinical finding from the meta-analysis is that children with some preintervention joint attention skills had better communication outcomes with joint attention interventions than with PECS (joint attention interventions were reviewed in a previous section of this chapter).

PECS has traditionally been used to increase interactions between a child and an adult but a few studies have documented the benefits of teaching children with ASD to use PECS with classroom peers (Cannella-Malone et al. 2010; Garfinkle and Schwartz 1994; Schwartz et al. 1998). The PECS with peers protocol (Garfinkle and Schwartz 1994) uses teaching techniques similar to the original manualized training. However, environmental arrangements are implemented so that the child receiving PECS training needs to initiate the picture exchange with a peer. For example, small group activities are set up so that a peer, rather than an adult in the room, controls the child's favorite material. If the child attempts to give the picture to the adult,

Table 14.2 Guidelines for implementing peer-mediated interventions (Adapted from Kamps et al. 2002; Strain et al. 2008; Thiemann and Goldstein 2004. Also see Ohio's Center for Autism and Low Incidence website at www.autisminternetmodules.org for technical training to implement peer mediation interventions)

Enlist key personnel. All personnel will assist in development of social communication goals (see # 2 below) for the child with ASD (hereafter, referred to as the "focus child") and the child's peers. Teachers will identify and recruit three to six peers to participate in intervention sessions and obtain parent permission as required by local school policies. Teachers will assist in scheduling across the day social activities, at least two 10–15-minute activities per intervention day. Speech-language pathologists and school psychologists will provide direct instruction to the focus child and the recruited peers
Identify social communication goals. Collect baseline data through observation of focus child and peers during social activities in the classroom or at recess. Specific behaviors to observe include the frequency of focus child's responses and initiations to peers, peers' responses and initiations to focus child, the appropriateness of the responses and initiations (e.g., Is the response relevant? Does the initiator attempt to get the other person's attention before making a statement?), and the duration of focus child and peer interactions. Note behaviors that facilitate and detract from interactions. Use these data to develop goals for both the focus child and the peers. The behaviors of the peers should be used to set criteria for goals (e.g., how many times do peers initiate with other children?)
Teach peers to facilitate interactions with the child with ASD. Encourage peers to play/interact close to the focus child, to persist in initiations to the focus child even if these initiations are ignored, and to respond to the initiations of the focus child (if the focus child uses idiosyncratic or repeats the utterances of his peers, teach peers to accept these utterances as a real "turn" by the focus child). Use modeling and rewards to teach and encourage interaction
Teach focus child to initiate and respond to peers. Use verbal, picture, or text supports as needed to prepare child to participate in an activity that the focus child prefers and that will be of interest to the peers (e.g., board games, building activities such that the group must work together to build one structure, "Tag" or other popular recess activities). If needed, model and rehearse appropriate comments and questions to "say" in the activity (e.g., "It's your turn." "Way to go.")
Conduct joint intervention session with focus child and trained peers. Introduce activity (see # 4 above). Discuss mutual goals in the activity (e.g., "stay close," "take turns," "talk to each other"). Ask children to set personal goals for the activity (e.g., "I will say five things"). Give children the activity materials and let them play. Provide prompting as needed to sustain the interaction. When activity is finished, discuss what everyone accomplished, provide corrective feedback as needed, and give rewards if personal goals were met
Support participation in classroom social activities. Share prompts with classroom teacher. Develop plan with classroom teacher for monitoring children's (focus child and peers) interactions in selected social activities. Plan should include nonintrusive strategies for corrective feedback and delivery of rewards

the adult redirects the child's attention to the peer who has the desired material, by stating, "I don't have it. Ask (peer's name)." If this verbal prompt is unsuccessful, the adult provides a physical prompt by guiding the child's hand and picture, to the peer with the material. Some peer training is needed to increase the effectiveness of the PECS with peers' protocol. The peer must be taught the purpose of the exchange; that is, that the child with ASD is requesting the object or activity represented in the picture and that the peer should honor this request (Cannella-Malone et al. 2010).

Social Stories™

Social Stories™ are a visual and text-based intervention developed by Gray (1995, 2000). The purpose of the social story™ is to describe a social situation including what the child could say or do to appropriately manage the situation. Examples and comprehensive directions for developing social stories™ are available in a curriculum guide (Gray 2000). Ideally, a social story™ should be individualized for a specific child and written from a first person "child" perspective, be relatively brief, and written at the child's comprehension level. The story should include positive statements about feelings and actions and avoid or limit negative statements (e.g., "don't do this"). Gray (1995) recommends that the story comprises one directive statement for every two other types of statements so that the story is not a list of "should do's" for the child. Other statements include descriptive (facts about the situation), perspective (the reactions, feelings, and responses of others), and cooperative statements (what others will do in the situation). For example, Ozdemir (2008) developed social stories™ to decrease disruptive behaviors in three children with ASD. Examples of descriptive, perspective, and directive statements in the study's stories included: "People talk quietly when they are in class. If I talk quietly, my friends and teachers can still hear me. I will try to use a quiet voice while I am in class."

Social story™ intervention sessions usually comprise two parts. First, the story is presented to the child by an adult who remains near the child as the child reads the story or listens to the story if the child is unable to read it. Stories can also be presented via audio recordings or computers. Then the child is placed in the situation described in the story. For example, if the social story™ is about using a quiet voice in class, the story is presented to the child just immediately before the child is to sit in the class. The story can be introduced several times a day across several weeks. When the child begins to demonstrate a stable change in the desired behaviors, procedures to fade the presentation of the story can be initiated. Fading procedures include reducing the number of times that the story is read to the child or reducing the number of directive sentences in the story (Wallin 2004). If changes in the targeted social behaviors are not observed after several weeks, Gray (1995) recommends rewriting and reintroducing the story. Once the skills of a story are mastered, the stories can be kept in a binder so that the child can review them as needed. Social stories™ should be a "team" intervention. All the child's teachers and caregivers should be aware of the specific social communication targets in the story so that they will reinforce those behaviors when they observe them.

Story-based intervention packages including the use of social stories™ as described here are classified as established evidence-based interventions for children with ASD (National Autism Center 2009). A recent meta-analysis of six controlled trial social story™ dissertation studies revealed positive changes in children's game-playing skills, story comprehension, labeling of facial emotions, social communication skills, and reduction of aggressive behaviors (Karkhaneh et al. 2010). The intensity of the social story interventions varied from two presentations of the story during a single intervention session to ten presentations across the school day with the duration of the interventions lasting from 2 days to 1 month. Studies that demonstrated the most positive outcomes were those that presented the stories in highly structured and predictable settings with well-controlled environments and well-trained personnel.

Script Training

Script training interventions comprise verbal, pictorial, and/or written scripts of explicit statements or questions to be used in a small group in vivo activity or a role-play. Scripts for role-play have also been called sociodramatic scripts (see Goldstein et al. 2007 for review). Scripts are usually introduced and practiced repeatedly just before the child with ASD and his or her peers will engage in the activity or the role-play. An important component of a comprehensive script training intervention is systematic procedure for fading the use of the script so that the child's production of the statements and questions becomes independent of script availability. Fading can be accomplished by systematically omitting parts of the script.

Krantz and McClannahan (1993) introduced script training to four children, ages 9–12, with ASD. The intervention was implemented because the children did not spontaneously initiate interactions with peers unless verbally prompted to do so by their teachers. Written scripts of ten statements and questions to be used during classroom activities were developed in collaboration with the children's teachers. As the scripts were written, the children's oral reading accuracy for the scripts was tested prior to the start of the intervention. The scripts were introduced during classroom art activities when talking among students was allowed. As children began the art class, they were prompted nonverbally (via pointing by their teacher) to read instructions posted at their desks: "Do your art." and "Talk a lot." These statements were followed by the script statements such as "{Name—the names of children in the group activity} do you want to use my {pencils/crayons/brushes}?" "{Name} won't it be fun to go to the {park/store/farm} on Fun Friday?" "{Name} I like your picture." No verbal prompts were used to encourage the children to read the script. Instead, the teacher stood behind the child and manually guided the child to pick up a pencil, pointed to a scripted statement or question, and then moved the pencil word-by-word below the text. If the child did not read or say the statement/question within 5 seconds, the manual guidance procedure was repeated. In some cases, the teacher also manually guided the child's head to face the peer who was being addressed. If the child did read the script, the child placed a check mark next to the statement or question each time he or she produced it. Manual prompts were eliminated as soon as the children began to read without the prompts (across the four children, 15–27 intervention sessions were needed before the prompting was discontinued). As soon as the manual prompts were eliminated, script-fading procedures were initiated. Scripts were faded word-by-word beginning with the end of the statement or question (e.g., "{Name} won't it be fun to go to the {park/store/farm} on . . . . .?") until the statement was reduced to {Name} and quotation marks. By the end of the intervention phase, children were producing scripted and unscripted spontaneous initiations to peers. Children's responses to the initiations of their peers also increased.

Script training interventions have recently been classified as emerging evidence-based interventions (National Autism Center 2009). Effective script training requires a collaborative effort among children's teachers, speech-language pathologists, and other service providers. Script development requires this team effort so that script statements and questions are individualized and appropriate for multiple situations to facilitate generalization of statement and question use across settings and partners. A potential disadvantage of script training interventions is that children can become dependent on the script if systematic fading procedures are not programmed within the intervention. McClannahan and Krantz (2005) provide practical guidelines, scripts templates, and script-fading techniques to assist with the implementation of script training.

Video-Based Instruction

Video-based instruction (VBI) is an intervention strategy that involves the demonstration of one or more social communication behaviors. Alternative names for this intervention strategy include video instruction, video modeling, and video-taped modeling. A video-based intervention session usually consists of the child watching a short video of himself or herself (i.e., self-modeling) or others (peer modeling) performing a sequence of social communication behaviors. After watching the video, the child is given immediate access to an identical set of materials, communication partners, the activity, and the setting that were presented in the video. Little, if any, verbal explanation is provided; rather the expectation is that the child will imitate the words and actions that he or she has just observed.

For example, Nikopoulos and Keenan (2003) made short 35-second videos to teach social initiation and play behaviors to seven children, ages 9–15 years, with ASD. The scenario of each video was as follows: the experimenter was shown entering a room with another individual; this individual served as the "actor" model, whom the child was to imitate. Three videos were made for each of the children using different actor models: a same-age typically developing peer, a familiar adult, and an unfamiliar adult. Once the experimenter and the actor model entered the room, the experimenter sat down opposite a number of toys; the model actor spent a few seconds wandering around the room, and then approached the experimenter, taking his hand, saying, "Let's play," and bringing the experimenter to a toy. The experimenter and the model then played with the toy for approximately 15 seconds. The intervention sessions consisted of two parts. First, the child watched a video. No introduction or explanation about the video was provided to the child. When the video was finished, the second part of the intervention session began. The experimenter and the child immediately walked into a second room in which the experimenter sat in a chair opposite an identical set of toys as presented in the video. The experimenter then waited for the child to initiate an interaction. If the child initiated an interaction, the experimenter played with the child and the toy for approximately 5 minutes. The children received two to five intervention sessions per day for multiple weeks. Outcome data for this study included latency to social initiation and time spent in appropriate play with the toys. Four of the seven participants in this study demonstrated significant increases in social initiations and appropriate play behavior. Two of the children who did not make changes engaged in disruptive behaviors that prevented them from closely viewing the entire video. Another child watched the video but changes were not observed in his social interactions. The experimenters made another video for this child. The new video was recorded with the child himself as the "model actor." To make this video, the child was recorded while he received verbal prompting to imitate another child in the room who performed the desired words and actions. Although not stated in the study, self-modeling videos are typically edited so that the verbal prompts and reinforcement are omitted and the child is able to view himself/herself performing the desired social communication behaviors without prompts or cues (to make the execution of the behavior appear as natural as possible). Unfortunately, the child did not make changes with the self-video. However, self-modeling videos have been used successfully to change social engagement of children with ASD (Bellini and Akullian 2007; Bellini et al. 2007).

The study by Nikopoulos and Keenan (2003) reveals important considerations for use of video-based interventions including child characteristics, the advantages of video instruction relative to "live" (in vivo) modeling, the ability to have the child view himself or herself doing a series of social communication behaviors, and the brevity of video-based instruction. One prerequisite for this intervention strategy is that children should enjoy watching videos, particularly videos of themselves if self-modeling will be used. Children who are visual learners, i.e., children who respond to visual schedules and are more likely to follow directions when visual prompts are provided, are good candidates for this intervention (Sherer et al. 2001). The benefits of video modeling relative to "live" in vivo modeling are that children seem to attend more closely to videos than to live models, clinicians can edit out irrelevant stimuli and other distractions from videos, and video modeling may reduce anxiety for children who find live social interactions stressful (Bellini and Akullian 2007). If self-modeling is used, videos should be edited so that the child views himself or herself performing the skill without prompts or cues. If a clinician wishes to teach a series of social communication behaviors that the child is able to do but unable to perform sequentially (e.g., looking at someone, saying hi, and then asking a question), the clinician can splice segments of short video clips together so that the skill is executed in the proper sequence. Effective videos are usually short in duration, approximately 3 minutes or less (Bellini 2006). Moreover, children who respond to video-based instruction do so in a relatively brief period of time (i.e., a few weeks to several months; see Bellini 2006; Bellini and Akullian 2007; Kagohara 2010).

Video-based instruction has a growing evidence base. A recent meta-analysis of 48 single-subject design studies and one group study revealed that approximately half of the studies reported that children demonstrated positive increases in social communication skills within intervention settings. Perhaps more importantly, approximately half of these studies reported generalization of the children's positive changes in social behaviors to other settings, activities, and communication partners (Kagohara 2010). An important caveat for clinicians to consider is that many of these video-based instruction studies implemented additional intervention techniques, such as live modeling, social stories™, self-management techniques, verbal and visual instruction and feedback, and reinforcement. In summary, video-based instruction appears to be an effective method for teaching observable and measureable social communication skills especially when paired with additional intervention strategies.

Social Skills, Social Pragmatic, and Social Cognitive Intervention Packages

Researchers and clinicians frequently use multiple procedures and strategies to support the development and refinement of children's social communication skills. In the empirical literature, these comprehensive interventions are typically referred to as social skills, social communication, or social cognitive intervention packages. The use of the word "package" reflects the multiple components employed within these interventions including direct instruction to define and explain how to do the skill, modeling of the desired skill, role-play or practice of the skill, visual or verbal prompting to support the skill practice, a systematic plan to fade these prompts, corrective feedback, and praise or reinforcement for use of the skill (Timler et al. 2007). Table 14.3 provides examples from various intervention packages of social communication goals and teaching steps. Goals are included for teaching peer group entry, topic initiation, complimenting, and conversation skills (e.g., how to avoid asking too many questions, asking appropriate questions and producing relevant statements, and why and how to use eye contact to find out what someone is thinking so that you can make an appropriate comment in a conversation).

Although there is substantial overlap among the components used in social skills, social pragmatic, and social cognitive interventions, some important distinctions exist, particularly in the choice of social communication targets and procedures used to teach these targets. Social skill interventions typically target basic social communication skills such as initiations, turn-taking, and responding. Specific social communication situations may also be targeted including teaching children to greet others, enter peer groups, and to reduce negative disruptive behaviors in small group and classroom settings (e.g., see Beilinson and Olswang 2003; Leaf et. al 2009; Liber et al. 2008). Effective social skill interventions use predetermined methods

Table 14.3 Examples of social communication goals and teaching steps

Social communication goal	Teaching steps
Enter a peer play group in the classroom using nonverbal means (Beilinson and Olswang 2003)	Clinician uses modeling, role-play, and visual prompts to teach student to do the following steps: Walk over to your friend Watch your friend (to see what he/she is doing) Get a toy like your friend is using Do the same thing as your friend Say something about the toy (if the child is verbal)
Initiate a conversation with a peer (adapted from Liber et al. 2008)	Clinician uses modeling and role-play to teach student to do the following steps: Student approaches the peer and uses the peer's name The student waits for the peer to look at him or her, then the student turns his or her shoulders or face towards the peer The student produces a statement, request, or asks a question of the peer
Show appreciation to a peer (adapted from Leaf et al. 2009)	Student faces a peer and uses at least 2 seconds of eye contact Student says, "thank you" Student produces an appreciative comment such as, "I like it" Student maintains positive tone throughout conversation (e.g., smiles, uses intonation that is appropriate for the comment)
Decrease question asking in conversations by increasing the student's awareness of the intrusiveness of asking too many questions (adapted from Adams 2008)	Clinician and the student have a conversation whereby the clinician asks the student lots of questions about a topic without allowing the student time to answer Clinician and student talk about what just happened in the conversation including how the conversation made the student feel Clinician and student have another conversation; this time, the student role-plays asking too many questions Student and clinician discuss what happened in the conversation (e.g., too many questions, conversation not interesting, questions too difficult to answer, or did not need an answer because the information was already known to clinician and student, etc.) Student and clinician repeat the conversation activity using puppets—(example role-play: a detective who is asking questions about a stolen bike) Student and clinician discuss the role-play (e.g., "Did the detective ask too many questions?" "Were the questions relevant and useful?" "Did the detective ask you questions that you knew the answer to?" "Did he ask you things you couldn't possibly know?" "How many questions did he ask?") Student and clinician develop a set of rules about asking questions based on the discussions of the role-plays
Use eye contact to predict what someone is thinking and use this prediction to say something appropriate in a conversation (adapted from Winner 2006)	Clinician explains the purpose of "eye contact" including why you should look towards someone's face (e.g., to get more information about what the person is thinking and saying); In addition, the clinician contrasts "looking" versus "staring into someone's eyes"

Table 14.3 (continued)

Social communication goal	Teaching steps
	Student then practices eye contact while in a conversation with another communication partner; student uses the following steps during this practice: Student looks in the direction of the communication partner's face Student observes partner's facial expressions and interprets the meaning of those expressions Student listens to the words that the partner says Student says something that relates to the partner's facial expressions and words
Produce topic-relevant comments and questions in conversations (adapted from Brennan 2011)	Student brainstorms responses to the question, "What could you say to this person?" or "What do you think this person might enjoy talking about?" when presented with pictures of people engaged in an activity or with an object; student responses should include questions to ask the other person and relevant comments about the activity/object Student observes others at school and brainstorms potential conversation topics using the questions described above Student has a conversation with a person who he or she has observed using a previously "brainstormed" topic that the student believe the peer will find interesting

for prompt fading and reinforcement, reflecting the behavioral principles that are the foundation for these interventions (Adams 2008).

Social pragmatic intervention packages focus specifically on the linguistic and paralinguistic skills needed for topic management, reading of emotional and situational cues, and understanding social situations. The targets for these interventions include introducing new topics, maintaining topics, reading emotions in facial expressions, identifying emotions associated with a particular situation, using pronouns appropriately so that a listener clearly understands who or what is being discussed, monitoring listener interest in a conversation, and recognizing and repairing breakdowns in conversation (Adams 2008; Brennan 2011; Hoskins and Noel 2011; Thiemann and Goldstein 2004). Social pragmatic interventions are typically implemented by speech and language pathologists because these service providers have extensive training in the development and management of conversation skills (Paul 2008). Children with limited verbal skills as well as children who are highly verbal have been the recipients of social pragmatic interventions.

Social cognitive interventions address similar targets as social skills and social pragmatic interventions, but these interventions include additional procedures to teach older school-age children, adolescents, and young adults "why" a skill is needed. Immediate, explicit, and extensive feedback is provided for not only the skills that an individual is trying to learn but also how inappropriate or ineffective use of that skill will negatively influence the perceptions of their communication partners. Social cognitive interventions teach individuals with ASD to "read" the social cues of communication partners including interpretation of body language, facial expressions, and tone of voice. Because much of the instruction is verbally mediated, social cognitive interventions are best suited for highly verbal individuals with ASD who have intact language comprehension skills. Alternative names for these interventions include teaching interaction procedures (Dotson et al. 2010), cognitive behavioral interventions (National Autism Center 2009), and Social Thinking® interventions (Crooke 2008; Winner 2006).

In addition to teaching the rationale for use of various social communication skills, many social cognitive interventions include a counseling component to change negative or unrealistic thought patterns and behaviors (National Autism Center 2009). Adolescents and young adults with ASD frequently report higher levels of loneliness and social anxiety than their peers without ASD (Bauminger et al. 2003; Locke et al. 2010; Müller et al. 2008). The counseling component of social cognitive interventions aims to change individual's self-perceptions and increase self-esteem (Laugeson et al. 2009; National Autism Center 2009; Solomon et al. 2004; White et al. 2010). Relaxation strategies may also be taught to address anger management and social anxiety (Beaumont and Sofronoff 2008). For example, Laugeson et al. (2009) have developed a manualized parent-assisted intervention to improve friendship quality and social skills in teens with ASD (ages 13–17). The teen and parents receive 90 minutes of intervention for 12 weeks. The intervention targets include a diverse set of social skills and social pragmatic skills including conversational skills, peer entry and exiting skills, development of friendship networks, and good sportsmanship and host behaviors. In addition, teens are taught strategies for changing bad reputations and how to manage teasing, bullying, arguments and social anxiety.

Effective Social Communication Supports: Insider Perspectives

Qualitative interviews and biographies of adults with ASD reveal anecdotal support for the social communication strategies and interventions summarized in this chapter (Grandin 1995; Tammet 2006; Müller et al. 2008). When asked to describe effective supports for teaching social communication skills, adults with ASD report that the most helpful teachers were those who provided explicit explanation and procedures for "why" a particular social communication skill was important, "when" to use that skill, and "how" to use the skill. As one adult stated, "Just going to need you to spell it out literally. Not metaphorically. Not in a roundabout way. They're going to need a literal explanation" (Müller et al. 2008, p. 184). In addition to learning from teacher instruction, adults with ASD recall that watching others—siblings, peers, and colleagues at work—helped them to learn the nuances of managing social situations. Peer-mediated interventions, social stories™, script training, video-based instruction, and the comprehensive social communication intervention packages described in this chapter focus on explicit instruction, visualization, peer models, and explanation for the importance of the skill.

Most children and adolescents with ASD spend countless hours in intervention settings throughout their school careers. It is important to remember that participation in "normal" community activities with typically developing peers is as important as intervention participation. Adults with ASD report finding value and a reprieve from social isolation in community activities that provide an opportunity to explore shared interests with others (Grandin 1995; Müller et al. 2008; Tammet 2006). Such activities include scouting, intramural sports, 4-H, hiking and gaming clubs, and community service organizations. All children and adolescents learn social communication skills from interacting with others and individuals with ASD deserve opportunities to have this interaction in fun "nonintervention" activities. At the same time, respect for an individual's desire for "alone" time is needed as participation in social activities might be more taxing for individuals with ASD than those without ASD (Müller et al. 2008).

Most social communication interventions place the impetus for change on individuals with ASD (peer-mediated interventions are a notable exception here). Certainly, a more balanced approach is to promote awareness, acceptance, and celebration of the unique visions and contributions that individuals with ASD bring to everyday interactions. As one adult with ASD put it, "Someday, I hope people will realize what richness we have in our community" (Müller et al. 2008, p. 186).

References

Adams, C. (2008). Intervention for children with pragmatic language impairments. In C. Norbury, J. B. Tomblin, & D. Bishop (Eds.), *Understanding developmental language disorders: From theory to practice* (pp. 189–204). New York: Psychology Press.

American Psychiatric Association. (2010). *Diagnostic and statistical manual of mental health disorders* (5th ed.). Washington, DC: Author. http://www.dsm5.org/.

Bauminger, N., Shulman, C., & Agam, G. (2003). Peer interaction and loneliness in high-functioning children with autism. *Journal of Autism and Developmental Disorders, 33,* 489–507. doi:10.1023/A:1025827427901.2003-08460-00310.1023/A:1025827427901

Beaumont, R., & Sofronoff, K. (2008). A multi-component social skills intervention for children with Asperger syndrome: The junior detective training program. *The Journal of Child Psychology and Psychiatry, 49*(7), 743–753. doi: 10.111/j.1469-7610.2008.01920.x.

Beilinson, J., & Olswang, L. (2003). Facilitating peer-group entry in kindergartners with impairments in social communication. *Language, Speech, and Hearing Services in Schools, 34,* 154–166.

Bellini, S. (2006). Building social relationships: A systematic approach to teaching social interaction skills to children and adolescents with autism spectrum disorders and other social difficulties. Shawnee Mission: Autism Asperger Publishing Co.

Bellini, S., & Akullian, J. (2007). A meta-analysis of video modeling and video self-modeling interventions for children and adolescents with autism spectrum disorders. *Exceptional Children, 73*(3), 264–287.

Bellini, S., Akullian, J., & Hopf, A. (2007). Increasing social engagement in young children with autism spectrum disorders using video self-modeling. *School Psychology Review, 36*(1), 80–90.

Brennan, L. C. (2011). *Teaching perspective-taking skills to children with autism spectrum disorders.* Austin: Pro-ED.

Cannella-Malone, H., Fant, J., & Tullis, C. (2010). Using the picture exchange communication system to increase the social communication of two individuals with severe developmental disabilities. *Journal of Developmental and Physical Disabilities, 22*, 149–163. doi:.1007/s10882-009-9174-4.

Crooke, P., Hendrix, R., & Rachman, J. (2008). Brief report: Measuring the effectiveness of teaching social thinking to children with Asperger syndrome (AS) and high function autism (HFA). *Journal of Autism and Developmental Disorders, 38*, 581–591. doi:.1007/s10803-007-0466-1.

Dotson, W., Leaf, J., Sheldon, J., & Sherman, J. (2010). Group teaching of conversational skills to adolescents on the autism spectrum. *Research in Autism Spectrum Disorders, 4*, 199–209. doi: 10.1016/j.rasd.2009.09.005.

Flippin, M., Reszka, S., & Watson, L. (2010). Effectiveness of the picture exchange communication system (PECS) on communication and speech for children with autism spectrum disorders: A meta-analysis. *American Journal of Speech-Language Pathology, 19*, 178–195. doi: 10.1044/1058-0360(2010/09-0022).

Frost, L., & Bondy, A. (1994). *PECS training manual*. Newark: Pyramid Educational Consultants.

Garfinkle, A., & Schwartz, I. (1994, November). *PECS with peers: Increasing social interaction in an integrated preschool*. Paper presented at the annual convention for The Association for the Severely Handicapped, San Francisco.

Girolametto, L., Weitzman, E., & Sussman, F. (2007). Using case study methods to investigate the effects of interactive intervention for children with Autism Spectrum Disorders. *Journal of Communication Disorders, 40*(6), 470–492.

Grandin, T. (1995). *Thinking in pictures*. New York: Doubleday.

Goldstein, H., Schneider, N., & Thiemann, K. (2007). Peer-mediated social communication intervention: When clinical expertise informs treatment development and evaluation. *Topics in Language Disorders, 27*, 182–199.

Gray, C. (1995). Teaching children with autism to read social situations. In K. A. Quill (Ed.), *Teaching children with autism: Strategies to enhance communication and socialization* (pp. 219–242). New York: Delmar.

Gray, C. (2000). *The new social story book: Illustrated edition*. Arlington: Future Horizons.

Hoskins, B., & Noel, K. (2011). *Conversations framework: A program for adolescents & young adults*. Verona: Attainment Company, Inc.

Individuals with Disabilities Education Improvement Act. (2004). P.L. 108–446, 118 Stat. 2647.

Kagohara, D. (2010). Is video-based instruction effective in the rehabilitation of children with autism spectrum disorders? *Developmental Neurorehabilitation, 13*(2), 129–140.

Kamps, D., Kravits, T., & Ross, M. (2002). Social-communicative strategies for school-age children. In H. Goldstein, L. Kaczmarek, & K. English (Eds.), *Promoting social communication* (pp. 239–278). Baltimore: Brookes Publishing.

Karkhaneh, M., Clark, B., Ospina, M. B., Seida, J. C., Smith, V., & Hartling, L. (2010). Social stories™ to improve social skills in children with autism spectrum disorder. *SAGE Publications and The National Autistic Society, 14*(6), 641–662. doi: 10.1177-1362361310373057.

Kasari, C., Gulsrud, A. C., Wong, C., Kwon, S., & Locke, J. (2010). Randomized controlled caregiver mediated joint engagement intervention for toddlers with autism. *Journal of Autism and Developmental Disorders, 40*, 1045–1056. doi: 1007/s10803-010-0955-5.

Krantz, P. J., & McClannahan, L. E. (1993). Teaching children with autism to initiate to peers: Effects of a script-fading procedure. *Journal of Applied Behavior Analysis, 26*(1), 121–132

Laugeson, E., Frankel, F., Mogil, C., & Dillion, A. (2009). Parent-assisted social skills training to improve friendships in teens with autism spectrum disorders. *Journal of Autism and Developmental Disorders, 39*, 596–606. doi: 1007/s10803-008-0664-5.

Leaf, J., Taubman, M., Bloomfield, S., Palos-Rafuse, L., Leaf, R., McEachin, J., & Oppeneheim, M. (2009). Increasing social skills and pro-social behaviors for three children diagnosed with autism through the use of a teaching package. *Research in Autism Spectrum Disorders, 3*, 275–289. doi: 10.1016/j.rasd.2008.07.003.

Liber, D., Frea, W., & Symon, J. (2008). Using time-delay to improve social play skills with peers for children with autism. *Journal of Autism and Developmental Disorders, 38,* 312–323. doi: 10.1007/s10803-007-0395-z.

Locke, J., Ishijima, E., Kasari, C., & London, N. (2010). Loneliness, friendship quality and the social networks of adolescents with high-functioning autism in an inclusive school setting. *Journal of Research in Special Educational Needs, 10*(2), 74–81. doi: 10.1111/j.1471-3802.2010.01148.x.

McClannahan, L., & Krantz, P. (2005). *Teaching conversation to children with autism: Scripts and script fading*. Bethesda: Woodbine House.

McDuffie, A., & Yoder, P. (2010). Types of parent verbal responsiveness that predict language in young children with autism spectrum disorder. *Journal of Speech, Language, and Hearing Research, 53,* 1026–1039. doi: 10.1044/1092-4388(2009/09-0023).

Müller, E., Shuler, A., & Yates, G. B. (2008). Social challenges and supports from the perspective of individuals with Asperger syndrome and other autism spectrum disabilities. *SAGE Publications and The National Autistic Society, 12*(2), 173–190. doi: 10.1177136236130708664.

National Autism Center. (2009). *The national standards project.* Randolph: Author.

Nikopoulos, C. K., & Keenan, M. (2003). Promoting social initiation in children with autism using video modeling. *Behavioral Interventions, 18*(2), 87–108.

Ohio Center for Autism and Low Incidence (OCALI). *Peer-mediated instruction and intervention.* Retrieved October 10th, 2011 from www.autisminternetmodules.org.

Ozdemir, S. (2008). The effectiveness of social stories on decreasing disruptive behaviors of children with autism: Three case studies. *Journal of Autism and Developmental Disorders, 38,* 1689–1696.

Paul, R. (2008). *Social skills development in school-aged children with high-functioning autism spectrum disorders.* [Audio CD and manual]. Baltimore: American Speech, Language, and Hearing Association.

Sainato, D., Jung, S., Salmon, M., & Axe, J. (2008). Classroom influences on young children's emerging social competence. In W. Brown, S. Odom, & S. McConnell (Eds.), *Social competence of young children* (pp. 99–116). Baltimore: Brookes Publishing.

Schwartz, I., Garfinkle, A., & Bauer, J. (1998). The picture exchange communication system: Communicative outcomes for young children with disabilities. *Topics in Early Childhood Special Education, 18*(3), 144–159.

Sherer, M., Pierce, K. L., Paredes, S., Kisacky, K. L., Ingersoll, B., & Schreibman, L. (2001). Enhancing conversational skills in children with autism via video technology. Which is better, 'Self' or 'Other' as a model? *Behavior Modification, 25*(1), 140–158.

Shumway, S., & Wetherby, A. M. (2009). Communicative acts of children with autism spectrum disorders in the second year of life. *Journal of Speech, Language, and Hearing Research, 52,* 1139–1156.

Smith, T., Scahill, L., Dawson, G., Guthrie, D., Lord, C., Odom, S., Rogers, S., & Wagner, A. (2007). Designing research studies on psychosocial interventions in autism. *Journal of Autism and Developmental Disorders, 37*(2), 354–366.

Solomon, M., Goodlin-Jones, B. L., & Anders, T. F. (2004). A Social adjustment enhancement intervention for high functioning autism, asperger's syndrome, and pervasive developmental disorder NOS. *Journal of Autism and Developmental Disorders, 34,* 649–668.

Strain, P., Schwartz, I., & Bovey, E. (2008). Social competence interventions for young children with autism. In W. Brown, S. Odom, & S. McConnell (Eds.), *Social competence of young children* (pp. 253–272). Baltimore: Brookes Publishing.

Tammet, D. (2006). *Born on a blue day.* London: Free Press.

Thiemann, K. S., & Goldstein, H. (2004). Effects of peer training and written text cueing on social communication of school-age children with pervasive developmental disorder. *Journal of Speech, Language, and Hearing Research, 47,* 126–144. doi: 10.1044/1092–4388(2004/012).

Timler, G., Olswang, L., & Coggins, T. (2005). Social communication interventions for preschoolers: Targeting peer interactions during peer group entry and cooperative play. *Seminars in Speech and Language, 26*(3), 170–180.

Timler, G., Vogler-Elias, D., & McGill, F. (2007). Strategies for promoting generalization of social communication skills in preschoolers and school-aged children. *Topics in Language Disorders, 27,* 167–181.

Wallin, J. M. (2004). *Social Stories*. http://www.polyxo.com/socialstories/.

White, S. W., Albano, A. M., Johnson, C. R., Connie, K., Thomas, O., Klin, A., Scahill, L. (2010). Development of a cognitive-behavioral intervention program to treat anxiety and social deficits to teen with high-functioning autism. *Clinical Child and Family Psychological Review, 13,* 77–90. doi:1007/s10567-009-0062-3.

Winner, M. (2006). *Inside out: What makes a person with social cognitive deficits tick?* San Jose: Michelle Garcia Winner.

Yoder, P., & McDuffie, A. (2006).Treatment of responding to and initiating joint attention. In T. Charman & W. Stone (Eds.). *Social & communicative development in autism spectrum disorders* (pp. 117–142). New York: Guilford Press.

Chapter 15
Interventions in School, Home, and Community for Individuals with Autism Spectrum Disorders

Brenda Smith Myles

Over the past several years, society has been witness to attempts to quantify effectiveness. Triggered, in part, by federal and state governments and funding agencies as a means of assessing accountability, the term "evidence-based" has been applied to multiple entities, including medicine, management, mental health, and education. The area of autism spectrum disorders (ASDs) has also experienced this phenomenon as illustrated by the publication of four reports that have attempted to identify evidence-based practice (EBP) for children and youth with this exceptionality. This chapter will briefly (a) review the criteria used in these publications, (b) overview and describe interventions identified across the various reports, (c) briefly describe the interventions, and (d) provide a context for using EBPs.

Review of Criteria Used to Identify EBPs

The National Professional Development Center on ASD (NPDC on ASD 2009), the National Autism Center (NAC 2009), the Centers for Medicare and Medicaid Services (CMS 2010) independently conducted reviews of literature to identify interventions for individuals with ASD. Each identified specific criteria to identify interventions and support as EBP.

In order to determine whether studies on interventions were scientifically rigorous, the NPDC on ASD used the following criteria for articles on interventions used with individuals with ASD (excluding intervention packages): (a) at least two experimental or quasiexperimental group design studies carried out by independent investigators, (b) at least five single-case design studies from at least three independent investigators, or (c) a combination of at least one experimental/quasiexperimental study and three single-case design studies from independent

B. S. Myles (✉)
Ziggurat Group and Ohio Center for Autism and Low Incidence Disabilities,
11400 W. 155th Terrace Overland, Park, KS 66221-2606, USA
e-mail: Brenda_myles@mac.com

S. Goldstein, J. A. Naglieri (eds.), *Interventions for Autism Spectrum Disorders*,
DOI 10.1007/978-1-4614-5301-7_15,

investigators. Nomination of strategies was secured from NPDC on ASD staff and their advisory board. Searches by NPDC on ASD staff using educational and psychological databases were conducted for the targeted practices until the aforementioned number of single-case or group design studies were identified. Studies included individuals with ASD at the preschool, elementary, and secondary levels.

The authors of the second report (NAC 2009) conducted a search for EBP that included search engines, conference proceedings and abstracts, book chapters, and identification of abstracts by an expert panel. Identified practices were not initially excluded because of design or sample size and were inclusive of practices used with individuals with ASD from ages 0 to 21 years. The NAC developed a Scientific Merit Rating Scale that analyzed the following within an article: (a) research design, (b) measurement of the dependent variable, (c) measurement of the independent variable or procedural fidelity, (d) participant ascertainment, and (e) generalization. Each of these elements was subsequently rated on a 5-point Likert scale with scores of 3, 4, or 5 indicating scientific rigor. Articles were reviewed independently by field reviewers who were recognized leaders in ASD.

The third report, commissioned by the CMS (2010), sought to determine scientific evidence of the efficacy, effectiveness, safety, and availability of ASD-related psychosocial services and supports for children, transitioning youth, and adults with ASD. Manuscripts were identified through environmental scanning of health care literature databases, books, integrated reviews of literature, meta-analyses, unpublished reports, and conference proceedings. The process included an analysis of study quality using a modified Campbell Collaborative Rating System (Schuerman et al. 2002). Interventions were classified as evidence-based using the criteria adopted by the NPDC on ASD and the categories identified by the NAC.

Evidence-Based Interventions for Students with ASD

Table 15.1 lists interventions identified as effective in the NPDC on ASD, NAC, and CMS reports. As one of the three documents used different intervention terminology and descriptions, verbiage describing the practice from each report is included so that the reader can determine the level of overlap among the reports. A brief overview of the interventions follows. It should be noted that functional behavior assessment was identified as an EBP, but as it is not an intervention per se, it is not reviewed here.

Antecedent-Based Interventions

Antecedent-based interventions are those that are put into place prior to the occurrence of a behavior to increase the likelihood of success and/or to reduce the occurrence of problem behavior. There are multiple interventions in this category, including incorporating students' special interests into activities and priming. These are not discussed below.

Table 15.1 Evidence-based practices (EBP)

Intervention	CMS	NAC	NPDC
Antecedent-based interventions			
Antecedent package	0–16, 17–21	3–18	EC-MH
Behavioral interventions			
Behavioral package	0–16	0–21	
Comprehensive behavioral treatment for children	0–16	0–9	
Differential reinforcement			EC-MH
Discrete trial training			EC-E
Extinction			EC-MH
Prompting			EC-MH
Reinforcement			EC-MH
Response interruption and redirection			EC-MH
Task analysis			EC-MH
Time delay			E
Modeling			
Modeling	0–16	3–18	
Video modeling			EC-MH
Multicomponent interventions			
Joint attention intervention	0–16	0–5	
Multicomponent package	0–16		
Naturalistic teaching strategies	0–16	0–9	EC-MH
Parent-implemented interventions			EC-E
Peer training package	0–16	3–14	EC-E
Pivotal response treatment	0–16	3–9	EC-E
Structured teaching	0–16		EC-MH
Picture Exchange Communication System			
Picture Exchange Communication System	0–16		EC-E
Self-management			
Self-management	0–16	3–18	EC-MH
Social groups-based interventions			
Social communication intervention	0–16		
Social skills package		0–16	
Social skills groups			EC-MH
Social narratives			
Social narratives			EC-MH
Story-based intervention package	0–16	6–14	
Speech generating devices			
Speech generating devices			EC-MH
Technology-based interventions			
Technology-based treatment	0–16		
Computer-aided instruction			E-MH
Visual supports			
Visual supports			EC-MH
Schedules	0–16	3–14	

EC early childhood, *E* elementary, *MH* middle/high school, *CMS* Centers for Medicare and Medicaid Services, *NAC* National Autism Center, *NPDC* National Professional Development Center

Incorporating Special Interests into Activities

Special interests have been broadly used with students with ASD to increase social interactions, decrease behavior problems, and increase task performance (Vismara and Lyons 2007). Winter-Messiers (2007), evaluating the impact of special interest areas on individuals on the spectrum, found strong positive relationships between special interests and improvements in social, emotional expression, sensory-motor, and executive function.

Priming

Wilde et al. (1992) introduced priming for learners with ASD. The purposes of priming are to (a) familiarize the student with schedules, activities, and/or materials before their use and (b) introduce predictability into the information or activity in an attempt to reduce anxiety and behavioral challenges while increasing student success (Koegel et al. 2003). Priming can take place in the classroom or at home; however, it is most effective when built into the learner's routine (Schreibman et al. 2000). Priming typically involves showing the actual materials that will be used in a lesson the day or morning before the lesson. In some cases, priming may occur right before the activity, such as when a peer mentor overviews what will occur during the science experiment just prior to the beginning of the science class (Wilde et al. 1992).

Behavioral Interventions

Skinner introduced modern behaviorism in the early 1900s to address issues of behavior. Behavioral interventions are systematically applied interventions based on an analysis of antecedents (events prior to a behavior) and consequences (events occurring after a behavior). The purpose of these interventions is to improve socially significant behaviors, including reading, academics, social skills, communication, and adaptive living skills, to a meaningful degree and to demonstrate that the interventions are responsible for the improvement in behavior (Baer et al. 1968). Behavioral interventions include, but are not limited to, prompting, fading, shaping, chaining, reinforcement, differential reinforcement, response interruption and redirection, and contingency contracting. It is not uncommon that these interventions are used in tandem with one another (Troutman and Alberto 2009).

Modeling

Modeling involves learning skills through either real time (in vivo) or video observations (Stahmer et al. 2010). Based on Bandura's (1977) social learning theory that posits that individuals learn from watching each other, different types of modeling exist, including "*direct modeling* (simply copying the model), *synthesized modeling* (combining several observations to create a new behavior), and *symbolic modeling* (copying fictional characters from television, books, etc.)" (Aspy and Grossman 2012, p. 205).

A more recent form of modeling is video modeling. Several types of video modeling exist: (a) self as model, (b) adult as model, and (b) visual point of view. The latter is structured such that the learner observes the target behavior as if she were engaged in it. A meta-analysis found that video modeling was successful in teaching a variety of skills, including self-help, social, transition behaviors, play, on-task, and speech and language skills (Bellini and Akullian 2007). A recent review indicated that all types of video modeling resulted in successful acquisition of skills (McCoy and Hermansen 2007).

Multicomponent Interventions

Multicomponent interventions involve a combination of supports and strategies that can be based on one or more theoretical orientations. These include (a) naturalistic teaching strategies, (b) parent-implemented interventions, (c) peer-implemented interventions, and (d) pivotal response training (PRT). Comprehensive behavioral strategies, which can also be considered a multicomponent, are discussed under behavioral interventions.

Naturalistic Teaching Strategies

These strategies are developed from concerns related to applied behavior analysis (ABA) instruction resulting in (a) lack of spontaneous use and generalization of skills and (b) behavior instruction divorced from communication (Schreibman and Ingersoll 2005). Their focus is to provide functional skills that can be used in the learner's natural environments. Typically, short instructional sessions that are child directed are embedded into play sessions. The four most commonly used instructional strategies in naturalistic teaching are (a) modeling a response and correcting or expanding a child's interaction (see Modeling), (b) providing a verbal label that is supported in a desired object or activity, (c) providing time delay, and (d) incidental teaching that emphasizes intentionality by arranging the environment around preplanned learning objectives that include student preferences and "teachable moments" initiated by the learner (McGee and Daly 2007).

Parent-Implemented Interventions

The history of autism intervention contains multiple examples of parents as teachers for their children on the spectrum (Schopler and Reichler 1971). In fact, research has demonstrated repeatedly that parents can be effective instructional agents for their children (Meadan et al. 2009), highlighting the importance of home-based programs. Caregivers have taught their children (a) communication (Green et al. 2010), (b) joint attention (Jones et al. 2006), (c) social (Laugesen et al. 2008), (d) academic and preacademic (Rogers et al. 2006), (e) developmental (Ingersoll and Gergans 2007), and (f) environmental (Kashinath et al. 2006) skills.

Peer-Implemented Interventions

Involving neurotypical peers as instructors and facilitators for individuals with ASD is collectively known as peer-mediated interventions (Chan et al. 2009). Peer-mediated interventions, which incorporate myriad instructional strategies, occur when trained peers teach or support the use of academic or social skills for learners with special needs, including those with ASD. Interventions, which can occur in school or community, include (a) peer networks, (b) classwide peer buddy programs (Kamps et al. 1994), (c) peer buddy assignment (Bellini 2006), and (d) friendship clubs (Carter et al. 2004).

Pivotal Response Training

Developed by Koegel et al. (1999b), pivotal response training (PRT) is a naturalistic child- and family-centered intervention that is based on ABA. Through PRT, the individual with ASD learns (a) how to respond to multiple cues and stimuli, (b) how to self-regulate and manage behavior, and (d) how to initiate with others. Motivation of learners is critical in all instructional opportunities, thus reinforcement is built into the model. Although PRT focuses primarily on young children in early intervention, it is suitable for individuals with autism across age range and can be implemented by general and special education teachers, therapists, parents, or other professionals (Koegel et al. 1999a).

Structured Teaching

Structured teaching, the principle program of the Treatment and Education of Autistic and Communication handicapped Children (TEACCH) founded by Eric Schopler, was one of the first strength-based instructional approaches for learners with ASD (Mavropoulou et al. 2011). Program elements include the following:

1. *A structured and predictable environment and activities.* The physical environment is carefully arranged to minimize distractions, to create physical boundaries, and to create a predictable series of events.
2. *Visual supports.* Myriad visual structures, such as written directions, photographs, and pictures, are used to create organized work and living spaces,

3. *Meaningful, functional social communication.* TEACCH encourages the use of communication systems such as signs, pictures, and speech to facilitate expressive language.
4. *Special interests.* Special interests are incorporated throughout the learner's program as instructional materials and reinforcers to increase motivation and encourage learning.

Structured teaching is founded on research-based principles and is appropriately considered to be an EBP because of the multiple studies that have been conducted on the model (for a review of these studies, see Aspy and Grossman 2012).

Picture Exchange Communication System

Picture exchange communication system (PECS) is a behavior-based augmentative and alternative communication (AAC) program that has been used to increase the communication skills of learners with ASD (Tien 2008). PECS requires learners to exchange a picture symbol(s) to communicate with others. Training includes six phases: (a) teaching the exchange of a picture symbol, (b) expanding spontaneity of the exchange and increasing the distance between the learner and his communicative partner, (c) discriminating between picture symbols, (d) making or using sentences, (e) responding to questions, and (f) commenting. PECS training begins with a reinforcer assessment that serves as the foundation for communication. Two instructors are involved in the process: one is the learner's communicative partner and the other prompts the learner. Physical prompts are used and are faded as quickly as possible (Bondy and Frost 1994).

Self-Management

Self-management procedures are designed to teach learners to self-initiate, select reinforcers, monitor performance, evaluate performance, and deliver reinforcers (Aspy and Grossman 2012). Many components have become a part of the self-management process: peer training, contingency contracts, token economy, pictures, and video (Southall and Gast 2011). Designed to teach choice making and self-advocacy (Paradiz 2008), self-management encourages independence. It also addresses a common concern experienced by individuals with ASD—generalization (Deitchman et al. 2010). These procedures have been used to address (a) time on task (Agran et al. 2005), (b) appropriate behavior (Mruzek et al. 2007), (c) task completion (Ganz and Sigafoos 2005), (d) communication (Delano 2007), and (e) social skills (Palmen et al. 2008). A review of studies on self-management revealed that these procedures have been successful regardless of components, learner's age, and learner's cognitive level (Southall and Gast 2011).

Table 15.2 Promising components to include in social skills instruction. (Adapted from White et al. 2007)

Focus on self-awareness and self-esteem	Use natural reinforcers
Develop a motivating environment	Model and role-play strategies
Start with easily learned skills	Use clear, concrete social rules
Provide practice opportunities in natural settings	Differentially reinforce positive behaviors or attempts
Teach social scripts for common situations	Review socially appropriate and inappropriate behaviors
Use a structured format	Use behavior charts
Including multiple trainers, peers, and parents in training	Intersperse new skills, homework, and previously mastered skills

Social Interventions

Interventions that target social skills in a group or individual format have been shown to positively impact the functioning of learners on the spectrum. Social interventions have included the use of social narratives, peers, technology, naturalistic procedures, video modeling, reinforcement, self-management, PRT, and incidental teaching (see discussion of each in this chapter). From an analysis of the research on social skills, White et al. (2007) identified strategies that appear promising for learners on the spectrum. These are included in Table 15.2. According to Koenig et al. (2009), "... the most successful [social skills group] interventions used multiple training sessions, modeling, and naturally occurring and direct reinforcement" (p. 1165). Manualization, a quality indicator in social skills and other intervention research (Smith et al. 2007), is becoming increasingly apparent. Two types appear in the social skills research: treatment manuals developed specifically for individuals on the spectrum (Koenig et al. 2009; White et al. 2007) and those adapted for use with other populations (Webb et al. 2004).

Social Narratives

Social narratives provide learners with information about social situations, such as what may occur or what to expect, when something may occur, what the learner can do in a given situation, what the learner should try not to do in a given situation, and so forth. Typically they (a) are written in the first person; (b) provide for flexibility and the possibility of change using words such as *may*, *probably, usually, will try to*, and *might*; and (c) are developed and presented in a manner appropriate to the learner, whether through the use of words only, pictures only, or a combination of the two. Comic Strip Conversations™ (Gray 1994), Power Cards (Gagnon 2001), social autopsies (LaVoie 1994), social scripts (Wichnick et al. 2010), Social Stories™ (Gray 1995), and social scripts (Wichnick et al. 2010) are all social narratives. Table 15.3 describes these social narratives.

Table 15.3 Descriptions of types of social narratives

Type	Brief description
Comic strip conversations™	This intervention uses thought bubbles, conversation bubbles, cartoon, or stick figures to illustrate people's thoughts and words during interactions in a comic strip format. Gray (1994) developed guidelines for this intervention, including the use of colors to illustrate emotions
Power Card Strategy	Based on a student's special interest, the Power Card Strategy contains two components: (a) a text-based scenario that describes a target behavior associated with a special interest area and how that individual addresses the target behavior and encourages the student to use the strategy employed by the person of special interest, and (b) a small card, the size of a baseball or business card, that synthesizes the text-based scenario (Gagnon 2001)
Social autopsies	An adult-directed exchange between a student and mentor in which a social error is defined and methods of (a) making amends and/or (b) interacting successfully in future events are discussed (LaVoie 1994)
Social Stories™	Developed by Gray (1995), these written stories inform or describe an activity and the anticipated behavior associated with it. They also provide information to teach appropriate social behaviors. Gray developed specific guidelines regarding types of sentences, language level, audience, and use
Social scripts	Written sentences or paragraphs that contain brief descriptions and text that can be used verbatim in academic and/or nonacademic settings

Speech Generating Devices

Programmable devices with a voice output function have become increasingly available in school settings for learners with speech production challenges, including those with ASD. Using digitized or synthesized speech, speech generating devices (SGDs) have distinct advantages in which they approximate the communication style of potential communicative partners and thus can readily obtain the attention of and responses from others (Trottier et al. 2011). Underlying the effectiveness of SGD are prerequisite skills. According to Kagohara et al. (2010), "First, users must be able to visually discriminate among icons so as to be able to select the correct one from a visual display. Second, the user must also be able to select icons with a response topography that will result in activation of the associated speech output" (p. 334). A variety of instructional strategies, including prompting, modeling, and reinforcement have been shown effective in teaching both skills (Rispoli et al. 2010; Van der Meer and Rispoli 2010). In addition, an emerging literature base reports that peer-mediated instruction may be effective in supporting SGD use of learners with ASD in school settings (Trottier et al. 2011). Similarly, family support of SGD has resulted in children with ASD increasing communication skills (Thunberg et al. 2009). Rispoli et al. (2010), in their review of studies that involved the use of SGDs, found that they were successful in teaching communication skills to children with ASD. Ganz et al. (2012) reported that these ACC supports were effective in increasing requesting, conversational skills, labeling, and receptive language of learners with ASD.

Technology-Based Interventions

The term "assistive technology" appears in the Individuals with Disabilities Education Amendment (2004) and refers any item, piece of equipment, or product system that is used to increase, maintain, or improve the functional capability of an individual with special needs. Assistive technology (AT) devices can be electronic or nonelectronic. Nonelectronic strategies typically include low-cost and easy-to-use equipment, such as dry-erase boards, laminated photographs, photo albums, natural aided language boards (Cafiero 2001), and so forth. Electronic technology devices can range from simple electronic devices, such as tape recorders, voice output devices, timers, and calculators to more complex and costly, such as computers, digital cameras, video cameras, and complex voice output devices (Texas Statewide Leadership on Autism Training 2011).

Recent advances have made the latter more accessible to learners with ASD and, in fact, are compatible with the way that children with ASD learn (Moore et al. 2000). Electronic technology can change instructional pace and highlight and repeat critical information, thus providing instruction in a controlled format (Doyle and Arnendillo-Sánchez 2011). Not only is technology compatible with the learning style of those with ASD, it may be the preferred manner to receive instruction. Research has shown that the learners on the spectrum may prefer electronically presented information, may learn more quickly with technology, and may be more motivated than when accessing traditional adult-directed instruction (Stromer et al. 2006).

Increasingly more popular for learners on the spectrum (and neuroytpical individuals, alike) are computers and personal digital assistants, including iPods. These can contain multiple prompt levels to increase various skills, including task completion, transitioning between tasks, social skills, communication, and following a schedule (Mechling and Savidge 2011; Wainer and Ingersoll 2011). Pennington (2010), in a review of the literature on using computer-assisted instruction to teach academic skills to learners on the spectrum, concluded that its results were promising but did not meet the criteria for evidence based. Similarly, Reed et al. (2011) reviewed technology applications to teach social skills and found that half of the 20 technology studies centered on video/DVD use and reported that "there is little research focusing on the efficacy and efficiency of the use of technology in this context, particularly within schools" (p. 1008).

A new technology is virtual reality (VR) that provides a computer-generated, three-dimensional, interactive environment. Based on the idea that multimodal processing is more effective than single mode, VR creates a computer-generated environment that resembles the real world and promotes a sense of presence for the user. Thus, people can visualize, manipulate, and interact with simulated environments. The research on VR appears promising (Cheng et al. 2010).

Visual Supports

Numerous types of visual supports have been used with students with ASD, including visual schedules, lists, signals/cues, labels, boundary markers, and maps. The most commonly used visual support is the visual schedule. Similar to all visual supports, the complexity of schedules varies across student need. "The use of schedules may be as simple as (1) placing pictures/texts on the board at the time of the activity, (2) pointing to the activity while engaging in the activity, (3) taking the picture off the board, and (4) placing it in a done/completed/finished bin/bucket/box/pile. More advanced schedules may involve the student crossing out the activity she has completed, much as you would do with your own 'to do' list. Some schedules also include photos of the staff involved in the activity, location details, and materials that are needed" (NAC 2009, pp. 61–62). Visual supports have been introduced to learners with ASD as a means of positively impacting behavior challenges, communication, leisure activities, daily living skills, social behavior, and vocational skills (Wheeler et al. 2006).

Comprehensive Planning

An understanding of EBPs in isolation has been established. However, in order to maximize educational benefit, "... evidence-based practices must be carefully selected to meet student needs AND they must be implemented well" (Fixsen et al. 2009, p. 5) in all educational settings. It takes cohesive team planning, clearly defined objectives, and professional development of all personnel to ensure that the chosen evidence-based strategies are implemented with fidelity and across all settings. This can best be accomplished by using two linked comprehensive planning models—the Ziggurat Model (Aspy and Grossman 2012) and the Comprehensive Autism Planning System (CAPS; Henry and Myles 2007)—that meets these goals. The CAPS, as well as the Ziggurat Model, is applicable from early intervention to adulthood across home, school, employment, university or postsecondary training, and community. Figure 15.1 depicts the process of comprehensive planning.

The Ziggurat Model

The Ziggurat Model is a comprehensive planning model for individuals with ASD based on the premise. In order for a program to be successful for an individual with ASD, his unique needs and strengths must be identified and then directly linked to interventions (Aspy and Grossman 2012). This model utilizes students' strengths to address true needs or underlying challenges in the context of the underlying ASD that result in social, emotional, and behavioral concerns. In doing so, the Ziggurat Model approach centers on a hierarchical system consisting of five levels: Sensory

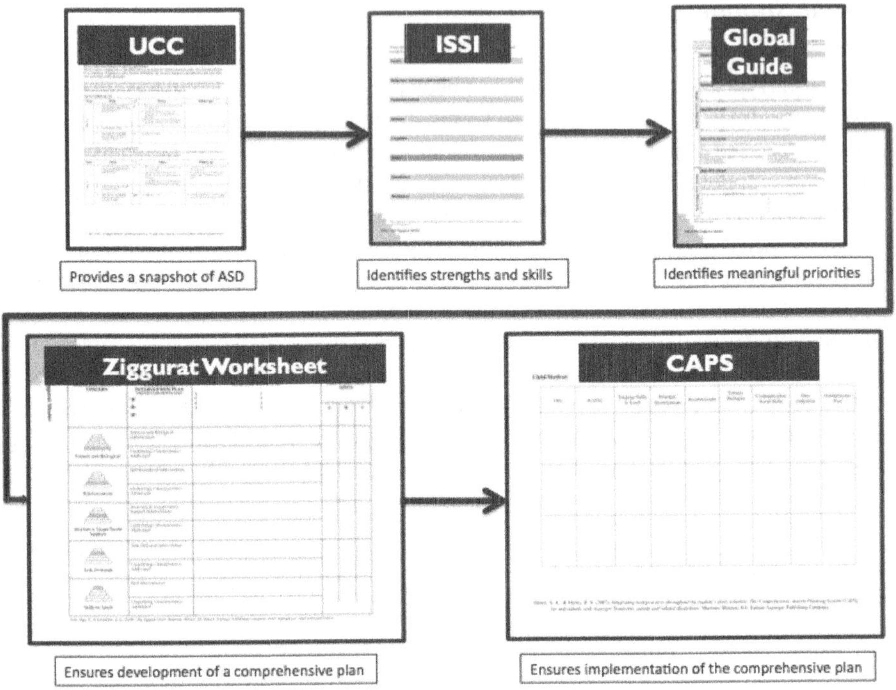

Fig. 15.1 Process of comprehensive planning using the Ziggurat Model and CAPS (Used with permission: www.aapcpublishing.net)

Differences and Biological Needs, Reinforcement, Structure and Visual/Tactile Supports, Task Demands, and Skills to Teach that must be addressed for an intervention plan to be comprehensive.

Underlying Characteristics Checklist (UCC)

Aspy and Grossman's (2012) Ziggurat Model approach targets an individual's specific needs as defined by ASD characteristics. This leads to interventions that are proactive and effective. The UCC in its three forms (CL for classic autism, HF for high functioning ASD, and EI for early intervention) offers a comprehensive perspective as a basis for program planning. Designed to be completed by parents, teachers, or other service providers, individually or as a team, the UCCs target eight areas. The first three represent the traditional autism spectrum triad: social, restricted patterns of behavior interests and activities, and communication. Characteristics associated with ASD are addressed in the next five areas: sensory differences, cognitive differences, motor differences, emotional vulnerability, and known medical and other biological factors.

Individual Strengths and Skills Inventory

Completed concurrently with the UCC is the Individual Strengths and Skills Inventory (ISSI), which ensures that an individual's underlying strengths and skills are incorporated in the intervention design process. The ISSI parallels the areas addressed in the UCC (Aspy and Grossman 2012).

Global Intervention Plan

The global intervention plan helps users complete a person-centered plan by identifying short- and long-term goals and targeting the UCC areas and items that would have the greatest impact on the individual's ability to be an independent self-advocate and experience a sense of well-being across multiple environments. Thus, the learner's educational plan is tied directly to leading a self-determined life as an adult replete with opportunities, happiness, and other aspects related to a high quality of life (Wigham et al. 2008).

Intervention Ziggurat

The centerpiece of the Ziggurat Model is the Intervention Ziggurat (IZ). Designed to help parents and educators avoid overlooking critical areas that impact the effectiveness of any intervention plan as they build a comprehensive program, the IZ comprises five critical levels structured into a hierarchy: (a) Sensory Differences and Biological Needs, (b) Reinforcement, (c) Structure and Visual/Tactile Supports, (d) Task Demands, and (e) Skills to Teach. The first level, Sensory Differences and Biological Needs, addresses basic internal factors that impact functioning. The second level, Reinforcement, addresses motivational needs prerequisite to skill development. The third level, Structure and Visual/Tactile Supports, draws on visual processing strengths and the fundamental need for order and routine in ASD. The final two levels of the IZ, Task Demands and Skills to Teach, emphasize the importance of expectations and skill development relative to the characteristics of individuals with ASD. Each level is essential and contributes to the effectiveness of the others. Thus, if needs on all levels are not addressed, the intervention will not be as effective and skills will not develop. Using the aforementioned information, the team uses the Ziggurat Worksheet to guide them through the development of a comprehensive intervention plan, matching prioritized ASD-related needs indentified with the UCC, strengths and skills listed on the ISSI, and long- and short-term goals described on the Global Intervention Plan to interventions across the levels of the Ziggurat. After completion of the Ziggurat Worksheet, the team is ready to discuss how these interventions will be embedded throughout the school day. While the Ziggurat Worksheet allows a team to know that the intervention plan is thorough and targeted, the CAPS provides a structure for implementation, as detailed further below.

Comprehensive Autism Planning System

CAPS provides an overview of a student's daily schedule by time and activity and specifies supports needed during each period. Based on information developed using the Ziggurat Model, CAPS provides a framework for listing a student's tasks and activities and the times they occur, along with a delineation of the supports needed for success. In addition, it includes a place for recording the results of ongoing data collection and consideration of how skills are to be generalized to others settings. CAPS contains the following components:

1. *Time*. This section indicates the clock time of each of the learner's activities.
2. *Activity*. Academic periods (e.g., reading), nonacademic times (e.g., recess, lunch) as well as transitions between classes are all considered activities.
3. *Targeted Skills to Teach*. This may include Individualized Education Program goals, state standards, and/or skills that lead to school success for a given student.
4. *Structure/Modifications*. Structures/modifications can consist of a wide variety of supports, including placement in the classroom, visual supports, and peer networks.
5. *Reinforcement*. Student access to specific types of reinforcement and reinforcement schedules are listed here.
6. *Sensory Strategies*. Sensory supports and strategies listed in this CAPS area.
7. *Communication/Social Skills*. Specific communication and social supports are delineated in this section.
8. *Data Collection*. This space is for recording the type of data as well as the behavior to be documented during a specific activity.
9. *Generalization Plan*. This section of the CAPS was developed to ensure that generalization of skills is built into the child's program.

Applicability of the Ziggurat Model and CAPS: A Brief Case Study

The following study describes how the Ziggurat Model and CAPS were used with Derek, a 15-year-old with ASD who is in the third quarter of his freshman year of high school. He attends all general education classes, including biology, history, English literature, algebra, composition, and physical education (PE). His schedule also includes a daily support period where he is given assistance with organizational and social skills. Derek, a visual learner, has a special interest in sports statistics and memorabilia. He has memorized a plethora of statistics of almost every Major League baseball player and often cites those statistics in conversation. Derek does well when expectations, directions, and schedules are presented in a written as opposed to a verbal form. He is extremely sensitive to sound and has difficulty reading facial expressions and body language. Although Derek has an intelligence quotient in the above-average range, he receives primarily C's and D's because a significant

Global Intervention Plan: Guide to Establishing Priorities: Derek
Ruth Aspy, Ph.D., and Barry G. Grossman, Ph.D.

Directions: Following completion of the UCC and ISSI, the next step is to identify UCC **areas** and **items** that will result in a *meaningful* Global Intervention Plan. Consideration of priorities and strengths for an individual facilitates selection of UCC areas and items. The following questions are provided as a guide.

Selecting UCC Areas

Vision "Begin with the end in mind" – Stephen R. Covey

- What is the short and long-term vision of/for the individual?

Note that "short-term" and "long-term" may be defined differently in order to be meaningful.

Short term:
Play independently (currently requires prompting); pretend play; increase communication skills – follow two-part directions; use four-word sentences; communicate with same-age peers
Long term (3 years):
Attend junior college; have at least good friend; drive; go out with friends

◉ Which UCC **areas** would have the greatest impact on achieving this vision?

Social, Communication, Sensory, Cognitive, Emotional Vulnerability

Settings

- In what settings does the individual participate?

School, home, family,

◉ Which UCC **areas** have the greatest impact on the individual's ability to function in multiple settings?

Communication, Sensory Differences, Social Emotional Vulnerability

Quality of Life

- What is most important to the individual? What provides a sense of well-being?

Consider independence, relationships, play/leisure activities, safety, health, etc.

Sports information, having a match between his and others' perspectives, predictability, a friend

◉ Which UCC **areas** have the greatest impact on the individual's quality of life?

Social, Cognitive, Emotional, Vulnerability, Sensory, Communication

Key UCC Areas

Based on your answers to the questions above, place a check **X** next to the key UCC **areas**.
*Transfer to the **Areas of Concern** section of the Ziggurat Worksheet.*

☒ Social	☒ Cognitive Differences
☐ Restricted Patterns of Behavior Interests, and Activities	☐ Motor Differences
☒ Communication	☒ Emotional Vulnerability
☒ Sensory Differences	☐ Known Medical or Other Biological Factors

Selecting UCC Items

Key UCC Items

Select key UCC **items** for *each* of the UCC **areas** listed above. Choose items that are essential (necessary for progress) and developmentally appropriate. Emphasize items that are more pivotal (building blocks for additional skills). Avoid selecting redundant items.
Write key item numbers and descriptions below. These items will be used to develop interventions keeping strengths and skills (identified on the ISSI) in mind.
*Transfer items to the **Selected UCC Item** section of the Ziggurat Worksheet. Develop interventions.*

# 1 Mindblindness	# 42 Responds in unusual manner to sounds, pain, and touch
# 9 Difficulty understanding others' nonverbal communication	# 53 Has poor organizational skills
# 25 Difficulty with rules of conversation	# 89 Difficulty managing stress and anxiety
# 28 Has difficulty starting, joining, and/or ending a conversation	
# 39 Difficulty talking about others' interests	

Fig. 15.2 Global Intervention Plan: guide to establishing priorities: Derek (Used with permission: www.aaapcpublishing.net)

portion of his grades is based on homework assignments that he forgets to record in his planner and, as a result, fails to complete and turn in. Derek also experiences challenges in PE, where he becomes increasingly anxious where the noise level is loud. When participating in team sports, he removes himself from the game and sits on the sidelines. When his teacher approaches him to discuss the situation, Derek

ZIGGURAT WORKSHEET: DEREK (PARTIAL)
RUTH ASPY, PH.D., AND BARRY GROSSMAN, PH.D.

AREAS OF CONCERN	SPECIFIC INTERVENTION PLAN	PRIORITIZED UCC ITEMS		CHECK ALL THAT APPLY		
				A	B	C
Social, Communication, Sensory, Cognitive, Emotional Vulnerability	Operationalized Behaviors	# [1] Mindblindness # [9] Difficulty understanding others' nonverbal communication # [25] Difficulty with rules of conversation # [28] Has difficulty starting, joining, and/or ending a conversation	# [39] Difficulty talking about others' interests # [42] Responds in unusual manner to sounds, pain, and touch # [53] Has poor organizational skills # [89] Difficulty managing stress and anxiety			
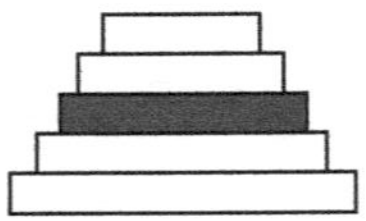 Structure & Visual/Tactile Supports	Structure and Visual/Tactile Supports Interventions:	*Antecedent Based:* Use stress thermometer to teach Derek about anxiety and to recognize signs that indicate that he needs to use coping strategies. Prompt Derek to monitor/recognize his stress level. *Visual Support:* Use coping cards. Provide reinforcement for prompted and unprompted use of cards. Fade prompts. Provide written rules. Provide a problem solving flow chart as a visual support for Derek. Create task cards that break assignments/activity steps into smaller segments. Provide Derek with a list of conversation cues in his binder. Reinforce use. Use homework checklist to assist Derek in keeping up with assignments and materials required to complete his homework. Use calendar to break down large assignments into smaller parts with separate due dates. Provide copies of notes for lectures; Derek will highlight items covered during lecture. Use a Travel Card to track (a) assignment completion, (b) homework turned in, (c) emotional regulation, (d) bringing supplies in class. Fade from teacher responsibility to student responsibility. *Social Narrative:* Use narratives to teach Derek about interrupting and about how people have different interests. Use cartooning to help Derek understand what the listener (whole class) is thinking and feeling when he interrupts or dominates a conversation. *Video Modeling:* Use video to help Derek learn conversational manners and related skills.		√	√	√
	Underlying Characteristics	[1] Mindblindness, [25] Difficulty with rules of conversation, [28] Has difficulty starting, joining, and/or ending a conversation, Difficulty talking about others' interests, [53] Has poor organizational skills, [89] Difficulty managing stress and anxiety				

Fig. 15.3 Ziggurat Worksheet: Derek (partial) (Used with permission: www.aapcpublishing.net)

COMPREHENSIVE AUTISM PLANNING SYSTEM: Derek
Shawn Henry and Brenda Smith Myles

Activity	Targeted Skills to Teach	Structure/ Modifications	Reinforcement	Sensory Strategies	Communication/ Social Skills	Data Collection	Generalization
PE	Participation in group sports Accepting loss	Calendar of competitive events Written sportsmanship rules Task cards	Social reinforcement 15 minutes on the computer for accepting loss and participating	Ear plugs Coping cards Stress thermometer Breaks	Game statistician Trained peer buddy Social narrative on accepting loss	Time in PE (min daily) Number of meltdowns (daily)	Task cards in Scouts

Fig. 15.4 Comprehensive Autism Planning System: Derek (Used with permission: www.aapcpublishing.net)

insists that his peers are intentionally trying to hurt him. Recently, these situations have increased in both number and intensity. His teacher thinks that Derek is a "sore loser." Derek's multidisciplinary team, including his parents, met to develop his program. Presented here is only one aspect of this program related to PE. His complete program can be viewed at www.texasautism.com. Following completion of a UCC-HF and ISSI, then team finalized a Global Intervention Plan to prioritize areas of need (see Fig. 15.2). Using information from these activities, Derek's team completed the Ziggurat Worksheet (see partial copy in Fig. 15.3). Finally, they created a CAPS to embed interventions and supports throughout Derek's school day (Derek's CAPS for PE class appears in Fig. 15.4).

Summary

To maximize educational benefit, practices must be used competently and consistently (Fixsen et al. 2009). Lastly, measurement of those skills with a vision of the effect on the student now and in the future is a final critical step, if sustained change is to be achieved (National Research Council 2001). Such implementation usually requires changes in the daily activities of staff, related service providers, administrators, and even parents. It takes cohesive team planning, clearly defined objectives, and professional development of all personnel to ensure that the chosen evidence-based strategies are implemented with fidelity and across all settings. EBPs combined with the Ziggurat Model and CAPS provide a vehicle by which this can occur.

References

Agran, M., Sinclair, T., & Alper, S. (2005). Using self-monitoring to increase following direction skills of students with moderate to severe disabilities in general education. *Education and Training in Developmental Disabilities, 40,* 3–13.

Aspy, R., & Grossman, B. G. (2012). *The Ziggurat model: A framework for designing comprehensive interventions for individuals with high-functioning autism and Asperger Syndrome (2.0)*. Shawnee Mission: Autism Asperger.

Baer, D. M., Wolf, M. M., & Risley, T. R. (1968). Some current dimensions of applied behavior analysis. *Journal of Applied Behavior Analysis, 1,* 91–97.

Bandura, A. (1977). *Social learning theory*. Englewood Cliffs: Prentice Hall.

Bellini, S. (2006). *Building social relationships: A systematic approach to teaching social interaction skills to children and adolescents with autism spectrum disorders and other social difficulties*. Shawnee Mission: Autism Asperger.

Bellini, S., & Akullian, J. (2007). A meta-analysis of video modeling and video self-modeling interventions for children and adolescents for children and adolescents with autism spectrum disorders. *Exceptional Children, 73,* 264–287.

Bondy, A. S., & Frost, L. A. (1994). The Picture Exchange Communication System. *Focus on Autistic Behavior, 9*(3), 1–19.

Cafiero, J. (2001). The effect of an augmentative communication intervention on the communication, behavior, and academic program of an adolescent with autism. *Focus on Autism and Other Developmental Disabilities, 16,* 179–189.

Carter, C., Meckes, L., Pritchard, L., Swensen, S., Wittman, P., & Velde, B. (2004). The friendship club: An after-school program for children with Asperger syndrome. *Family & Community Health, 27,* 143–150.

Centers for Medicare and Medicaid Services. (2010). *Autism spectrum disorders: Final report on environmental scan.* Washington DC: Author.

Chan, J. M., Lang, R., Rispoli, M., O'Reilly, M., Sigafoos, J., & Cole, H. (2009). Use of peer mediated interventions in the treatment of autism spectrum disorders: A systematic review. *Research in Autism Spectrum Disorders, 3,* 876–889.

Cheng, Y., Chiang, H., Ye, J., & Cheng, L. (2010). Enhancing empathy instruction using a collaborative virtual learning environment for children with autistic spectrum conditions *Computer & Education, 55,* 1449–1458.

Deitchman, C., Reeve, S. A., Reeve, K. F., & Progar, P. R. (2010). Incorporating video feedback into self-management training to promote generalization of social initiations by children with autism. *Education and Treatment of Children, 33,* 475–488.

Delano, M. (2007). Improving written language performance of adolescents with Asperger syndrome. *Journal of Applied Behavior Analysis, 40,* 345–351.

Doyle, T., & Arnedillo-Sanchez, I. (2011). Using multimedia to reveal the hidden code of everyday behavior to children with autistic spectrum disorders (ASDs). *Computers and Education, 56,* 357–369.

Fixsen, D., Blasé, K., Horner, R., & Sugai, C. (2009). *Concept paper: Develop the capacity for scaling up the effective use of evidence-based programs in state departments of education.* Unpublished document, University of North Carolina, Chapel Hill.

Gagnon, E. (2001). *Power cards: Using special interests to motivate children and youth with Asperger Syndrome and autism.* Shawnee Mission: Autism Asperger.

Ganz, J. B., & Sigafoos, J. (2005). Self-monitoring: Are young adults with MR and autism able to utilize cognitive strategies independently? *Education and Training in Developmental Disabilities, 40*(1), 24–33.

Ganz, J. B., Earles-Vollrath, T. L., Heath, A. K., Parker, R. I., Rispoli, M. J., & Duran, J. B. (2012). A meta-analysis of single case research studies on aided augmentative and alternative communication systems with individuals with autism spectrum disorders. *Journal of Autism and Developmental Disorders, 42*(1), 60–74. doi: 10.1007/s10803-011-1212-2. http://www.springerlink.com/. Accessed 3 Jan 2012.

Gray, C. A. (1994). *Comic strip conversations: Illustrated interactions that teach conversation skills to students with autism and related disorders.* Texas: Future Horizons.

Gray, C. (1995). *Writing social stories with Carol Gray.* Arlington: Future Horizon.

Green, J., Charman, T., McConachie, H., Aldred, C., Slonims, V., Howlin, P., LeCouiteur, A., Leasbitter, K., Hudry, K., Byford, S., Barrett, B., Temple, K., MacDonald, W., & Pickles, A. (2010). Parent-mediated communication-focused treatment in children with autism (PACT): A randomized controlled trial. *Lancet, 375,* 2152–2160.

Henry, S. A., & Myles, B. S. (2007). *The comprehensive autism planning systems (CAPS) for individuals with Asperger Syndrome, autism and related disabilities: Integrating best practices throughout the student's day.* Shawnee Mission: Autism Asperger.

Individuals with Disabilities Education Act Amendments, (2004) § 300.5.

Ingersoll, B., & Gergans, S. (2007). The effect of a parent implemented imitation intervention on spontaneous imitation skills in young children with autism. *Research in Developmental Disabilities, 28,* 163–175.

Jones, E. A., Carr, E. G., & Feeley, K. M. (2006). Multiple effects of joint attention intervention for children with autism. *Behavior Modification, 30,* 782–834.

Kagohara, D.M., van der Meer, L., Achmadi, D., Green, V.A., O'Reilly, M.F., Mulloy, A., Lancioni, G.E., Lang, R., & Sigafoos, J. (2010). Behavioral intervention promotes successful use of an iPod-based communication device by an adolescent with autism. *Clinical Case Studies, 9(5),* 328–338.

Kamps, D. M., Barbetta, P. M., Leonard, B. R., & Delquadri, J. (1994). Classwide peer tutoring: An integration strategy to improve reading skills and promote peer interactions among students with autism and general education peers. *Journal of Applied Behavior Analysis, 27*(1), 49–61.

Kashinath, S., Woods, J., & Goldstein, H. (2006). Enhancing generalized teaching strategy use in daily routines by parents of children with autism. *Journal of Speech, Language, Hearing Research, 49,* 466–485.

Koegel, R. L., Koegel, L. K., & Carter, C. M. (1999a). Pivotal teaching interactions for children with autism. *School Psychology Review, 28,* 576–594.

Koegel, L. K., Koegel, R. L., Harrower, J. K., & Carter, C. M. (1999b). Pivotal response intervention I: Overview of approach. *Journal of the Association for Persons with Severe Handicaps, 24,* 174–185.

Koegel, L. K., Koegel, R. L., Frea, W., & Green-Hopkins, I. (2003). Priming as a method of coordinating services for students with autism. *Language, Speech, and Hearing Services in School, 34,* 228–235.

Koenig, K., Reyes, A. D. L., Cicchetti, D., Scahill, L., & Klin, A. (2009). Group interventions to promote social skills in school-age children with pervasive developmental disorder: Reconsidering efficacy. *Journal of Autism and Developmental Disorders, 39,* 1163–1172.

Laugesen, E. A., Frankel, F., Mogil, C., & Dillon, A. R. (2008). Parent-assisted social skills training to improve friendships in teens with autism spectrum disorders. *Journal of Autism and Developmental Disorders, 39*(4), 596–606.

LaVoie, R. D. (1994). Learning disabilities and social skills with Richard Lavoie: Last one picked. . . First one picked on [Video and Teacher's Guide]. (Available from PBS Video, 1320 Braddock Place, Alexandria, VA 22314-1698).

Mavropoulou, S., Papadopoulou, E., & Kakana, D. (2011). Effects of task organization on the independent play of students with autism spectrum disorders. *Journal of Autism and Developmental Disorders, 41*(7), 913–925. doi:10.1007/s10803-010-1116-6. Accessed 1 Oct. 2012.

McCoy, K., & Hermansen, E. (2007). Video modeling for individuals with autism: A review of model type and effects. *Education and Treatment of Children, 30,* 183–213.

McGee, G. G., & Daly, R. (2007). Incidental teaching of age-appropriate social phrases to children with autism. *Research and Practice for Persons with Severe Disabilities, 32,* 112–123.

Meadan, H., Ostrosky, M. M., Zaghlawan, H. Y., & Yu, S. Y. (2009). Promoting the social and communicative behavior of young children with autism spectrum disorders: A review of parent-implemented intervention studies. *Topics in Early Childhood Special Education, 29*(2), 90–104.

Mechling, L. C., & Savidge, E. J. (2011). Using a personal digital assistant to increase completion of novel tasks and independent transitioning by students with autism spectrum disorder. *Journal of Autism Developmental Disorders, 41*(6), 687–704.

Moore, D., McGrath P., & Thorpe, J. (2000). Computer-aided learning for people with autism: A framework for research and development. *Innovations in Education and Training International, 37,* 218–228.
Mruzek, D., Cohen, C., & Smith, T. (2007). Contingency contracting with students with autism spectrum disorders in a public school setting. *Journal of Developmental and Physical Disabilities, 19,* 103–114.
National Autism Center. (2009). *National standards report: Addressing the need for evidence-based practice guidelines for autism spectrum disorders.* Randolph: Author.
National Professional Development Center on Autism Spectrum Disorders (2009). *Evidence based practice briefs.* Retrieved from http://autismpdc.fpg.unc.edu/content/briefs. Accessed 10 April 2010.
National Research Council. (2001). *Educating children with autism.* Washington: National Academy.
Palmen, A., Didden, R., & Arts, M. (2008). Improving question asking in high-functioning adolescents with autism spectrum disorders. Autism, 12, 83–98.
Paradiz, V. (2008). *The Integrated Self-Advocacy Curriculum: A Program for Emerging Self-Advocates with Autism Spectrum and Other Conditions (Student Workbook).* Shawnee Mission: Autism Asperger.
Pennington, R. C. (2010). Computer-assisted instruction for teaching academic skills to students with autism spectrum disorders: A review of literature. *Focus on Autism and Other Developmental Disorders, 25,* 239–248.
Reed, F. D., Hyman, S. R., & Hirst, J. M. (2011). Applications of technology to teach social skills to children with autism. *Research in Autism Spectrum Disorders, 5,* 1003–1010.
Rispoli, M. J., Franco, J. H., Van Der Meer, L., Lang, R., & Camargo, S. P. H. (2010). The use of speech generating devices in communication interventions for individuals with developmental disabilities: A review of the literature. *Developmental Neurorehabilitation, 13,* 276–293.
Rogers, S. J., Hayden, D., Hepburn, S., Charlifue-Smith, R., Hall, T., & Hayes, A. (2006). Teaching young children with autism useful speech: A pilot study of the Denver model and PROMPT intervention. *Journal of Autism and Developmental Disorders, 36,* 1007–1024.
Schopler E., & Reichler, R. J. (1971). Parents as cotherapists in the treatment of psychotic children. *Journal of Autism and Childhood Schizophrenia, 1*(1), 87–102.
Schreibman, L., & Ingersoll, B. (2005). Behavioral interventions to promote learning in individuals with autism. In F. R. Volkmar, A. Klin, & D. Cohen, (Eds.), *Handbook of autism and pervasive developmental disorders* (pp. 882–896). Hoboken: Wiley.
Schreibman, L., Whalen, C., & Stahmer, A. C. (2000). The use of video priming to reduce disruptive transition behavior in children with autism. *Journal of Positive Behavior Interventions, 2,* 3–11.
Schuerman, J., Soydan, H., MacDonald, G., Forslund, M., de Moya, D., & Boruch, R. (2002). The Campbell Collaboration. *Research on Social Work Practice, 12,* 309.
Smith, T., Scahill, L., Dawson, G., Guthrie, D., Lord, C., Odom, Rogers, S., & Wagner, S. (2007). Designing research studies on psychosocial interventions in autism. *Journal of Autism and Development Disorders, 27,* 354–366.
Southall, C. M., & Gast, D. L. (2011). Self-management procedures: A comparison across the autism spectrum. *Education and Training in Autism and Developmental Disabilities, 46*(2), 155–171.
Stahmer, A. C., Suhrheinrich, A., Reed, S., Bolduc, C., & Schreibman, L. (2010). Pivotal response teaching in the classroom setting. *Preventing School Failure: Alternative Education for Children and Youth, 54,* 265–274.
Stromer, R., Kimball, J. W., Kinney, E. M., & Taylor, B. A. (2006). Activity schedules, computer technology, and teaching children with autism spectrum disorders. *Focus on Autism and Other Developmental Disabilities, 21,* 14–24.
Texas Statewide Leadership on Autism Training. (2011, March 31). TARGET: Texas Autism Resource Guide for Effective Teaching. Retrieved from http://www.txautism.net/manual. Accessed 14 Oct. 2012.

Tien, K. (2008). Effectiveness of the Picture Exchange Communication System as a functional communication intervention for individuals with autism spectrum disorders: A practice-based research synthesis. *Education and Training in Developmental Disabilities, 43,* 61–76.

Thunberg, G., Ahlsen, E., & Sandberg, A. D. (2009). Interaction and use of speech-generating devices in the homes of children with autism spectrum disorders: An analysis of conversational topics. *Journal of Special Education Technology, 24*(2), 1–16.

Trottier, N., Kamp, L., & Mirenda, P. (2011). Effects of peer-mediated instruction to teach use of speech-generating devices to students with autism in social game routines. *Augmentative and Alternative Communication, 27,* 26–39.

Troutman, A. C., & Alberto, P. A. (2009). *Applied behavior analysis for teachers* (9th ed.). New York: Pearson.

van der Meer, L. A., & Rispoli, M. (2010). Communication interventions involving speech-generating devices for children with autism: A review of the literature. *Developmental Neurorehabilitation, 13,* 294–306.

Vismara, L. A., & Lyons, G. L. (2007). Using perseverative interests to elicit joint attention behaviors in young children with autism. *Journal of Positive Behavior Interventions, 9,* 214–228.

Wainer, A. L., & Ingersoll, B. R. (2011). The use of innovative computer technology for teaching social communication to individuals with autism spectrum disorders. *Research in Autism Spectrum Disorders, 5,* 96–107.

Webb, B. J., Miller, S. P., Pierce, T. B., Strawser, S., & Jones, W. P. (2004). Effects of social skill instruction for high-functioning adolescents with autism spectrum disorders. *Focus on Autism and Other Developmental Disabilities, 19,* 53–62.

Wheeler, J. J., Baggett, B. A., Fox, J., & Blevins, L. (2006). Treatment integrity: A review of intervention studies conducted with autism. *Focus on Autism and Other Developmental Disabilities, 21,* 45–55.

White, S. W., Koenig, K., & Scahill, L. (2007). Social skills development in children with autism spectrum disorders: A review of the intervention research. *Journal of Autism and Developmental Disorders, 37,* 1858–1868.

Wichnick, A. M., Vener, S. M., Pyrtek, M., & Poulson, C. L. (2010). The effect of a script-fading procedure on unscripted social initiations and novel utterances among young children with autism. *Research in Autism Spectrum Disorders, 4,* 290–299.

Wigham, S., Robertson, J., Emerson, E., Hatton, C., Elliott, J., Mcintosh, B., . . . Joyce, T. (2008). Reported goal setting and benefits of person centered planning for people with intellectual disabilities. *Journal of Intellectual Disabilities, 12,* 143–152.

Wilde, L. D., Koegel, L. K., & Koegel, R. L. (1992). *Increasing success in school through priming: A training manual.* Santa Barbara: University of California.

Winter-Messiers, M. A. (2007). From tarantulas to toilet brushes: Understanding the special interest areas of children and youth with Asperger Syndrome. *Remedial and Special Education, 28,* 140–152.

Chapter 16
Changing the Mindset of Children and Adolescents with Autism Spectrum Disorders

Robert Brooks and Sam Goldstein

In our therapeutic work with children and adolescents with autism spectrum disorders (ASD), a major goal is to change the negative, self-defeating mindset that directs their lives. The concept of *mindsets* has become an increasingly prominent area of study, especially with the emergence of the field of "positive psychology." As examples, Carol Dweck authored a book titled *Mindset* (2006) in which she distinguished between a "fixed" and a "growth" outlook; the research and writings of Martin Seligman and his colleagues about "learned helplessness" and "learned optimism" as well as resilience (Reivich and Shatte 2002; Seligman 1990) have roots in attribution theory, which is basically a theory about mindsets, examining how we understand the reasons for our successes and setbacks (Weiner 1974).

A major focus of our collaboration has been to elaborate upon the concepts of both *mindsets* and *resilience* (Brooks and Goldstein 2001, 2004, 2007, 2012; Goldstein and Brooks 2005, 2007). We proposed that all people possess a set of assumptions about themselves and others that influence their behaviors and the skills they develop. In turn, these behaviors and skills impact on their assumptions so that a dynamic process is constantly operating. We labeled this set of assumptions a *mindset* and sought to identify the features of the mindset possessed by hopeful, resilient people, including:

- Feeling in control of one's life.
- Being empathic and displaying effective communication and other interpersonal skills.
- Possessing solid problem-solving and decision-making skills.
- Establishing realistic goals and expectations.

R. Brooks (✉)
Department of Psychiatry, Harvard Medical School, 60 Oak Knoll Terrace, Needham, MA 02492, USA
e-mail: contact@drrobertbrooks.com

S. Goldstein
Neurology, Learning and Behavior Center, School of Medicine, University of Utah, 230 South 500 East, Suite 100, Salt Lake City, UT 84102, USA
e-mail: info@samgoldstein.com

S. Goldstein, J. A. Naglieri (eds.), *Interventions for Autism Spectrum Disorders*,
DOI 10.1007/978-1-4614-5301-7_16,

- Learning from both success and failure.
- Being a compassionate and contributing member of society.
- Living a responsible, self-disciplined life.

Our interest in resilience slowly emerged in our clinical work. Similar to other therapists trained in the 1960s and 1970s, we came to believe that too much time and effort were expended on approaches that focused on fixing deficits rather than building on assets. A deficit model may serve to identify how and why some children are developmentally behind their peers in different domains of functioning and may even prescribe particular interventions for addressing these problems. However, we concluded that if we were to improve the future of children, we must direct our attention toward identifying and harnessing their strengths.

The shortcomings of a deficit model, especially when working with or raising children with ASD, reside in the multifaceted problems these children display. If clinicians and other caregivers spend most of their time in a reactive mode, constantly and frenetically moving from one problem to the next, it is difficult to have an opportunity to reflect upon and adopt a proactive approach that asks, "What are the strengths and interests that this child possesses, strengths that can be nurtured to bring this child a realistic sense of accomplishment and dignity?"

It has been well-documented that children with ASD require much more assistance than other youngsters if they are to transit successfully into adult life (Adams 2009; Atwood 2008; Bondy and Frost 2008; Grandin and Sullivan 2008; Janzen 2009; Robinson 2011; Shumaker 2008; Sicile-Kira and Sicile-Kira 2012; Siegel 2007). Symptom relief though essential is not the equivalent of changing long-term outcome. This is not to suggest that symptom-relieving medication, therapies, or educational interventions in and of themselves cannot assist youngsters with ASD to transit into adult life. However, if our goal is to raise children with ASD to be resilient, we must not only provide symptom relief, but also experiences that develop those skills that will help them to negotiate the many challenges that will appear in their life's journey.

A Social Resilient Mindset

In our work with children with ASD, we expanded upon our earlier writings about a *resilient mindset*, especially given the specific challenges that these youngsters face. Social impairments have been found to be the strongest predictors of the risk of a child receiving a diagnosis of ASD (Brooks and Goldstein 2012). Children with ASD struggle to develop normal, satisfying, and appropriate social connections and relations with others. They often do not understand how to initiate interactions. They have noticeable difficulty in developing appropriate play skills, in modulating facial and emotional responses, and in responding effectively to social cues. They can be self-absorbed, shutting off interactions with peers and adults alike. Many display odd interests and routines, often demonstrating rigid, obsessive–compulsive behaviors that isolate them even further from meaningful relationships.

Children with ASD typically lag in social language or pragmatics, so that a give and take discourse with others is difficult to achieve. They misread social cues, failing, for example, to comprehend the messages and jokes of others while being far off the mark with their own attempts to communicate. They may appear disinterested in interacting with others, preferring instead to interact with objects. Their dilemma is twofold. Not only do they fail to begin to develop the skills and abilities necessary for functional and satisfying social relations and connections, but along the way they fail to have experiences and opportunities to develop what we refer to as a *social resilient mindset*. Our expansion of the concept of *resilient mindset* to *social resilient mindset* with youngsters with ASD is to capture the key developmental problems they experience in the social domain.

Collaboration Among Professionals and Parents

We believe that therapists who work with children with ASD will be most effective if: (a) they collaborate closely with the child's parents, teachers, and other professionals involved in the child's care to insure a comprehensive treatment program and (b) their interventions and consultations are guided by a strength-based model that views the nurturing of a *social resilient mindset* as a central goal.

Ongoing collaboration among professionals and parents should be the norm for all clinicians who work with children and adolescents, but assumes even greater urgency when youngsters face the multitude of developmental issues housed within an ASD diagnosis. If all the significant adults in the lives of children with ASD possess an understanding of the child's functioning and the characteristics of a social resilient mindset, then any interactions with the child can be directed toward developing this mindset.

A Strength-Based Approach

Therapists are in an excellent position to convey information about and implementation of a strength-based approach. To do so, the therapist must articulate guideposts for raising a social resilient child with ASD. Prior to our identifying eight key guideposts, we wish to emphasize that there is neither one "fixed set" of operating guidelines nor one direct course to follow in treating, educating, or raising children with ASD. Children with a diagnosis of ASD not only share some common features with each other, but they also share many characteristics with children who do not display developmental lags. Each youngster with ASD should be seen as possessing unique strengths and vulnerabilities.

Guideposts for Nurturing a Social Resilient Mindset

Though each child's journey in life is shaped by a variety of factors, including inborn temperament, family style and values, educational experiences, and the broader society or culture in which the child is raised, the eight guideposts we have selected provide principles and strategies for nurturing a social resilient mindset in children with ASD. Each of the guideposts involves reinforcing skills necessary for the development and maintenance of friendships, a difficult task for children with ASD. They can be reinforced by parents, therapists, teachers, and other professionals.

Guidepost 1: Teaching and Conveying Empathy

A basic foundation of any relationship, parent–child, teacher–child, therapist–child, child–child, is empathy. Empathy is the capacity to put oneself inside the shoes of other people and to see the world through their eyes. Empathy of adults toward children is influenced by a number of factors. It is easier to be empathic when children do as we ask and when they are warm and responsive in their interactions with us. It is more challenging to be empathic when we are angry, exasperated, or disappointed with a child's actions. It is important to note that when parents and other caregivers are confused and do not understand the reasons for a child's particular behaviors or problems, a situation that often transpires with children with ASD, maintaining an empathic view may be difficult.

The struggle for adults to be empathic, especially toward children with ASD, is paralleled by the difficulties that these children have in being empathic. Empathy involves both cognitive (e.g., taking the perspective of another person) and affective skills (e.g., identifying and understanding different emotions), skills that typically lag in children with ASD. Thus, it is important for parents to model and teach these skills to their children.

Questions to Promote Empathy

In our clinical work, we attempt to promote empathy in parents and professionals alike by posing the following questions (Brooks and Goldstein 2001):

- How would I hope my child (student, patient) describe me?
- What have I said or done that is likely to lead my child (student, patient) to describe me as I hope he or she would?
- How would my child (student, patient) actually describe and how close is that to how I hope he or she would describe me?
- When I talk or do things with my children (students, patients), am I behaving in a way that will make them most responsive to listening to me?
- Would I want anyone to speak to me the way I am speaking to my child (student, patient)?

When we pose these questions, we remind adults that children with ASD typically have difficulty "reading" the verbal and nonverbal messages of others. Thus, if children misperceive what we are attempting to communicate, we must do our best not to become annoyed or to disagree angrily with their perceptions, but instead consider how we can assist them to become more accurate in terms of their perceptions.

Richard, a 9-year-old with ASD, exemplified the gains that can be achieved when parents focus on reinforcing empathy. Richard failed to understand the ways in which his behaviors impacted on others, including their becoming upset or frustrated with him. In an effort to help Richard, his parents began a "family empathy project." They started with simple activities such as discussing the feelings of some of Richard's favorite cartoon characters after joining him to watch those programs. Then, as Christmas approached, they "adopted" a family with limited resources. During the course of shopping for gifts, they spoke with Richard about how the children in that family would feel not receiving much for Christmas and how they would now feel receiving gifts because of his actions. Though Richard struggled with this concept, he slowly began to improve his ability to identify the thoughts and feelings of others and the ways in which his behaviors triggered different feelings and reactions in others.

Laurie, also a 9-year-old with ASD, was described by her mother as obsessed with movie stars. Her mother observed that while Laurie does not like to read, she constantly looks at movie magazines from cover to cover. Laurie's parents used what they termed her "obsession" as a vehicle through which to help her develop empathy and improve her social skills. Since Laurie did not want to cut photos from the magazine, they made copies of the photos of the faces of different Hollywood stars and pasted them on index-sized cards. They designed a game that involved taking turns picking a card and then creating a brief story about what caused the stars to feel the way they looked in the photos.

Laurie's parents noticed that occasionally Laurie's story was discrepant from the photo (e.g., a star who was obviously angry was described by Laurie as happy). They used this discrepancy as an opportunity to teach Laurie about facial expressions and feelings. Laurie invited her two sisters to participate. Given Laurie's continued interest in the game, her parents added another dimension suggesting that each player had to say not only what events led a star to feel a certain way, but also to describe a time the player felt the same way. Although Laurie's answers could be repetitive (e.g., offering the same reason someone would feel happy), her parents varied their responses as a way of teaching Laurie about experiences that elicited different emotions.

Parental Assumptions to Enhance and Maintain Empathy

There are assumptions that therapists can identify for parents and other adults to help them to be more empathic with children on the autism spectrum. Three of the assumptions that we highlight in our clinical work include:

Knowledge is power: This is an often-stated phrase and deservedly so. It is imperative that parents of children with ASD understand what this diagnosis entails in terms of all dimensions of their child's development and functioning. It is equally important for parents to recognize a point we noted earlier, namely, children with ASD are not a homogeneous group and while the diagnosis can provide some common parameters, each child with ASD will differ. Such knowledge will provide parents with a more accurate portrait of their child, a portrait that will allow for more realistic, effective strategies. We advocate that parents as well as professionals keep as informed as possible with the burgeoning amount of information that is available about ASD. Of course, it is vital that parents become wise consumers of this information, separating spurious claims from scientifically based studies and interventions.

Your child has little control over thoughts or behaviors associated with ASD: Many parents of children with ASD, especially if their children are on the higher functioning side of the spectrum, may entertain the belief that their children could control their behavior if they "only wanted to do so." Some parents have told us that while they know their child has been diagnosed with ASD, they still wonder if their child could change if he or she were more motivated to do so. They view their child as lacking in "will" rather than in "skill." As Greene (1998, 2009) has emphasized in his work with challenging youngsters, such a view may contribute to adopting a more punitive approach that only serves to exacerbate the child's problems and weaken the parent–child and/or teacher–child relationship.

When we ask parents and teachers to consider the ways in which their response to their child or student would change if they shifted their perspective from will to skill, we have been impressed with the lessening of anger and the increase in empathy that ensues. As one parent of a child with ASD said, "Why punish a child for lacking a skill? When children are not able to do something, it's better to figure out how to teach them rather than how to punish them."

Another parent wondered at a workshop, "But what if the child has the skill but just isn't using it?" We replied, "If kids aren't using skills they have, there are obviously obstacles in the way. The obstacles may vary. Some kids may believe they can't do the task. Others may worry that they will fail and people will ridicule them. Regardless of the reasons for children backing away from a task, the best approach is to patiently teach these children the skills involved in the task. This will be more effective in addressing the obstacles than exhorting a child, 'You could do it if you wanted to do it!'"

Strive to become "stress hardy" instead of stressed out: The more stress and frustration we experience as parents and caregivers, the less likely we are to adopt an empathic stance toward our children. It is for this reason that we have been devoting an increasing amount of time in our clinical practices and workshops to highlight the work of psychologist Suzanne Kobasa and her colleagues (Kobasa et al. 1982; Kobasa and Puccetti 1983). Kobasa has described a *stress-hardy personality*, or what we prefer to call a *stress-hardy mindset*.

Kobasa identified the characteristics or mindset of individuals who deal effectively with stress and pressure. The mindset comprises three interrelated components: commitment, challenge, and control. *Commitment* is defined as being involved with, rather than alienated from, many aspects of life. When commitment is present, we possess a sense of purpose that provides us with a reason for why we are doing and what we are doing. This meaning is not confined to a single area, but is manifested in our personal relationships, our work, our charitable activities, and the causes we adopt. It is little wonder that parents of children with ASD report a feeling of gratification when they are involved in helping others through support groups or autism-related organizations.

The second feature, *challenge*, captures the belief that difficult situations are opportunities for learning and growth rather than reasons for despair and helplessness. People are less stressed when they have the ability to think outside the box, to consider new ways of solving problems. This is an especially important perspective when parenting or working with a child on the autism spectrum.

The third component is control or what we have titled *personal control*. Kobasa found that people are less stressed when they devote their time and energy to manage those situations over which they have some control or influence. A lack of personal control is associated with stress and a lessening of empathy. Personal control is evident when parents of a child with ASD can take the step of moving from a "Why me?" or "Why my child?" perspective to recognizing that while they had no control over their child having ASD, what they do have control over is their attitude and the services they can obtain to facilitate their child's development.

Famed football player Doug Flutie and his wife Laurie, noted in an interview that when they first learned that their son Dougie was autistic, they asked "why us?" but quickly realized that such an attitude was of little use. Instead, they applied all three features of a stress-hardy mindset. They focused on what they had control over, leading them not only to obtain services for their son, but also to establish a foundation in his name to assist other families with children with ASD, an activity that enriched a sense of purpose to their lives (Brooks and Goldstein 2012).

The stronger a stress-hardy outlook, the better-equipped parents and professionals are to be empathic with children with ASD and to help these children become more empathic themselves.

Guidepost 2: Using Empathic Communication and Listening Effectively

This is closely related to the first guidepost, but focuses specifically on communication. Effective communication has many features. It is not just speaking to another person with clarity. It also involves actively listening to others and understanding and validating what they are attempting to say.

Resilient children develop a capacity to communicate effectively, aided by parents capable of serving as important models in this process. The art of effective communication has significant implications for many components of behaviors associated with resilience including interpersonal skills, empathy, and problem-solving and decision-making abilities. Mastering these skills presents a challenge for children with ASD. They have difficulty in experiencing empathy, understanding or "reading" verbal and nonverbal messages, sharing their interests and experiences, and displaying flexibility in a back-and-forth conversation.

Given all the obstacles that exist when communicating with children with ASD, it is important to practice empathy in every interaction we have with them. We can use our empathic communications with them to model empathy, hope, problem-solving and coping skills, and a sense of control or ownership over one's life. Empathic parents and professionals are guided by the following kinds of questions, which are related to the questions outlined in Guidepost 1. These are the questions we ask parents of children with ASD to consider in our parent counseling sessions. The questions are just as relevant for teachers and for other professionals working with children with ASD.

Questions to Promote Empathic Communication

- Whenever I say or do things with my child, what is my goal, what is it that I hope to achieve?
- Am I doing or saying things in a way that will lead my child to be more responsive to listening to me?
- Would I want anyone to speak with me in the way I am speaking with my child?
- When I communicate with my child with ASD, do I take into consideration his or her unique way of understanding and responding to my message in order to lessen a disconnect between us?
- Even when I disagree with my child's point of view, do I *validate* my child's perspective, remembering that validation does not infer agreement, but rather reinforces that I have heard and am attempting to understand my child's message?

Although children with ASD perceive the world differently than we do and are not as skilled in social pragmatics and interpreting the feelings and thoughts being expressed by others, parents have found a couple of additional questions beneficial in strengthening effective communication. They are:

- What makes it easiest for me to listen to what others have to say without becoming defensive?
- What do others say and do that turns me off and keeps me from truly listening to their messages?

Stephen and Amanda, the parents of Grant, a 12-year-old boy diagnosed with Asperger's, found these questions very helpful in their communications with their son. Grant frequently blurted things out to strangers without thinking about the impact his words had on others. On one occasion, he saw a woman smoking in the parking lot of a mall and in a loud voice he informed her that she had a "bad habit and could die soon if she didn't stop smoking." Similarly, he told a man inside a store in the mall that he was "fat and fat people are not healthy."

Stephen and Amanda attempted to teach Grant not to say these things, but Grant responded that what he said is true and he was just trying to help people. His inflexibility triggered frustration in his parents that led to comments often accompanied with an angry tone such as: "You have to learn to listen to us," "You aren't helping people, you're hurting their feelings," "Why can't you remember what we tell you?"

In reflecting upon the questions we listed earlier in this guidepost, Stephen and Amanda recognized that their goal for Grant was to comprehend the situation and not offer comments that would be startling and offensive to strangers. They also realized that the way they were responding to Grant was resulting in his becoming more angry and confused. As a first step, they attempted to validate his viewpoint by noting, "It's really great that you want people to be healthy and stay alive. It's great you want to be so helpful."

Stephen and Amanda found that such a seemingly simple comment of validation lessened Grant's defensiveness when they brought up the delicate subject of when and how to say things to people. They discussed in a supportive way that even if he thought he was being helpful, speaking with strangers about their habits and health often made these people upset and less likely to want to listen. Although it was not easy for Grant to accept this position, he became more open to doing so, especially given his parents' empathic communication. In essence, they were also serving as models for communicating in ways in which the other person could listen.

Communication Through Play

Before leaving this second guidepost, it is important to appreciate that the communication of children is not always direct, but may be expressed through their play. For youngsters with ASD, play often assumes a repetitive quality that may prove bewildering to parents who are uncertain how to respond to their child's seemingly obsessive thoughts and behaviors. For example, a boy with ASD was preoccupied playing with cars in what seemed to be a purposeless fashion. His parents became concerned that this preoccupation contributed to his becoming increasingly isolated from others. They attempted to take the cars away, but this action led to a meltdown on their son's part.

When they discussed their problem at a parent support group, another father, Mike, described his son playing aimlessly and endlessly with cars, sometimes just crashing them together. Mike said that while he did not understand the reasons for his son's need to play with cars repetitively, he decided to "join" him by buying a couple of toy cars and playing with them next to his son. He described that at first his son moved away and seemed upset by his seeming intrusion. Mike persisted. He made a tunnel and road paths with blocks and bought some small stop signs. He even had his cars talk with each other about learning to stop and to stay on the road. After a while, Mike's son made his own road with blocks and soon the two roads intersected. The play permitted more focused interaction between father and son.

The late psychiatrist Stanley Greenspan and psychologist Serena Weider (2009) in their book *Engaging Autism*, which covers the entire autism spectrum, discussed the benefits of communicating effectively by entering the child's world through a technique developed by Greenspan called "Floortime." They wrote:

> The first step is engagement and the first principle of the Floortime technique is to follow the child's lead, regardless of where the interest lies. But what if a child's interests are unusual or peculiar or are not things we want to encourage? This should not be a concern at this point, because only by joining in the child's interest, by taking his lead, do we get a first clue about what he finds important. It may not remain important to him as we pull him into our shared world and new things come to his attention. But initially, the ticket to engaging the child's interest is joining him in his world. (Greenspan and Weider 2009, p. 70)

Empathic communication, via words or play, is essential if we are to create an environment in which children with ASD will learn from us and develop an optimistic, hopeful outlook.

Guidepost 3: Accepting Our Children for Who They Are: Conveying Unconditional Love and Setting Realistic Expectations

To truly nurture a social resilient mindset requires that we love our children unconditionally and help them feel appreciated. To accomplish this, we must learn to accept our children for who they are, not necessarily what we hope or want them to be. In our therapeutic interventions and our workshops, we examine the question of what does it mean to *accept* our children for who they are? Why is acceptance so integral to effective parenting (or teaching), perhaps even more so when a child with ASD is involved?

Illustrations of acceptance may be found in previous examples, including Richard's parents initiating a "family empathy project," Michael joining the car play of his son, Laurie's parents designing a social skills game using Laurie's interests in Hollywood stars, and Doug and Laurie Flutie establishing a foundation in the name of their son with autism. As we often discuss with parents, we all have dreams or hopes—whether well-articulated or not—about the lives our children will lead from the time they are born. Typically, these dreams are only partially realized or not realized at all since most children do not live up to all the expectations we have for them. Noticeable disappointment of children is present in many homes. If parents are to maintain a warm, loving relationship with their children, then acceptance and unconditional love are essential. We continue to be impressed by the number of parents who speak with us after our workshops and describe with both sadness and anger what they experienced growing up in a home in which they could not please their parents and in which love was conditional, based on such factors as their obtaining higher grades, performing better in sports, or being more sociable.

The process of acceptance and creating realistic expectations is rendered even more challenging when our children have ASD and/or other developmental difficulties. The presence of disabilities often widens the gap between the dreams parents have for their children and the probability of these dreams being realized. A time of "mourning" for the child one hoped for, but did not have is to be expected, eventually to be replaced by a belief housed within "stress hardiness," namely, while we did not have control over our child having autism, we do have control over our attitudes and actions in response to their condition.

The Impact of a "Charismatic Adult"

An essential factor in nurturing a social resilient mindset is the presence of at least one adult actively involved in a child's life, an adult who not only believes in the worth of the child, but also communicates that belief in ways the child can understand. Segal (1988) referred to that person as a "charismatic adult," an adult from whom a child "gathers strength." To assume the role of a charismatic adult is to practice acceptance and unconditional love. We know that Michael would have preferred if his son were not preoccupied with cars. We know Laurie's parents were frustrated by her obsession with Hollywood stars. However, by accepting that this is who their children are, they were able to join their children's world and nurture a more positive parent–child relationship.

We emphasize to parents that accepting children for who they are and appreciating their different temperaments, learning styles, and communication skills should not be interpreted as synonymous with excusing inappropriate or unacceptable behavior. It means that we appreciate that our child's behavior is not driven by malicious intent. It also suggests that we will strive to assist our child in ways that will strengthen his or her sense of worth and dignity.

The issue of acceptance was captured in our work with Emily and Jonas Spencer, the parents of 12-year-old Jill and 10-year-old Jeremy. Jill was on the autism spectrum. They described Jeremy as an easy child to raise, while Jill's behavior proved to be much more challenging and frustrating.

Jonas raised the question, "But in fact isn't it easier to love our kids when they do live up to what we want them to be or at the very least don't frustrate or embarrass us?" We concurred that it is easier, but in an empathic way noted that almost all parents with children on the autism spectrum will experience heightened levels of frustration, embarrassment, pessimism, and anxiety.

One issue that arose related to acceptance was Emily and Jonas' hesitation in allowing Jill to play with two younger girls who lived next door, one who was 7 and the other who was 5 years old. They felt that Jill should be playing with her own peer group. Emily and Jonas reported that the two girls have a very large dollhouse and while Jill was placing a little doll into a crib in the dollhouse she was also teaching the sisters a lullaby that had been sung to her when she was baby. Jill also played the board game Candyland with the girls.

Although at first disappointed by her playing more with younger children than children her own age, Emily and Jonas came to accept that these kinds of activities with the neighborhood girls were in keeping with Jill's cognitive level and that while the two girls were several years younger than she was, playing with them afforded her opportunities to relate with other children, opportunities she might not have otherwise. They also understood that playing with these girls did not preclude interacting with children her own age, but that such interactions had to be carefully planned with children who would be understanding of Jill's disabilities such as several of her cousins.

Jill's contact with the two younger sisters went very well. The sisters' mother, Lizzie, reported to Emily and Jonas how nicely Jill played with her daughters. This compliment had a noticeable impact on Emily and Jonas. They were accustomed to hearing about what "a great kid" Jeremy was, but they rarely, if ever, heard such accolades about Jill. Most friends and family refrained from saying anything, a silence that Emily and Jonas interpreted as "if you have nothing good to say, don't say anything."

Emily commented that Lizzie's positive remark took place in Jill's presence, which was a big boost to Jill's self-esteem. "It was obvious that Jill relished these compliments. When you have a child on the autism spectrum, a child who is having so many problems in so many areas of her life, it's easy to neglect things your child does well."

Accepting Jill's developmental delays permitted Emily and Jonas to allow her to engage in activities that were more in keeping with her level of functioning and provided her with opportunities to experience success and increase her sense of dignity and confidence.

Guidepost 4: Nurturing "Islands of Competence"

We have described that in the early part of our careers we focused on pathology. When involved in an evaluation of a child, we asked few, if any, questions of parents to elicit what they perceived to be the strengths of their children or what they considered to be their own assets as parents. We were more inclined to speak with parents as well as their children about their problems rather than invite them to elaborate upon their interests and strengths.

It may seem natural for psychologists and other mental health professionals to zero in on problem areas when meeting with parents. It is a reality that when parents request a consultation they do so because they have concerns about various aspects of their children's behavior and development. While it is crucial we address these problems, we have come to recognize that to place the emphasis on analyzing pathology and fixing deficits limits our ability to assist children and their parents to lead more satisfying, resilient lives. Wisely, we shifted our focus to identify and build on strengths, or what we call *islands of competence*.

Questions to Focus on *Islands of Competence*

The metaphor of *islands of competence* is the embodiment of a strength-based approach. To apply the essence of this metaphor to our clinical practices, we began to pose the following questions to parents, teachers, and other professionals as well as to the children themselves (we also offer a commentary in parentheses after each question):

What are two or three islands of competence or strengths your child possesses? (We clarify for parents of children with ASD that in identifying their children's strengths or interests, they should not do so in comparison with children who do not display developmental problems. The island of competence of a child on the autism spectrum may not appear to be a strength when compared with other children, but for the child with ASD it may represent the child's highest functioning area.)

If your child were asked to list his or her islands of competence or interests, would they be the same ones on your list? (Sometimes a discrepancy exists between the perceptions possessed by parents and those of their children about the latter's strengths. Such discrepancies are likely to prompt parents to steer their children into activities that are not of interest to them even though they may be to their parents.)

How do you acknowledge or celebrate your child's islands of competence? (Related to the previous question, some children report that they do not believe their parents value or encourage their strengths or interests. This parental absence to honor a child's strengths frequently occurs when there is a lack of acceptance, that is, the child's islands of competence are not in keeping with the parents' dreams.)

What activities appear to elicit positive emotions in your child? (We inform parents and teachers that it may be challenging to assess the level or kinds of positive emotions triggered in our children when they are engaged in particular tasks, but we must be vigilant to do so. Tapping into and encouraging expression of a child's islands of competence as Emily and Jonas Spencer did by allowing their daughter Jill to play with and teach younger neighborhood girls a lullaby, proved to be an invaluable opportunity for Jill to experience a sense of accomplishment.)

A number of parents have reported a problem when complimenting their children with ASD, namely, their words often appear to fall on "deaf ears," resulting in parents becoming frustrated and reducing positive feedback. Parents may assume that since children with ASD at times seem to be unresponsive to the praise of others, they should refrain from expressing positive statements. However, we advise parents to realize that when children possess low self-worth or fail to accurately evaluate their self-worth, as is true of many youngsters with ASD, they are less likely to accept positive remarks. Parents and other adults should continue to offer these remarks, but recognize that true self-worth, hope, and resilience are based on children experiencing success in areas of their lives that others deem to be important.

The islands of competence of children with ASD can be varied and sometimes perplexing. For example, 11 year old John, a child with ASD, loved cartooning. He would sit for hours drawing a cartoon series he titled "The Screaming Babies from Planet Mercury." Though adults did not always understand his humor, he proudly displayed his cartoons to anyone who would take time to look.

John was socially isolated in his classroom. The teacher was asked if she would consider initiating a cartooning club in the classroom, introducing children to the art of cartooning and asking John to be her assistant since he was already a "cartoonist." She was willing to do so. John assumed his new role with obvious joy. Although he had to be supervised at times as he attempted to teach or guide the other students, eventually a number of students also took an interest in cartooning and the cartooning club blossomed as did John's social interaction with his classmates. John's teacher and parents displayed his cartoons at school and home. This boosted his self-esteem and in a concrete fashion communicated to him that he had strengths that were appreciated by others and provided him a means to relate with others.

The Strengths of Parents

We also think it is important for parents of children with ASD to consider their own strengths. These parents typically experience day-to-day struggles and doubts. Many have reported that their efforts to help their children seem unsuccessful. Their children are slow to learn from them and show little affection. Many question whether they will ever be effective as parents. Doubts and insecurities permeate their psyches, often reinforced by family and friends who convey suggestions that intentionally or unintentionally are tinged with judgmental or accusatory overtones.

To begin the process of offsetting their own negativity, we ask parents of children on the autism spectrum the following question:

What are two or three of your strengths or islands of competence as a parent?

Interestingly, we frequently hear from parents an answer similar to what their children offer when we ask the latter what they view as their strengths, namely, "I don't know" or "I can't think of anything." We use such responses as an opportunity to say, "We know that you may not be able to identify your strengths now, but it is something we can continue to discuss. It's important for us to realize we all have things at which we are good."

A mother who was the single parent of a 12-year-old boy with ASD initially viewed herself as a failure as a parent. In parent counseling sessions, she came to appreciate that her persistent and thoughtful efforts to obtain the best services for her son, even in the face of many obstacles, represented a strength that was of immeasurable benefit to her son's progress.

The more that parents, teachers, and therapists can identify the strengths of children with ASD, the more they can harness these strengths and help these children to recognize that their lives need not be constricted by their diagnosis. As Chantal Sicile-Kira, the mother of a young man with autism, eloquently observed:

> Autism is a spectrum, and the talents, strengths, and support needs are different.However keep in mind that being ready to work doesn't happen overnight for any of us.It is important to raise all children to believe that they have positive attributes and qualities, and this is done by focusing on the positive, not the negatives. As parents of children with IEPs (Individual Educational Plans) we lean to focus on the child's deficits, and this is not conducive to building one's confidence. Wherever possible, notice your child's strengths, reinforce them, praise him for them. It is the strengths that will help him as an adult, not the areas that he has trouble with (Sicile-Kira and Sicile-Kira 2012, p. 185).

Guidepost 5: Helping Children Learn from Rather than Feel Defeated by Mistakes

There is a significant difference in the ways by which resilient children view mistakes compared with children who do not possess a social resilient mindset. This difference may be understood through the lens of attribution theory (Brooks 1991; Brooks and Goldstein 2001; Weiner 1974). Resilient youngsters perceive setbacks as opportunities for learning. In marked contrast, children who lack confidence and hope attribute mistakes to variables that cannot be corrected or modified. In reaction to this pessimistic outlook, they are vulnerable to retreating from challenges, experiencing feelings of inadequacy, and/or projecting blame on others for their problems. We advise parents of children with ASD that it is imperative that they help their children develop a healthy outlook about mistakes from an early age and that they help their children to realize that mistakes are both *expected* and *accepted* and are important experiences for learning.

Strategies to Help Children Manage Mistakes and Setbacks

We discuss several strategies with parents and other adults to lessen the negative impact of mistakes on children with ASD. A very obvious one is to avoid comments that may be quickly interpreted by children as accusatory or judgmental. Well-meaning parents have told us of uttering things out of frustration that they quickly realized were counterproductive. One mother of a daughter on the autism spectrum reported that on several occasions she yelled at her daughter, "Why can't you just stop and think about what you should and shouldn't do?"

This mother continued, "One day it broke my heart, but it opened my eyes, when my daughter cried and said, 'Don't you think if I was able to I would think more about what I should and shouldn't do?'"

A second strategy we describe is for parents to serve as models for managing mistakes and setbacks effectively. As we have often stated to parents, whether they intend to or not they serve as primary models for their children. If children witness us backing away from challenges, offering excuses for mistakes, becoming frustrated and angry at our own setbacks or the setbacks of our children, it is more likely that our children will do the same.

To help parents remember their important role as models, we ask them, "How would your children describe what you do when you make a mistake? How would you hope they described you?"

When we have actually asked youngsters this question, we have heard some not so pleasant responses including, "They scream and yell at each other," They blame everyone else," or "They say mean things to me." In contrast, one child replied, "When my parents make a mistake, they talk to each other and they ask each other what they can do differently next time."

We advise parents of children with ASD that when they (the parents) make mistakes, they should when possible verbalize aloud in the presence of their children what has occurred and how they plan to remedy the situation. This kind of constructive modeling, which we often use as a therapeutic strategy in our sessions with patients with ASD, helps to reinforce a problem-solving approach that will be discussed under Guidepost 6.

A third technique to assist children to deal more constructively with mistakes overlaps with Guidepost 3 and involves setting realistic expectations for what our children are capable of doing. What is determined to be realistic will vary from one child to the next and as we emphasize with parents, developmental milestones are very different for children on the autism spectrum compared with youngsters who are not beset with developmental issues. This does not imply that we do not challenge children to meet certain goals, but rather that we do not throw children in 10 feet of water if they are not yet capable of swimming.

If the expectations of parents are consistently too high, leading youngsters to experience failure on an ongoing basis, the child's mindset will be dominated by the idea, "I am a failure, I cannot succeed, there is something wrong with me." As one patient plaintively said, "I think I was born with half a brain. Do you know how to fill in the other half?"

A fourth strategy to assist children with ASD to manage setbacks is to provide positive feedback and encouragement for appropriate behaviors and accomplishments. We have described this factor to some extent in previous guideposts, but we want to highlight it here for a couple of reasons. First, when we are engaged in correcting the behaviors of children on a seemingly hourly basis, we may neglect to notice and/or provide positive feedback when they are handling situations effectively. This should not be construed to mean that we compliment children every few minutes, but rather that there will be opportunities to let children with ASD know that we recognize what a nice job they are doing. Under Guidepost 3, we described how pleased Jill was to hear Lizzie, the mother of the two young girls with whom Jill was playing, tell Jill's parents how nicely their daughter played with her children.

A basic premise of this fourth strategy is that children are more likely to develop a constructive attitude toward mistakes if they have built up a reservoir of positive experiences and accomplishments, a task that is reinforced with genuine, realistic praise.

Guidepost 6: Teaching Children to Solve Problems and Make Sound Decisions

If Guidepost 5 is to be successful, it is imperative for parents and professionals to model and teach a problem-solving approach that their children with ASD can use when encountering setbacks. The attitude of resilient youngsters is that mistakes serve as catalysts for problem solving. They believe they have control over what transpires in their lives rather than being victims of events. In describing to parents the actions involved in the process of effective problem solving, we acknowledge the contributions of our friend and colleague Dr. Myrna Shure, who was instrumental in developing the I Can Problem Solve (ICPS) program (1996, 2000). The process of solving problems includes identifying and acknowledging problems, articulating short- and long-term goals, considering several possible options for dealing with the problem and reaching the goals, selecting and applying the option that appears to have the greatest probability for success, assessing how effectively the option is working, and learning from the outcome if changes have to be made to the goals or the strategies used.

Children on the autism spectrum struggle to problem solve. They lack many of the prerequisite skills required to engage in this process. They have difficulty identifying problems, planning ahead, establishing short- and long-term goals, and considering options or choices for addressing the problems. In many ways, they are adrift, similar to captains lost at sea without a compass, following one course or another, but without any sound judgment to guide their actions. In such a scenario, some children may freeze up not knowing what to do, while others may act impulsively without considering the consequences of their behavior. Still others may not even realize there is a problem, although their parents and others seem distressed.

We emphasize to parents that teaching problem-solving skills to children with ASD may, at times, feel like a Herculean task, but it represents one of the most important responsibilities they have if their children are to develop a social resilient mindset. What adds to the difficulty of the task is the tendency for parents (and even therapists) to jump in and tell their children with ASD what to do rather than involving them as much as possible in arriving at the solution. When we too quickly offer the answers, we rob our children of opportunities to learn how to solve problems. In addition, they often experience our advice as intrusive, intensifying tension in the parent–child relationship. The challenge is to apply empathic communication and validation so as to teach without lecturing.

Teaching Problem-Solving Skills

As an initial step in developing a child's problem-solving capacity, we suggest that parents of children with ASD provide choices that are in keeping with their child's cognitive abilities. A number of parents hesitate to give choices, reporting that their child can be very rigid and get stuck. One mother, describing her 7-year-old son with autism observed, "If I give him even a simple choice of two things to eat, he can become paralyzed about which to choose or he can become very stubborn and declare he doesn't like either choice."

The problem reported by this mother is not unusual, but we believe clinicians can assist parents to manage it effectively. Parents of Lucy, an 8-year old girl on the autism spectrum, were distressed by Lucy obsessing about what clothes to wear to school. They noted that they thought they had a good solution by offering Lucy the evening before a choice of one of two outfits to wear the next day. Unfortunately, when morning came Lucy often complained that she did not like the choice she made the prior evening and began to rummage through the closet for other outfits. The parents found themselves having to step in and dictate to Lucy what she had to wear lest she be late for school.

To address this behavior, a "fall-back choice" was introduced. The parents were instructed to continue to give Lucy a choice before bedtime of one of two items to wear the next day, but to tell her that sometimes children change their minds about the choice they made the evening before. If this occurred, Lucy could have a back-up choice that would also be taken out the night before. The back-up choice would be placed next to the choice that Lucy made so that she did not have to open the closet door and view all her other clothes.

The parents wondered if this strategy was just "adding one more choice for Lucy to obsess about." We responded that this could occur, but that for many children the presence of a back-up choice actually helped to set a limit on their wanting more choices. In this instance, the back-up choice proved an effective intervention and reinforced Lucy's feeling of having a sense of ownership.

After discussing choices, therapists can describe a problem-solving sequence for parents to use, one based on Shure's ICPS program. The sequence includes the following steps:

Articulate the problem and agree it is a problem: If a problem is not clearly defined and if children do not agree with parents that it is a problem, then all our efforts will be a waste of time. Children will not be motivated to change behaviors that they do not view as problematic. When this occurs, we suggest to parents that they validate their child's perception, but then cast the issue as a "family issue" that requires the input of all family members.

Consider two or three possible solutions and the likely outcome of each: The task of defining and agreeing about the problem leads naturally to the next step, arriving at possible solutions. Parents can engage children in this task by considering various courses of action. We do the same when conducting therapy with these youngsters. Given the overriding goal of nurturing a social resilient mindset, we suggest to parents with children with ASD that they encourage their child as much as possible to generate the solutions. In addition, we note that children with ASD may have more difficulty considering different options than peers without developmental problems, requiring parents to be more active in helping them arrive at possible solutions. If a child with ASD offers a solution that is unrealistic, it is important for parents not to summarily reject the child's idea, but rather to use it as an opportunity for further discussion.

Put into action the strategy that seems to have the highest likelihood of success: After considering different courses of action, it is time to implement the option that seems to offer the best outcome. Many of the problems that parents of children with ASD have discussed with us concern their child's difficulties with interpersonal relationships and developing friendships. Consequently, we often recommend to parents that in reinforcing problem-solving skills in their children, a main focus should be on their child applying these skills to improve friendships and develop more satisfying relationships.

Develop a way to remind each other if someone forgets to follow through on the selected plan: Not surprisingly, what seems to be an excellent plan hatched in one's office does not always prove successful in the "real world." If children with ASD forget to follow through, the natural reaction of parents is to remind them of what they neglected to do. Not surprisingly, the child experiences these reminders as "nagging." Consequently, we have recommended to parents that after a strategy is selected they can say, "This strategy sounds great, but any of us might forget a strategy. So how can we remind each other so that none of us feels we're nagging each other?" Many parents have attested that asking children how they would like to be reminded helps minimize the impression that parents are on their backs since the children helped to suggest the "reminder plan."

What to do if the selected solution does not work: This step is closely related to helping children deal with setbacks. When potential trouble spots are defined in advance, children and their parents are better prepared to avoid them, deal with them, and/or switch to a back-up intervention. In working with many parents with children on the autism spectrum, we learned the value of anticipating possible roadblocks to success. Not only did this anticipation lessen the likelihood of a defeatist attitude emerging if a strategy proved ineffective, but also it encouraged both parents and children to consider in advance other future strategies that might be applied.

As therapists, we have found that we are in a unique situation to teach parents of children with ASD ways to assist their children to develop those skills that will help them to solve problems, especially many that occur in the social domain. When working directly with the children, we actively use the problem-solving sequence as part of our therapeutic strategies.

Guidepost 7: Disciplining in Ways That Promote Self-Discipline and Self-Worth

One of the most frequently asked questions by parents in our clinical practices and our workshops focuses on discipline. We have stated that one of the main responsibilities of a parent is to be a disciplinarian in the true sense of the work (Brooks and Goldstein 2007). The word *discipline* relates to the word *disciple* and is best understood as a teaching process. We explain to parents that if discipline is placed within the context of an educational process, we must ask, "What is it that we are attempting to teach?" We believe that discipline has several key functions, two of which we always highlight. The first, which most parents readily identify, is to make certain that we provide a consistent, safe, and secure environment in which children not only learn that reasonable rules, limits, and consequences exist in the household, but also that they exist for a reason.

A second equally important function of discipline, but not one as readily identified by parents, is to nurture self discipline or self-control in children. Goleman (1994, 2006) has asserted that self-discipline is one of the pillars of both emotional and social intelligence, predictors of satisfying interpersonal relationships and successful activities in life, qualities that are frequently limited in individuals on the autism spectrum.

Self-discipline implies that a child possesses an internalized set of rules so that even if a parent is not present, the child will act in a thoughtful, reflective manner. Self-discipline may be understood as a significant component of a social resilient mindset in which a sense of responsibility for one's behavior flourishes. This view of self-discipline encourages parents to develop disciplinary practices that reinforce *comfortable* and *flexible* self-control within a safe and secure environment rather than generating feelings of resentment and anger in children. When we explain our position about self-discipline to parents, we emphasize *comfortable* and *flexible*, especially when considering the difficulties displayed by children on the autism spectrum whose thinking and behavior are often marked by the seeming polarities of impulsivity and rigidity.

The Mindset of Effective Disciplinarians

In helping parents of children with ASD to become more effective disciplinarians, we highlight five main points. They include:

View your child's inappropriate or counterproductive actions as predicated on a lack of skills rather than intentional behavior: This is a point we emphasized under Guidepost 1. We know that it is often difficult for parents to appreciate that particular behaviors displayed by their children with ASD are not within their children's control. However, it is essential they do so. If parents interpret the behaviors of their children as intentional, they are less likely to be empathic or understanding and more apt to adopt a punitive approach. In contrast, if parents view problematic behaviors as a lack of skills their focus will be on teaching these skills rather than on implementing negative consequences.

When Stephen and Amanda, the parents of 12-year-old Grant whom we described under Guidepost 2, shifted their thinking about their son's blurting out embarrassing comments to strangers as a lack of skills, they moved from being punishers to being teachers.

Remember that a major goal of discipline is to promote self-discipline and self-control: This is a position we offered earlier in this guidepost that invites the following questions for parents to ask themselves: "When I discipline my child with ASD, does it help my child to develop self-discipline? Does it help my child to appreciate the importance of limits and consequences? Does it help my child to adhere to a more balanced, flexible style?" Empathy, empathic communication, and problem-solving skills are critical dimensions that parents can use to assist their children to consider the consequences of their actions and strategies for adopting more constructive behaviors.

Focus on prevention, not just intervention: In our clinical practices, we have seen many examples of well-intentioned parents who put their children with ASD in situations that you can predict will lead to behavior problems, including meltdowns. It is essential for parents to become proactive rather than reactive in their disciplinary style. Given the developmental lags their children with ASD demonstrate, parents should be careful not to place them in situations that are beyond their ability to handle.

As one example, a mother told us of her 4-year-old son with ASD who was hypersensitive to noise. Although she prepared him on numerous occasions when they went to the supermarket, he always became agitated and started to throw things. We advised that at some point he would be able to handle such an environment, but he was not capable of doing so at the present time. This mother wisely refrained from taking him shopping with her or bringing him into other noisy places. Another example of prevention involved an 8-year-old boy on the autism spectrum who had meltdowns in restaurants as he obsessed about what to order. One intervention that his parents applied that proved successful was to review the menu with their son prior to going to the restaurant and calling in the order in advance so that it was ready when they arrived.

Understand that if discipline is viewed as a teaching process it should not be harsh or belittling, especially in the form of spanking or verbal assaults: As parents ourselves, we empathize with parents in our practices and workshops about the frustrations involved with the parenting role. Even empathic, caring parents, when tired and exhausted, can say and do things under the umbrella of discipline that are counterproductive and result in greater resentment and anger rather than respect, responsibility, and resilience. This frustration and confusion are much more intense for parents who have children on the autism spectrum, leading to a higher probability of engaging in harsh and belittling acts of so-called discipline. Thus, parents must plan ahead and develop coping strategies to use when they recognize that they are becoming very angry. This is why we describe techniques for stress hardiness to parents. One mother decided she should take a time-out when very frustrated with her oppositional daughter, realizing that this was a far more effective approach than attempting to place her daughter in time-out.

Remember that positive feedback and encouragement are often the most powerful forms of discipline: We discussed this under Guidepost 5, but it deserves special mention when considering the theme of discipline. In our work with parents of children on the autism spectrum, we encourage them to shift their disciplinary practices from a reliance on punishment to using positive feedback. These parents love their children, but when children are consistently displaying what are considered to be inappropriate behaviors, the focus can easily turn to relying on punitive actions.

This last point was captured in the poignant observations of a father whose child is on the autism spectrum. Following a discussion of discipline, he lamented, "I feel I' m constantly telling my son what not to do. I just don't want him to behave in ways that are embarrassing and will lead to more trouble or rejection. But in thinking about what you said about positive feedback I realize that sometimes I'm so focused on stopping his behaviors that I neglect to provide encouragement and to build up his self-esteem."

Given the cognitive, language, and social lags of children on the autism spectrum, we emphasize to parents that any feedback, whether positive or negative, should be very specific. Saying, "You're a good boy" or "You're a good girl" or "You're not acting nice" is much too vague. Jill's parents were more specific when they said to her, "It was really nice how you taught the girls a lullaby. Now they know a new lullaby they didn't know before."

Guidepost 8: Developing Responsibility, Compassion, and a Social Conscience

A frequently asked question from parents concerns how best to teach their children to be more caring and more responsible. Many researchers have demonstrated that from a young age children are not only empathic, but also enjoy helping others. We have asserted that there appears to be an inborn need to help others (Brooks and Goldstein 2001). Observe young children, even those on the autism spectrum. They take great pleasure in helping as evidenced by their smiles when we compliment and appreciate their contributions.

Our belief in the inborn need to help was reinforced when we asked a large group of adults to complete a questionnaire about their positive and negative memories of school (Brooks 1991; Brooks and Goldstein 2001). We asked specifically about positive events that included something a teacher said or did that enhanced their self-esteem and motivation. The most frequently cited positive memory was one that we would not have predicted at the time, but seems more evident now, namely, being asked to help others in some manner (e.g., tutoring a younger child, taking messages to the office, or running the film projector).

Introducing "Contributory Activities"

Our experience has found that similar to all children, youngsters with ASD are very receptive to contributing to the welfare of others, especially if the words are phrased as an invitation to help and the task is within the developmental level of the child (Brooks and Goldstein 2012). Since the strengths of children with ASD are often eclipsed by their problems, it is especially important to provide them with opportunities to help others. Such experiences reinforce a key belief within a social resilient mindset: I can make a positive difference in the lives of others. We should note that what we call "contributory activities" are important factors not only in childhood, but also in leading a resilient lifestyle at any age (Brooks and Goldstein 2004; Post and Neimark 2007).

Given the lifelong influence of contributory activities, it is a strategy that we consistently recommend to parents and teachers of children with ASD. One 9-year-old boy on the autism spectrum was given the responsibility by his teacher of going down to the kindergarten class at the end of the day to assist students to get ready to leave. He helped them to put on their coats and made certain they had packed their belongings in their backpacks. When we interviewed this child's teacher, she remarked that the "glow on his face" indicated how much he enjoyed this responsibility, an observation confirmed by the kindergarten teacher as well. An added benefit was that in helping the kindergarten children be more organized at the end of the day, he became more organized about his own possessions.

Earlier, we reported other instances of children with ASD becoming increasingly responsible when enlisted to help others. As examples, we have Jill teaching two younger girls to sing a lullaby, Richard's "family empathy project" leading to "adopting" at Christmas time a family with limited resources and giving them family gifts, and John becoming the teacher's assistant in a "cartooning club." These endeavors boosted the self-esteem of all three children, provided a means through which to interact more effectively, and in a concrete fashion communicated to them that they possessed strengths that were appreciated by others.

Similar to the other guideposts, we frequently use Guidepost 8 in our therapy sessions with children on the autism spectrum. We have enlisted their advice to use with other children with ASD or with their own parents and teachers, we have conferred upon them the title of "assistant psychologist," and we have in a genuine way thanked them for the ways in which they have increased our understanding of youngsters with ASD.

Responsibility and a Social Resilient Mindset

Although the link between responsibility and a social resilient mindset may seem apparent, in our work with parents and teachers, we find it beneficial to articulate the nature of these bonds. We emphasize that when children are requested to assist others and engage in responsible behaviors that are within their cognitive and social abilities, we communicate our trust in them and faith in their ability to manage a variety of tasks. In turn, involvement in these tasks reinforces several key characteristics of a social resilient mindset in children with ASD, including:

- The ability to be empathic and understand the needs of others.
- The ability to demonstrate caring and moving away from a seemingly self-centered position.
- The capacity to see oneself as an accepted contributing member of the family and of society.
- The capacity to solve problems that may arise in the helping role.
- A feeling of ownership of one's behavior.
- A more confident outlook as islands of competence are recruited in the service of helping others.

We have also suggested to parents that when possible, they participate with their child with ASD and other children in the family in contributory or charitable activities. These can be undertaken through their places of worship or through such endeavors as "Walks for Hunger" or "Walks for AIDS" or a designated charity.

In keeping with our belief that children possess an inborn need to help and that they receive much satisfaction when they are altruistic, we would contend that one of the most effective ways to encourage compassion and responsibility in children with ASD is to provide them with ample opportunities to engage in contributory activities. The benefit for these children will be significant.

Concluding Remark

Therapists who work with children with ASD as well as with their parents, teachers, and other professionals are in a powerful position to have a significant impact on the present and future lives of these children. We believe that this impact should be guided by a strength-based approach that has a major goal as the nurturance of the different components of a social resilient mindset. When adults in the life of a child with ASD provide this nurturance, they assume the role of a "charismatic adult," an adult from whom children "gather strength" (Segal 1988). Jeremy Sicile-Kira, a young man with autism, succinctly summed up the power of adults to influence the course of one's life:

> I just have to tell everyone that getting out of the darkness was not a miracle. It was a team effort of lots of work over a long period of time. The real reason for my success is frankly that my mom got good people to work with me and professionals who believed in me..... I think I have a bright future ahead. I know life will not be easy but I look forward to doing my best (Sicile-Kira and Sicile-Kira 2012, pp. 210–211).

References

Adams, L. W. (2009). *Parenting on the autism spectrum: A survival guide*. San Diego: Plural Publishing.

Atwood, T. (2008). *The complete guide to Asperger's syndrome*. London: Kingsley.

Bondy, A., & Frost, L. (2008). *Autism 24/7: A family guide to learning at home and in the community*. Bethesda: Woodbine House.

Brooks, R. (1991). *The self-esteem teacher*. Loveland: Treehaus Communications.

Brooks, R., & Goldstein, S. (2001). *Raising resilient children*. New York: McGraw-Hill.

Brooks, R., & Goldstein, S. (2004). *The power of resilience: Achieving balance, confidence, and personal strength in your life*. New York: McGraw-Hill.

Brooks, R., & Goldstein, S. (2007). *Raising a self-disciplined child*. New York: McGraw-Hill.

Brooks, R., & Goldstein, S. (2012). *Raising resilient children with autism spectrum disorders*. New York: McGraw-Hill.

Dweck, C. (2006). *Mindset: The new psychology of success*. New York: Random House.

Goldstein, S., & Brooks, R. (Eds.) (2005). *Handbook of resilience in children*. New York: Springer.

Goldstein, S., & Brooks, R. (2007). *Understanding and managing children's classroom behavior: Creating resilient, sustainable classrooms*. New York: Wiley.

Goleman, D. (1994). *Emotional intelligence*. New York: Bantam Books.

Goleman, D. (2006). *Social intelligence*. New York: Bantam Dell.

Grandin, T., & Sullivan, R. (2008). *The way I see it: A personal look at autism and Asperger's*. Arlington: Future Horizons.

Greene, R. W. (1998). *The explosive child: A new approach for understanding and parenting easily frustrated, "chronically inflexible" children*. New York: Collins.

Greene, R. W. (2009). *Lost at school: Why our kids with behavioral challenges are falling through the cracks and how we can help them*. New York: Scribner.

Greenspan, S. I., & Weider, S. (2009). *Engaging autism: Using the Floortime approach to help children relate, communicate and think*. Philadelphia: Da Capo Lifelong Books.

Janzen, J. D. (2009). *Autism handbook for parents: Facts and strategies for parenting success*. Waco: Prufrock Press.

Kobasa, S., & Puccetti, M. (1983). Personality and social resources in stress resistance. *Journal of Personality and Social Psychology, 45,* 839–850.

Kobasa, S., Maddi, S., & Kahn, S. (1982). Hardiness and health: A perspective inquiry. *Journal of Personality and Social Psychology, 42,* 168–177.

Post, S., & Neimark, J. (2007). *Why good things happen to good people: How to live a longer, healthier, happier life by the simple act of giving*. New York: Broadway Books.

Reivich, K., & Shatte, A. (2002). *The resilience factor: 7 keys to finding your inner strength and overcoming life's hurdles*. New York: Random House.

Robinson, R. G. (2011). *Autism solutions: How to create a healthy and meaningful life for your child*. Don Mills: Harlequin.
Seligman, M. E. P. (1990). *Learned optimism: How to change your mind and your life*. New York: Pocket Books.
Shumaker, L. (2008). *A regular guy: Growing up with autism*. Lafayette: Landscape Press.
Shure, M. B. (1996). *Raising a thinking child*. New York: Pocket Books.
Shure, M. B. (2000). *Raising a thinking preteen*. New York: Holt.
Sicile-Kira, C., & Sicile-Kira, J. (2012). *A full life with autism: From learning to forming relationships to achieving independence*. New York: Macmillan.
Siegel, B. (2007). *Helping children with autism learn: Treatment approaches for parents and professionals*. Oxford: Oxford University Press.
Segal, J. (1988). Teachers have enormous power in affecting a child's self-esteem. *Brown University Child Behavior and Development Newsletter, 10,* 1–3.
Weiner, B. (1974). *Achievement motivation and attribution theory*. Morristown: General Learning Press.

Index

S. Goldstein, J. A. Naglieri (eds.), *Interventions for Autism Spectrum Disorders,*
DOI 10.1007/978-1-4614-5301-7,

CPSIA information can be obtained at www.ICGtesting.com
Printed in the USA
LVOW01*1348260114

371021LV00009B/123/P

9 781461 453000